*The Extraordinary Life and Historic Adventures
of a Servant called*

# LITTLE,

*containing travels across three countries, lost children, lost parents,
ghosts of monkeys, tailor's dummies, wooden dolls, an artificial
populace, one king, two princesses, seven doctors, the man who walked
all over Paris, the man who was sewn and stuffed with wadding, his
mother a mogul, the man who collected murderers, famous philosophers,
heroes and monsters, everyone of significance, several houses each bigger
than the last, progress, retreat, a large family, scenes of historical
import, famous people, ordinary people, love, hate, massacres of
innocents, murders witnessed, bodies taken apart,
blood on the streets, misery, prison,
loss of everything, marriage,
memories captured and contained,
calamity daily exhibited,
history owned.
Written by
herself.*

*ALSO:*

*Drawn by herself.*
*In graphite, charcoal, and black chalk.*

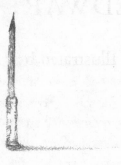

This being a likeness of her pencil

Edward Carey is a novelist, visual artist and playwright. He is the author of two acclaimed novels, *Observatory Mansions* and *Alva & Irva*. His YA series *The Iremonger Trilogy* is published in thirteen countries and has been optioned for film adaptation. Born in England, he teaches at the University of Austin, Texas.

*For Elizabeth*

# Little

by

## EDWARD CAREY

Illustrated by Edward Carey

Gallic Books
London

A Gallic Book

Copyright © Edward Carey, 2018
The moral right of the author has been asserted

First published in Great Britain in 2018 by Gallic Books,
59 Ebury Street, London, SW1W 0NZ

A CIP record for this book is available from the British Library

ISBN 978-1-910709-39-9

Typeset in Fournier MT by Palimpsest Book Production Limited,
Falkirk, Stirlingshire
Printed in the UK by CPI (CR0 4YY)

This is a work of fiction.

*Before*

1761–1767

# A Little Village

*From my birth until I am six years old.*

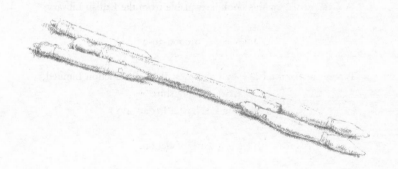

# Chapter One

*In which I am born and in which I describe*
*my mother and father.*

In the same year that the five-year-old Wolfgang Amadeus Mozart wrote his Minuet for Harpsichord, in the precise year when the British captured Pondicherry in India from the French, in the exact same year in which the melody for 'Twinkle, Twinkle, Little Star' was first published, in that very year, which is to say 1761, whilst in the city of Paris people at their salons told tales of beasts in castles and men with blue beards and beauties that would not wake and cats in boots and slippers made of glass and youngest children with tufts in their hair and daughters wrapped in donkey skin, and whilst in London people at their clubs discussed the coronation of King George III and Queen Charlotte: many miles away from all this activity, in a small village in Alsace, in the presence of a ruddy midwife, two village maids, and a terrified mother, was born a certain undersized baby.

Anne Marie Grosholtz was the name given to that hurriedly christened child, though I would be referred to simply as Marie. I was not much bigger, at first, than the size of my mother's little hands put together, and I was not expected to live very long. And yet, after I survived my first night, I went on, despite contrary predictions, to breathe through my first week. After that my heart still kept time, without interruption, throughout my first month. Pig-headed, pocket-sized thing.

My lonely mother was eighteen years old at my birth, a small woman, a little under five foot, marked by being the daughter of a priest.

3

This priest, my grandfather, made a widower by smallpox, had been a very strict man, a fury in black cloth, who never let his daughter out of his sight. After he died, my mother's life changed. Mother began to meet people, villagers who called upon her, and among them was a soldier. This soldier, a bachelor somewhat beyond the customary age, possessing a sombre temperament brought on by witnessing so many appalling things and losing so many soldier friends, took a fancy to Mother; he thought they could be happy, so to speak, being sad together. Her name was Anna-Maria Waltner. His name was Joseph Georg Grosholtz. They were married. My mother and my father. Here was loving and here was joy.

My mother had a large nose, in the Roman style. My father, so I would come to believe, had a strong chin that pointed a little upward. That chin and that nose, it seems, fitted together. After a little while, however, Father's furlough was over, and he returned to war. Mother's nose and Father's chin had known each other for three weeks.

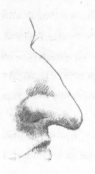

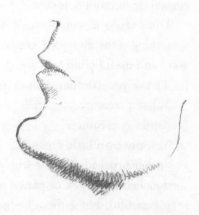

I was born of love. The love my father and mother had for each other was forever present on my face. I was born with both the Waltner nose and the Grosholtz chin. Each attribute was a noteworthy thing on its own, and nicely gave character to the faces of those two families; combined, the result was a little ungainly, as if I were showing more flesh than was my personal due. Children will grow how they will. Some distinguish themselves as prodigies of hair growth, or cut teeth at a wonderfully young age; some are freckled all over; others arrive so pale that their white nakedness is a shock to all who witness it. I nosed and chinned my way into life. I was, certainly, unaware then of what extraordinary bodies I should come to know, of what vast buildings I would inhabit, of what bloody events I would find myself trapped within, and yet, it seems to me, my nose and my chin already had some inkling of it all. Nose and chin, such an armour for life. Nose and chin, such companions. To begin with, for always, there was love.

Since girls of my stamp were not schooled, it was Mother who gave me education through God. The Bible was my primer. Elsewise, I brought in logs, looked for kindling in the woods, washed plates and clothes, cut vegetables, fetched meat. I swept. I cleaned. I carried. I was always busy. Mother taught me industry. If my mother was busy, she was happy; it was when she stopped that uncertainty caught up with her, only to be dispelled by some new activity. She was constantly in motion, and movement suited her well.

'Discover,' she would say, 'what you can do. You'll always find something. One day your father will return, and he'll see what a good and useful child you are.'

'Thank you, Mother. I shall be most useful; I do wish it.'

'What a creature you are!'

'Am I? A creature?'

'Yes, my own little creature.'

Mother brushed my hair with extraordinary vigour. Sometimes she touched my cheek or patted my bonnet. She was probably not very beautiful, but I thought her so. She had a small mole just beneath one of her eyes. I wish I could re-member her smile. I do know she had one.

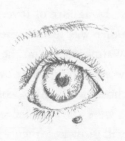

By the age of five I had grown to the height of the old dog in the house next to ours. Later I would be the height of door-knobs, which I liked to rub. Later still, and here I would stop, I would be the height of many people's hearts. Women observing me in the village were sometimes heard to mutter, as they kissed me, 'Finding a husband will not be easy.'

On my fifth birthday, my dear mother gave me a doll. This was Marta. I named her myself. I knew her little body, about a sixth the size of my own; I learned it entirely as I moved it about, sometimes roughly, sometimes with great tenderness. She came to me naked and without a face. She was a collection of seven wooden pegs, which could be assembled in a certain order to roughly resemble the human figure. Marta, save my mother, was my first intimate connection with the world; I was never without her. We were happy together, Mother, Marta, and me.

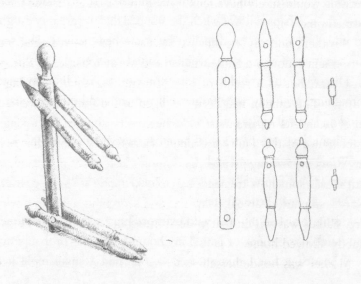

# Chapter Two

*The Family Grosholtz.*

Father was absent during those beginning years, his army finding ever more excuses to postpone his next furlough. And what could Father do about it? The poor dandelion seed must go wherever they blew him. To us, he was absent but not forgotten. Sometimes, Mother would sit me on the joint-stool by the fire and instruct me about Father. I took much enjoyment in saying that word, *Father*. Sometimes, when Mother was not about, I would address the stove in my private way as Father, or a chair or chest, or various trees, and bow to them or hug them, in rehearsal for my father's return. Father was everywhere about the village; Father was in the church; he was by the cowsheds. Father was an upright man, said Mother. And he would surely have remained so in our minds had he never come home.

But then, one day, he did. Actual Father had been forced into retirement – not by a battle, since there were no battles in Europe that year, but as a result of a malfunctioning cannon during a parade. The cannon had been damaged at the Battle of Freiberg in 1762 and its repairs must have been very shoddy, for a single appearance of that faulty instrument caused irrevocable change in my life. One Sunday parade, the cannon's last, it was lit as a salute, but it was somehow tremendously blocked, and it sprayed, backwards, sulphur, charcoal, saltpetre, and scorching metal in a wide arc. Father was within that wide arc, and because of that he was finally allowed home.

Mother was beside herself in worry and in joy. 'Your father is coming home to us! And very soon he will be quite recovered. I feel certain of it. Your father, Marie!'

The man who returned to our house, however, was pushed. The father who arrived was a father in a wheelchair. Father's yellow eyes were moist; they seemed to recognise nothing in the wife who stood before him; nor even did they show any change when the wife began to tremble and moan. There was no hair on top of Father; that erupting cannon had scalped him. Most of all, though, what was lacking about this poor bundle contained in its wheelchair was the inferior maxillary bone, the largest bone in the human face, commonly called the lower jaw.

Here and now I must make a confession: it was I who had credited my chin to Father. Otherwise, why else would I have such a proud, rude thing about me? I had never seen Father, but, not seeing him, I desired to have his mark upon my person, so that it was daily certain that I was his and he was mine. I cannot now say for certain — these early years being so far away and the other actors in them being no longer upon the stage — whether I declared my chin to be his only after his return, in some fit of longing, or whether I had always believed it. But its absence was the thing, and I longed to understand and to make a fuller picture of the man who was my father in distress. I wished to see him complete and fancied my face could complete the portrait, as the portrait before me was such an unhappy, ruined one.

With my father's arrival, a hint of my future had appeared to me. A small window opened up and called.

The man in the wheelchair may have been lacking his lower jaw, but in its place had been fitted a silver plate. This silver plate was moulded into the shape of the lowermost portion of a very average human face. This silver plate was taken from a mould, and so it would be fair to conclude that several tens of unfortunate people had exactly this same silver chin that Father had now. The silver plate could be detached. Father came in two pieces, which could be fitted together with a little pain.

8

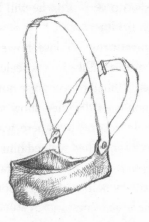

Poor Father had no idea where he was. He was incapable of recognising his wife, nor could he tell that the little girl silently watching him was his own daughter.

For assistance my mother rehired her midwife, a fond, breathless lady with thick arms who adapted herself to any paying occasion, and called often upon the doctor from the nearby village, Doctor Sander. Together they made up the little room beside the kitchen for Father, and once he was in he never left. He just lay there all day, sometimes looking out of the window, sometimes at the ceiling, but never, I think, exactly focusing on anything. I sat with Father very long hours, and when he did not talk to me I gave him some words, and imagined all the things he would want to tell me.

After Father's arrival, Mother climbed the stairs to her bedroom and closed the door. As days went on, she spent more and more time in bed. She stopped moving, and that was never good for her. Doctor Sander said that my mother was in a state of pronounced shock and must be slowly encouraged back to herself. Her whole body changed after Father's arrival; her skin grew shiny and yellow, like that of an onion. She gave off new smells. One morning I found her outside, barely clothed, lying on the ground, in winter, crying. I helped her back to bed.

I went from one parent to the other, from Mother upstairs to

Father downstairs, and read to them both from the Bible. I used the little joint-stool, my extension, to position myself at various stations around the perimeter of Father's bed, depending on his needs. I was present when Father was cleaned and washed. The midwife was very affectionate to me; she sometimes held me fast to her, and in those moments I was surprised at how very big bodies could be and held her in return with all possible force. We ate many meals together; I think she must have given me some of her food. When she spoke to me of my father she frowned in concern; when she spoke of my mother she shook her head.

One morning, as I sat beside him, Father died. It was a very small death, even gentle. I watched very carefully. He shook a little and rattled, only a tiny bit, and then very quietly, barely noticeably, left us. The last little noise was the sound of the last Grosholtz thought in his Grosholtz head making its way out. I was still seated beside him holding his hand when the midwife came in. She knew immediately that Father was no longer to be numbered among the living. Gently she put his hand on his chest and moved the other one beside it, then took my hand and led me to the house of her daughter. I must have slept there the night.

A few days later, Father was buried. But the father in the box, which we were invited to throw earth on top of, was not complete. Doctor Sander had given me Father's silver plate, which he said was worth money. It had a certain weight to it, about that of a tin mug filled with water. I could not help wondering if Father would miss it, and suspecting that it might better have remained with him. I wanted to dig up his grave and slip the jawplate in. How on earth otherwise could he talk in heaven? But then, when I thought it through, I realised: this plate was not Father's chin, not really. It was modelled after someone else. Only I had his true chin, keeping it always with me, a little beneath Mother's nose.

Father had left behind his military uniform, a silver plate, a widow, a half-orphan, and penury. His army pension would not suffice. For Mother and me to survive, she would need to find work. Taking the matter in hand, Doctor Sander discovered through his medical connections news of a doctor, one Philip Curtius of Berne Hospital, who was in need of domestic help. Employment and usefulness, said Doctor Sander, would save my mother's health.

Mother, with unhappiness displayed throughout her shining body, sat down to write to Doctor Curtius. Doctor Curtius wrote back. When the letter arrived, motion returned to Mother – more than even before, as if she feared terribly to stop.

'A very educated gentleman, Marie!' she exclaimed, her eyes wide. 'Of the city, Marie, a doctor of the city! Not for us any more the small, dark rooms of the countryside. We shall find instead tall places of light and air. My father, your grandfather, always said we were worthy of better places. Oh the city! Curtius of the city!'

Shortly afterwards, sometime in 1767, Mother and I found ourselves on a cart headed towards the city of Berne. I sat next to Mother in the cart, holding a corner of her dress in one hand, Father's jawplate in the other, and Marta in my lap pocket. The Family Grosholtz was on the move. We rattled away from the village of my birth, away from the pigsties, and the church, and Father's grave.

We would not be coming back.

## Book One

1767–1769

# A One-Way Street

*Until I am eight years old.*

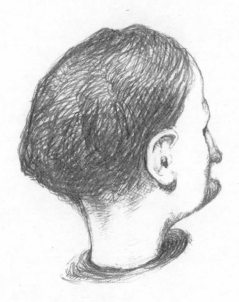

# Chapter Three

*In which my mother and I are introduced to many*
*wonderful things, some of them in rosewood cases,*
*and I come to witness my second death.*

A Berne night consists of gloomy rising buildings, narrow and
unlit streets, shadow people moving about them. Berne Hospital
appeared, helpfully enough, looming above the streets. We were
set down in front of the hospital, our single trunk, former possession of our priestly antecedent, placed beside us. The cart rattled
away, longing for the countryside.

At the centre of Berne Hospital was a great black gate, wide
enough for two carriages to pass at once, a great titan's mouth to
swallow patients into its vast and mysterious interior. It was this
black gate that Mother and I approached. There was a bell. Mother
rang it. The noise echoed all around the empty hospital square.
From somewhere nearby came a sound of coughing and spitting.
A tiny square of wood in the gate opened. A head appeared; we
could barely see it.

'No thank you,' said the head.

'If you please—' said Mother.

'Come back in the morning.'

'If you please, I've come for Doctor Curtius. He's expecting me.'

'Who?'

'Doctor Curtius. We're to live with him, my daughter and me.'

'Curtius? Curtius is dead. Five years since.'

'I had this letter from him,' Mother strained to insist, 'a week
ago.'

A hand stretched out, taking the letter; the hatch was closed again. We could barely hear people talking behind it before it opened once more and the head reappeared. '*That* Curtius! The *other* Curtius. No one has ever come asking for *that* Curtius before. He doesn't live on the grounds; he's off on Welserstrasse. You don't know where that is? Country people, is it? Ernst could guide you, I suppose.' We heard another voice behind the gate, and the head responded: 'You will, Ernst – yes, you will if I say. Ernst will show you. Go round the corner. You'll find a side door. In the side door will be a lantern, waving. Beneath that waving lantern will be Ernst.'

The hatch closed again and Ernst came out to greet us, wearing the black porter's uniform of the hospital. Ernst had a nose that twisted in the opposite direction of his face; his nose set forth one way, his face quite another. He had clearly been in many fights during his young life. 'Curtius?' asked Ernst.

'Doctor Curtius,' Mother said.

'Curtius,' said Ernst once more and off we went.

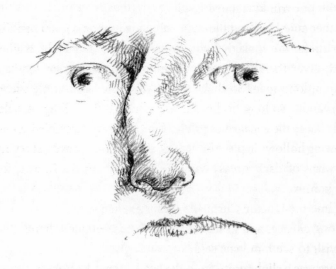

Only five minutes from the hospital was a small, mean street. This was Welserstrasse. Walking its length that night, I thought the houses seemed to be murmuring to us, *Don't stop here. Keep moving along. Out of our sight.* Ernst finally halted at a house thinner and smaller than the rest, squeezed in between two bullying neighbouring residences, poor and neglected.

'House of Curtius,' said Ernst.

'Here?' Mother asked.

'Even here,' confirmed Ernst. 'I came here once myself. Shan't ever again. What's inside, I won't say, but I will say I never liked it. No, I don't do Curtius. You'll forgive me if I leave before you knock.' And off went Ernst and his contrary nose, quicker than before, taking light with him.

We put down our trunk. Mother sat down on it and looked at the door, as if perfectly content to find it closed. And so it was I who stepped forward and knocked three times. Four. And finally the door opened. But no one came out into the night. It remained open, and no one came to meet us. I waited for a while with Mother, until I tugged on her hand and she at last gathered herself up and we, with our trunk, stepped inside.

Mother quietly closed the door behind us; I took a good handful of her dress. We looked about in the shadows. Suddenly Mother gasped: Over there! Someone was lurking in the corner. It was a very thin, long man. So thin he seemed in the last terrible stages of starvation. So long his head nearly touched the ceiling. A pale, ghostly face; the meagre candlelight in the room trembled about it, showing hollows in place of cheeks, showing moist eyes, showing small wisps of dark, greasy hair. We stood by our trunk, as if for protection.

'I came for Doctor Curtius,' Mother explained.

A long silence, and in that silence the head nodded, barely.

'I wish to see him,' she said.

There was a slight noise from the head. It may have been, 'Yes.'

'*May* I see him?'

17

Quietly, slowly, as if it were a coincidence, the head volunteered: '*My* name is Curtius.'

'I am Anna-Maria Grosholtz,' said Mother, trying to hold on to herself.

'Yes,' said the man.

The introductions exhausted, another silence followed. At last the man in the corner spoke again, very slowly. 'I . . . You see, I . . . I'm not so very used to people. I haven't had much practice lately. I'm very out of . . . practice. And you need to have people around you, you need to have people to talk to . . . or you might forget, you see, how they . . . *are* exactly. And, in truth, what to do with them. But that'll change now. With you here. Won't it?'

There was a longer silence.

'Shall I, perhaps, if you're ready – shall I show you the house now?'

Mother, a great unhappy look on her face, nodded.

'Yes, perhaps you'd like to see it. I'm so glad you're here. Welcome. I meant to say that before: Welcome. I meant to say that when you first arrived. I had the word ready, I was thinking of it all day. But then, ah, I forgot. I'm not used . . . you see, not *used*,' said the doctor and slowly unravelled himself from his corner. He seemed made of rods, of broom handles, of great lengths, tall and thin, unfolding the great length of himself as if he were a spider. We followed, keeping our distance.

'There's a room, at the top, just for you,' said Curtius, pointing the candle up the stairs, 'for you alone. I'll never go up there. I do so hope you'll be happy.' Then, with more confidence: 'Please, please, come this way.'

Doctor Curtius opened a door off the hall and we stepped into a small passageway. At the end of it was another door, a little light glowing from underneath. This was surely where the doctor had been when I knocked. 'This room,' said Curtius, 'is where I work.'

Curtius stopped in front of it, the great length of his narrow back towards us. He paused, straightened himself as much as he could, then spoke slowly and precisely: 'Please to come in.'

Ten or more shielded candles were burning inside the room, illuminating it wonderfully, showing us a place so cluttered it was impossible to understand at first. Long shelves were filled with corked bottles, inside them colours in powder. Other shorter shelves contained different, thicker bottles; these had more persuasive glass stoppers, hinting at the possibly fatal personality of the viscous liquids they contained, black or brown or transparent. There were boxes filled with hair; it looked like – wasn't it? – human hair. Positioned across the length of a trestle table were various copper vats and several hundred small modelling tools, some with sharp tips, others curved, some minute, no larger than a pin, others the size of a butcher's cleaver. In the centre of the table, upon a wooden board, was a pale, drying-out object.

It was difficult to identify this object precisely at first. A piece of meat? The breast of a chicken perhaps? But that wasn't it, and yet there was something so familiar about it, something everyday about it. It *was* a something . . . and the name of that something was on the tip of my tongue. And that – what a jolt – was it! It was a tongue! Very like a human one, upon a trestle table. And I wondered: if it was indeed a tongue, how did it get here and where was the someone who'd lost it?

There were other things besides tongues in this room. The most impressive part of the atelier, I saw now, was to be found in rosewood display cases, their clearly labelled shelves running up and down, left and right, till they covered most of one wall. Among the labels, inscribed in sepia by a fine calligraphic hand, were a host of words: *OSSA, NEUROCRANIUM, COLUMNAE VERTEBRALIS, ARTICULATIO STERNOCLAVICULARIS, MUSCUS TEMPORALIS, BULBUS OCULI, NERVUS VAGUS, ORGANA GENITALIA.* Near the tongue on that table was one more sign, this reading *LINGUA.*

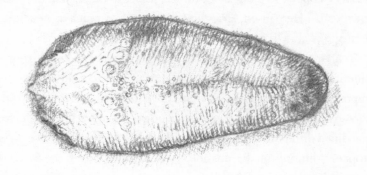

I was beginning to understand: body parts. A room filled with them. There I was, a little girl, looking at all the parts of the body. We were being introduced: Bits and pieces of the human body, this is a little girl called Marie. Little girl called Marie, this is the body in pieces. I hovered behind Mother, still grasping her dress, but peered out at the spectacle.

Curtius spoke now: 'Urogenital tract. With dangling bladder. Bones. From the femur, the strongest and largest, to the lachrymal, the tiniest and most fragile of the face.' He was surveying the contents of his room. 'Many muscles, too, all labelled. Ten group-ings of the head, from occipitofrontalis to the *pterygoideus internus*. Many of the ribbons of arteries, from the superior thyroid to the common carotid. Veins, too: the cerebellar, the interior saphenous, the splenic and the gastric, the cardiac and the pulmon-ary. I have organs! Individually, resting on a bed of red velvet, or displayed with their neighbours on the wooden boards. The impres-sive intricacy of the ear's osseous labyrinth. Or the long, thick clouds of intestines, both the small and the large – such long and winding ways.'

Mother was regarding the room, looking increasingly unwell. Curtius must have noticed her horror, for he continued now very hurriedly: '*I* made them. I made them. My osseous labyrinth, and my gall bladder and my ventricles. I made them. They are models

20

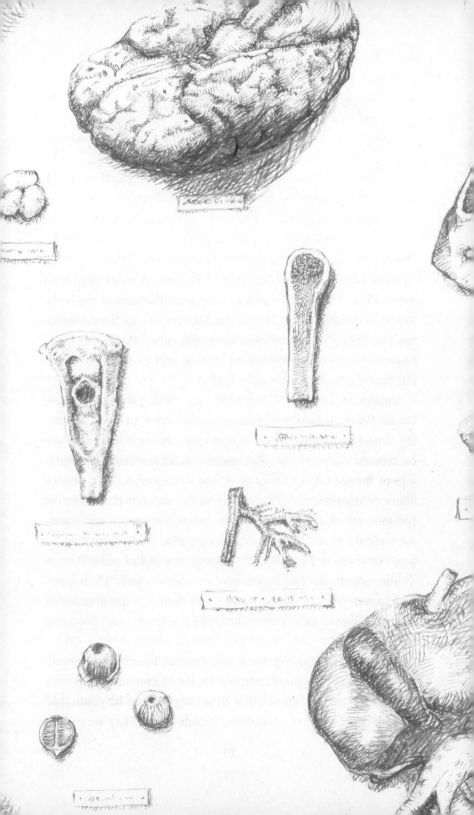

only, that is, replicas. I didn't mean . . . I'm not used . . . I do apologise. What can you think of me? Don't think them . . . *real*. They look real, of course. Don't they look real? You must say yes. You know you must say yes. Oh yes, very real, but they're not. No. Though they do look it. Yes. Because, in fact, you see, I made them.'

We turned to look at him. We had been so surprised at the objects all about this room that we had failed at first to study the most significant object of all: Doctor Curtius, in the light. Curtius was a young man, it now appeared, at least younger than Mother. When I had seen his long shadowy form move itself about in the darkness, I had assumed him to be old, but now I saw him both long and thin, shy and passionate, and young, breathing excitedly. Six feet or more of leanness, rising far above us in the corner of his atelier, his thin nostrils flaring slightly now. He was so clearly proud of his room, watching us looking at his work. His cheeks pulled inwards, never out, as he breathed; his nose stretched down his long face like a tightrope. Veins sprawled across the sides of his forehead, thickly and thinly. Finally, the enormous slender hands of this strange man met before his narrow chest. I thought he might be about to pray but instead he began to clap. It was not a loud noise but an excited little beating, as of a small pleased child at the promise of something sweet to eat, a happy noise that sounded out of place in this room. His upper body stooped over his clapping hands as if some pale bird were trapped there, flapping before his heart, and he was anxious that it should not escape.

'Me. I made them all. Every one. Out of wax. On my own! And many more besides, this being but a fraction. The great majority housed in the hospital, visited frequently!'

When Doctor Curtius had finished his introductions, I turned to Mother. Her face was very pale and sweaty. She did not say anything. We three stood together in silence until Curtius, disappointed I think, wondered if we needed to sleep after our long journey.

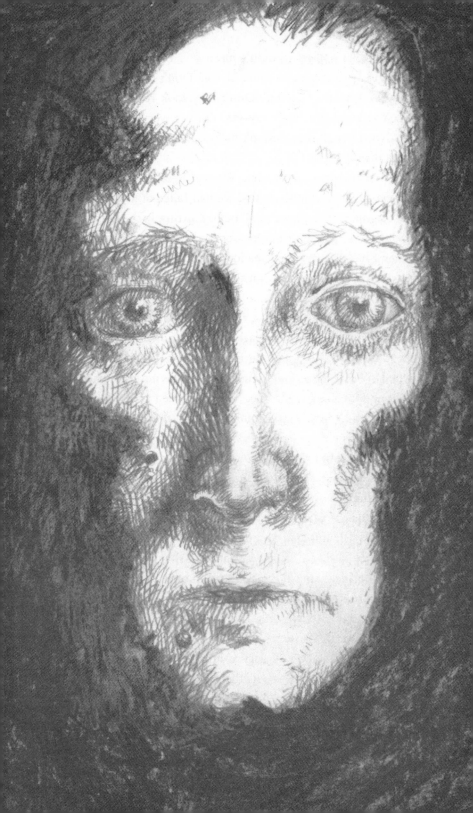

'Most tired indeed, sir,' she said.

'Good night then.'

'Oh, excuse me, sir,' Mother said. 'Our papers. I suppose you should take them.'

'No, no, I don't think so. Please to keep them yourselves.'

I followed Mother as she carried our trunk upstairs, closing the door to our small room behind us. Curtius could be heard wandering about downstairs. Mother sat by the window for a long time. She kept so still, I feared her illness had returned. In the end, I helped steer her towards our bed. We did not sleep at all that first night in this new place. Mother held on to me. I, in my turn, held on to Marta. In the morning we were still holding one another. Three small women, very anxious.

Before we went downstairs, Mother said to me, 'We are bound now, you and I. Do you understand? Our every action must be to please him. If he abandons us, we are lost. So long as we remain in Doctor Curtius's employ, so long do we persist. Be of good service, dear daughter.'

When I took a handful of Mother's dress, she said, quietly, sadly, 'No.'

Mother took the keys. We scrubbed floors. Mother cooked. We went to the market for food, but the market was frightening to her. The streets were filled with people, but it wasn't just that. The objects on sale – all that meat hung on hooks, cut open, all those animals divided in fractions or whole and strung up by their feet, whole birds with lazy necks and bloody beaks, hanging like felons – all these, and the eyes of fish, and the flies, and the meat of living people's hands, spotted with gore, all this recalled to Mother, again and again, what she'd seen in Doctor Curtius's atelier.

The doctor's house, at least, was quiet. Curtius himself spent the day in his atelier and rarely came out. When he did appear, he seemed surprised to see us there: 'Not used . . . not *used*,' he whispered, and retreated to his room. When it was time for his lunch,

Mother loaded the food on a tray, her Waltner nose flared in disapproval, and held the platter hovering above the kitchen table until she shuddered, causing the soup to spill a little. I led her to a chair, sat her down, then carried the food in to Doctor Curtius myself. He was bent over his table, a portrait of three tongues: the actual separated human tongue, his perfect wax duplicate, and his own tongue sticking out between his lips as he worked.

'Soup, sir,' I said.

He said nothing in response. I left the soup with him and closed the door. It was the same later that day, when I entered the atelier saying, 'Stew, sir.' It was the same in fact throughout the first week. Twice, Curtius came into the kitchen to say to Mother, 'I'm so pleased you're here, so pleased, so glad, so . . . *happy*.' Twice, Mother's hands sought her crucifix.

During the second week, when we had I thought grown a little more used to one another, Mother and I were startled by a knock at the door. It was a visitor from the hospital, dressed in a black uniform like Ernst, but called Heinrich. Heinrich had an unimpressive nose and other unremarkable features; I recall nothing of them now, indeed nothing of him at all beyond his unmemorable name. 'Delivery for Curtius,' Heinrich said, introducing himself. 'I do the bringing. We'll be seeing a lot of each other. What have we got today?' he said, lifting the lid a little and poking at a muslin-covered object within. 'Bit of a diseased gut, I reckon.'

Mother closed her eyes and crossed herself. I stepped forward, aiming to be useful, and held out my hands. Heinrich looked uncertain.

'Thank you,' I said, holding my hands out a little further. 'Thank you.'

When Heinrich reluctantly passed the box to me, Mother closed the door in a hurry. She looked at me for an instant as if I were no longer recognisable, then retreated to the kitchen. I followed to ask her if I should take the object in. She nodded fiercely, waving me and the box from the room. I carried it to the atelier.

'Bit of a gut, sir,' I said, leaving the box on the same portion of the table where I always left him his meals. This time Doctor Curtius did look up.

Mother found it increasingly difficult to work. She often sat in the kitchen with her hands on her small crucifix. Flies in Curtius's house, and there were always flies, caused her to panic utterly, for they could travel throughout the house, could get into the atelier and from there spread the news of the atelier everywhere about. Mother often sat still, eyes closed but perfectly awake, whilst I moved about to her instructions.

Two days after I delivered the parcel to Doctor Curtius, I was sitting in the kitchen by the fire, with Mother reading to me from the Bible, when Doctor Curtius knocked faintly and came in.

'Widow Grosholtz,' he said. My mother closed her eyes. 'Widow Grosholtz,' he said again, 'I would like, if it isn't too much trouble, Widow Grosholtz – and I'm so happy, by the by, at how happy we are, so, um, delighted, at all this . . . company, at how we are getting on so well, at what companions we are, at this community we have – I should like, yes, a little help in my atelier. Could I? Tomorrow would be best, I think. First thing would be perfect. I should like to teach you how to handle my work, so that you don't harm it. I should like you to get, you see, properly acquainted with it. I'm sure you shall come to love your new duties. You'll be an expert in a trice.'

Doctor Curtius saw Mother give a slight nod. But I was not taken in by it. Mother's nod was, rather, a flinch misinterpreted.

'Good night, then,' he said. 'Thank you.'

That night, back in our attic room, Mother kissed me on the forehead as she put me to bed. 'Be useful, Marie. You are a very good child,' she said. 'I'm sorry, I cannot. I have tried, but I cannot.'

'You cannot what, Mother?'

'Do be good now, quiet down. Good night, Marie.'

'Good night.'

Then Mother told me to close my eyes, that I must go to sleep

26

instantly. Keep your eyes shut, she told me, your face turned to the wall. I heard her busy arranging things, pulling a sheet from the bed, moving a chair. I went to sleep.

When I woke up, the candle was out. It was the early hours of the morning. Mother was not in the bed beside me. A faint blue light was coming into the room. I could just make out something dark suspended from the rafters. I couldn't recall seeing such an object before. More light slowly arrived and I began to understand what this object was. It was Mother. Mother had hanged herself.

Fretting, I took one of Mother's feet in my hand, but that naked foot gave me little comfort; it was a cold foot after all, and in that coldness was the awful confirmation of Mother's passing. A woman's death is a simple enough thing perhaps; women will always be dying about the place; no doubt several women have died as I have been writing this sentence; only this one woman who concerns me now, this one woman tied up to the rafters, unlike all the others in the world – this woman was my mother. Before, I had always had Mother to hide behind; now I was exposed. Her death was not a quiet, thinking-death like Father's had been, her death was about business; it was all hurried action; Mother had jolted herself out of life. Whose dress should I cling to now? There would be no more dress-clinging for me, not ever again. Her cold nose had swung away from me, the signpost of her rejection.

'Mother,' I said, 'Mother, Mother. *Mother!*' But Mother, or that hanging thing that was only partly Mother, kept herself very quiet. In my panic I flailed around for something, some solace or protection, and found only Marta.

Doctor Curtius must have heard me crying, for he called to me from the bottom of the stairs. 'Where's your mother?' he asked. 'It's time. It's time long since. It was agreed.'

'She won't come, sir.'

'She must, she must, it was agreed after all.'

'Please, sir. Please, Doctor.'

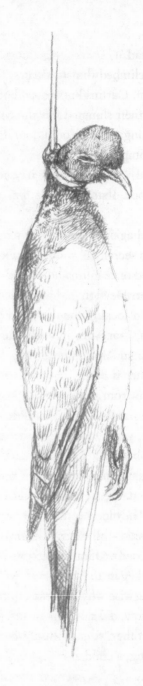

I have cast a wood pigeon to play the role of my mother.

'Yes?'

'I think she is dead.'

And so Curtius climbed the attic stairs. He opened the door; I followed behind him. Curtius knew dead bodies. He was an expert in dead bodies and their slumped faces. And here, he immediately recognised on opening our bedroom door, hanging up like a coat, was yet another example.

'Stopped,' he said, 'stopped, stopped . . . stopped.'

He closed the door. I stood beside him at the top of the attic stairs.

'Stopped,' he said again, bending down very close to me, whispering as if it were a secret. He walked down the stairs, then turned round to me, nodded once more and whispered, his face collapsing into a grimace of terrible sorrow, '*Stopped*,' and walked out of the building, closing and locking the door behind him.

After a long time, I sat halfway down the stairs with Marta. We sat very still and waited. Mother is upstairs, I thought. Oh, Mother is upstairs and Mother is dead.

At last men came from the hospital. Doctor Curtius was with them. 'I can't make people work,' he said. 'I can unwork them, I can take them apart, yes, I'm actually very good at that, considerably accomplished, but they'll never work with me. They won't. They refuse. They shut up. They stop.' The men from the hospital walked up the attic stairs, stepping around me and Marta, barely regarding us at all. The oldest of the hospital men opened the door, and let everyone inside – all except Curtius, that is, who was kept outside, the door closed on him. And so we both remained outside, and both, I think, began to wonder if we had done something terribly wrong, otherwise why wouldn't they let us in too? Doctor Curtius, very shy now, did not look at me, even though we were very close to one another, young Doctor Curtius and I. He seemed now extremely young, a child almost, his eyes fixed only upon the door.

Finally, the door opened. The oldest of the men, very serious, spoke quietly and slowly: 'Take the girl downstairs. Keep her there.'

Curtius shook his head, then spoke in a very small, very hurt voice. 'If you make me touch her, Surgeon Hoffmann, I think that she'll die too.'

'Nonsense. Come now, Philip. Philip Curtius, you can do this.'

'I'm not sure. I'm really not sure.'

'Take the child downstairs. Let us attend to matters here.'

'But what do I do with her?'

'It doesn't matter,' snapped the surgeon. 'Just get her away from here.'

The door was closed on us again.

After a moment, Curtius tapped me lightly on my shoulder. 'Come,' he said, 'please come,' and led me down the stairs to his atelier. I put Marta in my pocket so she would be safe, then stood up and slowly followed.

In the atelier, Curtius looked about him, as if unsure what to do with me. Then he seemed to find the answer. Taking a box of bones down from a shelf, he handed me, with great kindness I remember, a human scapula, the right, I think.

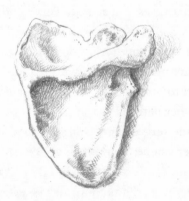

'It's a good bone,' he whispered to me, 'a great comforting bone. This part of the shoulder girdle is large and flat and triangular, and is excellent for stroking. Yes, a wonderful, soothing bone.'

After a time Surgeon Hoffmann came down to find us sitting together in the atelier, I on a stool, Curtius on the floor beside me, rummaging through a box of bones.

'And this, you see, is the temporal bone . . . And this, ah, the left parietal . . . And this, the sacrum – wonderful, isn't it? Wonderful, aren't they? All my old friends!'

'It is done,' said the surgeon.

I kept very still.

'Now,' continued the surgeon, 'what is to become of the child? Some place must be found for her.'

'Can I keep her?' asked Doctor Curtius quickly. 'The child. Can I keep her?'

I was the subject of a discussion. I did not move.

'Out of the question,' said the surgeon.

'Oh, I'd like to keep her.'

'Why on earth?'

'She isn't frightened.'

'Why should she be?'

'She holds bones.'

'And what does that signify?'

'She is quiet.'

'And so?'

'She may be wise, she may be stupid, I do not know. But for now, if you don't mind, I'll keep her.'

'Is she useful to you?'

'I shall train her perhaps.'

'Well,' said the surgeon, 'keep her for now, for all I care. Until something better can be thought of.'

# Chapter Four

*In which one becomes two.*

That first evening together, I stood in the kitchen while Curtius tried to cook. Aiming to be useful and working as Mother had shown me, I asked Doctor Curtius if I might assist him, for he was very agitated, and so I stopped the pans from burning and helped in the preparation of the food. Doctor Curtius said to me: 'I'm not frightened of you. You don't frighten me at all. You have nothing, do you? Nothing at all.' When we were finished, and it was time for bed, Curtius watched me walk up the attic stairs.

'Good night, little child.'

'Good night, sir.'

'What is your name? I should know your name, you know. I'm not certain what to do with children, I'm sure to make mistakes, but it is generally understood that they have names. What do you go by?'

'Anne Marie Grosholtz. But Mother always calls me . . . Marie.'

'Good night, then, Marie. Go to bed.'

'Good night, sir.'

And so I went upstairs into the attic, harbouring frail hopes that Mother would be there again, so that I might tell her about this most extraordinary day. And of course she was not there any more. But though they had taken Mother away, they had forgotten the sheet she had hanged herself with; it remained in one corner of the room, in a heap. And I thought then that she really would not be coming back. Not tomorrow, or the next day, not by the end of the week; the city of Berne, the house of Curtius, even I myself

32

would have to keep moving without Mother. I wondered where they had taken her.

I was very unsure of the attic room. When I looked away I could suddenly feel Mother still hanging from the rafters, with her bent neck and her head leaning to one side, but when I looked back she was gone. And that hanging person did not exactly seem to me to be Mother at all, but perhaps the person who had stolen Mother from me. I did not trust the room – I would rather be in any room, I thought, than the attic – and so when I felt certain that Doctor Curtius had gone to his bed I crept back down the stairs with a blanket, with Marta whom Mother had given me and with the jawplate that was Father's. I tried the kitchen, but in the kitchen I felt the hanging woman back again; I felt that twisted-necked mother sitting by the fireplace; I saw Mother's Bible still there upon the ledge and I was frightened of it now. I would rather be in any room, I thought, than the attic or the kitchen. But as I moved from the kitchen it seemed to me that the twisted-necked mother was following me about the house, and it occurred to me that the only place she would not follow me was the atelier. In the atelier, I knew, were kept all those terrible objects, all those secrets that were best undiscovered, but outside the atelier I felt the twisted-necked mother breathing nearby, and so I went very quickly there and closed the door hurriedly behind me. I was alone in a room full of body pieces, their characters crowding about me. But I could no longer feel the twisted-necked mother, and so I carefully made a little bed for myself under the atelier table, and begging the body parts to please be kind, and closing my eyes very tight, I finally fell asleep.

I had intended to be awake early enough to tiptoe back upstairs without Doctor Curtius hearing me, but all at once I was aware that Curtius was shaking me and that it was morning. 'And there you are! Asleep here!' he said. 'Come now, time to get up.' He said nothing more about my sleeping in the atelier, under his trestle table. I folded the blanket and placed it on a shelf, the remembrance of Mother's death rushing to me. 'Come on, come on,' he said. 'Hurry, hurry, you must hurry.'

Promptly at seven, my education began.

'You must remember,' he said to me, 'I am not used to people. I know only parts of people. Not whole people. I want to understand them; I want to know them. But the influence of my models upon me is too strong. I have begun to dream of myself in a rosewood display case backed with red velvet. Yes, and the worst of it is, what really terrifies me, what I can't get on top of, what I can't ignore, what I cannot seem to get over, is that in my dreams I feel so comfortable there. Let me out,' Curtius said, tapping my chest lightly with his fingers. 'Someone, let me out. Can't you hear me tapping on the glass? I'm in here. Who will let me out? I want to get to know people. I want to know you. Yes. Here we are. This is it. I'm not frightened of you. Not in the slightest.'

Doctor Curtius stood up suddenly and hurriedly went to work.

A short while later, he turned abruptly from what he was doing. 'I know!' he exclaimed. 'I know how to go about it! I know just the way!' He moved around the atelier collecting objects and positioning them upon the table.

'Let us, Marie – for that is your name, you know,' said Curtius when he was satisfied with his progress, 'let us, if you are ready and if you are willing, let us begin.'

'I am quite ready, sir.'

'These tools were once my father's,' he said. 'My father was the head anatomist at Berne Hospital, a very great man. When he died, these tools came to me.' He went over to a bin filled with plaster dust and took a measure of it, then poured this into a metal bucket and mixed it with a certain amount of water, stirring it thoroughly.

'To show you how it all works, so that you can get an understanding, so that you may follow the process, I shall take a cast. Not of any body piece, no, not today. Today I shall cast, for your education, if you do not object, your own head.'

'My head?'

34

'Your head, yes.'

'My head, sir?'

'I say again: your head.'

'If you wish it, sir.'

'I find I do.'

'Well then, sir, yes, my head.'

And so we began.

'First a very little oil' – he applied this oil to my face – 'so that afterwards,' he said, 'the plaster can be easily removed.' He began to apply it. 'Straws!' he suddenly called out. 'There must be straws! I almost forgot,' he said as he cautiously placed straws in my nose so that I might breathe. 'Close your eyes. Do not open them again until I say.'

He brought the plaster. I felt it dripping upon me in small layers, followed by more strips of cloth dipped in plaster. The strange warmth of the plaster seemed to lock into my face. All was dark and warm about my cheeks and eyelids and lips and neck, until I felt I was floating away somewhere and might even be dead already. In the darkness, once, I thought I saw Mother, but she was gone again and it was black and empty and no one was there at all.

At last the plaster was pulled away and light returned, and I was back inside the room. Doctor Curtius hurried with the cast to the table. Next he smoothed down my hair with oil, I was repositioned, and he took another cast of the back of my head, then further casts of my ears.

'Now,' he said, 'the stove must be laid, and lit. I shall do this but one more time only. The next: your turn.' He lit the stove. 'Now watch and follow.' He moved about placing tools upon the desk. At first he ground pigments. 'Madder lake,' he explained, 'cinnabar, together. And crimson dye. A little blue. And green. A touch. And crush. Very little yellow. And mix. Like this. Now this,' he said, marching to a large demijohn with a tap and pouring some out into a smaller container, 'turpentine oil, added all the time to the pigments. So: a mixture. So: your colour.'

He took from a shelf a large copper bowl, showed it to me, made me look into it. He placed the empty bowl upon the stove top.

'So far: nothing. Now, there is a stool, sit down upon it. Now, I think we are ready.' Picking up a large knife, he walked over to a locked cupboard, unlocked it, and very carefully, out of my sight, cut into something. Then he locked the cupboard again and returned.

'This,' said Curtius, holding up a slab of yellowish murky material, 'what I am holding, this substance, this is everything. And yet,' he continued, moving it lovingly around in his hands, 'and yet it is itself without character, without personality. In itself it is nothing, it is no one. And yet it can be friendly, it can be stand-offish, it can be beauty, it can be ugliness, it can be bone, it can be abdominal wall, it can be strings of arteries or of veins, it can be lymphatic nodes, it can be brainstems, it can be fingernails, it can be all, from the tiny stirrup we keep in our ears to the miles of intestines we keep curled up inside us. Anything! It can be anything! It can be: YOU!'

'But what is it, sir?' I asked.

'It is sight, it is memory, it is history. It can be grey lungs, and brown-red like a liver; it can be anything: it can be *you.*'

'Can it be Marta my doll?' I asked.

'It can be! Yes, it can! It can adopt the surface of any object with astonishing accuracy. Rough, smooth, serrated, shiny, flat, mottled, pitted, torn, scarred, crusted, slippery. Make your choice. There is not a surface it cannot be.'

'And can it then, can it be Mother?'

'No, child,' he said after a moment, 'this it cannot be. Nor can it be my father or mother. Dead also. It could have been. I wish that it had. But now it is too late. They have gone into the void. Can you understand? They cannot be taken out again, images of them we hold inside us, not precise images, flickers, little bits. There's not enough for it. There's no surface left, and it, you see, needs surface. That is its one rule. Too late for your mother.'

'I am sorry that it cannot be Mother.'

'It longs for personality,' he said, rushing on when he saw tears coming, 'it longs to be something. It just needs a little instruction. Shall we instruct it, little girl, Marie child? Shall you see what a wonderful servant it is, what a great actor?'

'Yes, sir.'

'Well then, why not hold it? Here, take it. Here, smell it.'

And I took it. And I smelt it.

'It is only wax,' I said, disappointed.

'No! Never! Never *only* wax! Not ever! All wax is sacred, and this, this here, is the aristocrat of waxes, the very prince among waxes. Greatest of detail collectors, finest of imitators, most honest of matters. This, even here, is a portion of finest beeswax.'

'Finest beeswax,' I repeated.

'Made by Asiatic honey bees of the genus *Apis*. Very good then, let us put it to work.'

'Of the genus *Apis*,' I said.

Wax was melted in the copper pan, the pigment was added, and also some resin. He explained how the heat must be watched, how the wax must be mixed very carefully. And then he was ready. First the mould of my face. He brushed its surface with a substance called 'soft soap,' so that afterwards the wax could be easily removed, and then the wax was poured in. At first only the tiniest amount, a very thin surface over the mould, carefully watched over by the doctor. He picked up the mould with his hands and moved it about so that the wax journeyed up and down the surface, so that all air bubbles might be gone; then after a while a second layer was added, and a while after that a third, a fourth, a fifth. For the last two layers, he said, he was only adding thickness to give the cast some strength. And then a few minutes' wait, only a few, and it was ready. It came away very easily from the mould.

'Is that my face?' I asked.

'Precisely,' he said.

37

He left me with it. It was still warm, as if it had a life of its own. But soon enough it was cold again. He poured wax into the remaining casts of my head. Each mould revealed its secret. There in front of us were different portions of my head in skin-toned wax, exactly my colour, just as he had said. My hair had been flattened down atop my head, and this he cast in wax coloured brown. Then began the business of fitting those pieces together, of joining the model up. Each bit connected to the next: at the joins the wax had to be attended to, chipped off or cut away, then new warm wax was smoothed over, eliminating the seams, and the neck made flat at the bottom so that the head could stand on its own. The wax head was hollow, the inside filled with old rags, with hemp waste and some wood chippings. 'For strength,' he said.

And there upon the worktable was my head.

'I put that all together,' Curtius said, 'not apart.'

I looked at my head: there I was in the atelier, with my eyes closed. A girl, with her father's chin and her mother's nose. It seemed to me now that I existed twice as much.

At the end of that first day we had soup in the kitchen.

'Excuse me, sir?' I said.

'Yes, what is it?'

'I have been wondering, sir, about my mother. Where they took her.'

'I cannot say,' he replied. 'But we may find out. Surgeon Hoffmann will surely know. We shall ask him when next he comes.'

'I should like to visit her grave.'

'Yes, yes. Of course. We shall ask.'

When we had finished the soup and I had cleared all away, he said, 'It is time to go to bed, Marie Grosholtz.'

'Yes, sir,' I said, fearing terribly to return to the attic room.

'You may sleep downstairs, if you wish. In the atelier. But don't touch anything! Though wait a moment. Tell me, you weren't frightened in that room alone?'

'I could feel them about the place. All those bits.'

'Yes?'

'And after a while I didn't mind.'

'Yes? Some people are repelled. Bed now. And sleep hard.'

I returned to the atelier and bedded myself down. There I was, under the table, and also there was my head, on the table. In the night, if I was very quiet, I thought I could hear all the body bits breathing. With my wax head in the room I felt I almost belonged.

I thought, also, that if I was very careful he would keep me.

# Chapter Five

*The surgeon again.*

Sometimes I was required at the stove, sometimes to pass Doctor Curtius his tools. To be of use to him, I must learn the names. There were compasses and spatulas, there were burnishers and finishers, there were rakes and wires, and paddles and gougers, there were plaster scrapers and catgut for cutting clay, there were whole battalions of different knives with different grooves upon their tips, some with curved noses, some twisted; there were tools made of iron and of lead and of different woods, of hardwood, and softwood, of rosewood and cherrywood, some smooth, some rough, some must be very sharp and others absolutely blunt; all these I must know by name. All these were the familiar business of the sculptor, but they were only a portion of the tools he used. Curtius had many surgeon's devices that he found essential for his work. They had been christened too and must never be referred to as 'this one' or 'that one', nor ever 'long tip with bend' or 'curved with hook' but the whole enormous genus must be learned and remembered. There was the family of scalpels, from the straight to the convex to the straight-buttoned to the fistula. There were many cousins of scissors, the straight and the fine-angled, the dilator-holders, the plate tenculums. Here was the cannulated stylet, there the cannulated probe. Do not forget the coin-shaped cautery, nor his brother the tapered cautery, nor their cousin the key-shaped cautery. Never confuse a pointed stylus with a seton needle. There are the simplified pelican pliers and those the tirtoir pliers. That there is a cataract knife, and that a nasal probe, this a tongue

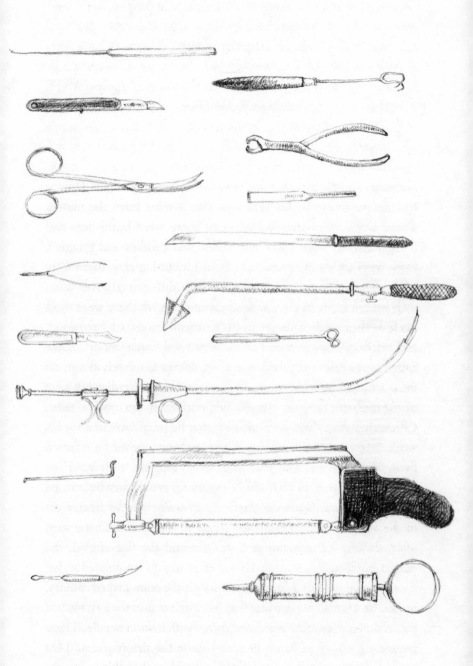

depressor, that a gorgeret. And all these odd-looking tools were made for the wheedling about inside of people, for the picking at this, for the plucking at that, here to scrape, there to cauterise. But Doctor Curtius did not use them for their original purposes; he had adapted them all for his specific modelling purposes. And it did seem to me they had a very deep thirst to enter inside humans. Whenever I picked one up by its handle, I was always absolutely sensible that it wished to change its direction and burrow into me. You had to be very strong with those tools; they had very determined personalities. You must always show them who was master, for the moment – the tiniest moment – you became relaxed with them, they were at your skin. Several times they had the better of me, grazing my fingertip or biting my palm, and always to Curtius's fury. For Curtius they always behaved; he had tamed them all. In his hands they were absolutely meek.

Heinrich from Berne Hospital came twice that first week with his boxfuls, loaded with pieces for Curtius to copy. I watched him and began to assist in minor tasks. Here I was among deep objects. Often those diseased pieces that were delivered to us had already been attacked by some anatomy student in the hospital, had been raked to shreds, a torso already riddled with student holes. What yellow and grey skins were heaved onto the worktable. The smell would wipe out all other scent. Long after the source of the stench had gone away it stayed with you very close, inside your mouth, up your nose, in eyes and skin. Body part, I would wonder, whose were you? A scar, a freckle, a mole, a crease in the cold flesh, hairs along an arm, were enough for wonder. It wasn't such a horror after a while; it became quite usual, something to expect. Curtius taught me that.

'It's just a little of a human body, Marie. Nothing to get worked up about. Human bodies are after all such an everyday thing.'

At the end of the week, Surgeon Hoffmann came. He stood before my wax head in wonder. 'Well, well, here you are all over again. It is a good likeness, Curtius. A very good likeness.'

42

'Thank you, sir,' he said.

'Of course, it is of little significance,' he mused, though he seemed unable to look away. 'I don't suppose, Curtius, but no . . . of course not.'

'Sir?'

'I was going to say something unnecessary, something foolish.'

'Sir?'

'Well, that is, Curtius, I was going to wonder, to suggest, that perhaps you could make such a likeness, such an exactitude, of me. Could you? Do you think?'

'Yes, sir. I could.'

'Really?'

'Certainly, sir.'

'You think me foolish?'

'Not at all. If you would like it, sir.'

'I *would* like it. I believe I deserve to be celebrated, after all. I've done very well. I cannot expect bronze statues, but this, one like this, of wax, well, why not? I should appreciate it.'

'It may be done, sir.'

'Good. Yes. Good.'

Curtius went away to the plaster bins. I stepped forward to the older man.

'Do sit down, sir.'

He sat, a nervousness about him now. I placed a sheet around him as if he were at the barber-surgeon's. Curtius came forward with the oil.

'I must open your shirt a little to expose the neck. Close your eyes, sir.'

'Yes,' he said.

'And keep them closed.'

My master smoothed some oil upon the face. The surgeon flinched.

'I shall be quite under your command, shan't I, Curtius?'

'You must keep absolutely still,' he said. 'It is very necessary that you do. I shall place these straws in your nostrils, and you

43

must breathe through these until I say. And your mouth must remain closed.'

Silence then from the surgeon, silence as we went about him. He had given himself over. His chest upped and downed, sole proof of his continued living. When Curtius pulled the plaster away, there was the man underneath, humbled and vulnerable, blinking, uncertain of us. It was then that I took my moment.

'Excuse me, sir?' I asked the surgeon.

'What is it, child?'

'I was wondering where it is that my mother was taken.'

'Your mother, I'm afraid, is dead.'

'Yes, sir, I do know that. But where is she? I should like to visit her.'

'Visit?' he marvelled. 'What a notion.'

'When my father died, there was a grave. Where, sir, please, is my mother's?'

'Child,' he said, 'there is no grave.'

'No grave, sir? None at all?'

'No, no, there's a pit. She will have been put in with many other unfortunates. But not for the students, not to the hospital, on account of Curtius. I would not allow that. Still a pauper's grave, you understand. A quick burial, not undignified. Some words said. Quicklime. Put alongside the rest of the day's moneyless dead.'

'But where is this pit? Where is my mother now?' I was by now quite desperate.

'You do not speak to me like that. You may not.'

'Please! Please.'

'Records of such matters are not kept. And the quicklime is . . . quick.'

'Oh, Mother!' I cried.

The surgeon went to Curtius.

'May I see my head?'

'It is in there,' said Curtius, showing the mould, 'in negative, in opposite space. But wax shall bring it out.'

44

'I should like to see it.'

'You may, in time. A couple of days. Come back later. We don't need you any more. Not now we have this.'

'I leave my head with you?'

'It is quite safe with us.'

That night, alone in the atelier, I wept into my blanket, for my mother had no grave to visit. Nothing of her, nothing left at all, save her Bible, which seemed to contain only a scrap of her unhappiness. But then, wiping my snotting nose, I came upon a great theory. Here was my nose – my mother's nose. Here she was then, still. Mother. My mother. Thus I stumbled upon my great nose system: she had left me her nose, and that was all I needed to remember her by. My twin air tunnels, from which I might breathe love and smell love. I was glad of these thoughts, proud of my theory. Here was Mother, here was Father, so I might go on.

# Chapter Six

*Heads.*

Curtius made a head of the surgeon. It was a wrinkled head, sagging down slightly at the mouth. A slight frown marked permanently upon the forehead. Thin lips.

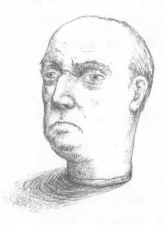

'With your head,' said Curtius to me, 'I felt a great discovery and contentment. With this new one, I feel an anxiety. I must behave in front of this head. I will not be sorry when it is taken away.'

Surgeon Hoffman returned and stood before his wax head. He was very taken with it; there was moisture in his eyes. He sighed very deeply, flared his nostrils.

'Yes,' he said, 'that is me, I admit. How strange to see myself from every angle, to walk around . . . me. As if I were not I at all, but someone else. I had not fully known myself before. Yes, well done.'

46

I do not know whether the last sentiment was delivered to Curtius or to the wax head; certainly he was looking at the head when he said it. He took the head and went back to Berne Hospital. We were neither of us sad to see them go.

Two days later, we had a visit from the hospital chaplain, requesting a head of himself. He was very eager for it, so Curtius took the commission, but when it was made and he came to collect it, he looked a little saddened, as if he had hoped to see some saint presented to him but found only a little balding man with a dimpled chin.

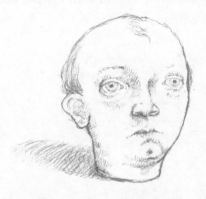

We worked very well together in Welserstrasse, I thought, Doctor Curtius and I. Though on occasion, I admit, I was in his way.

'Sir? Please, sir, do you mind?'

'What?'

'All those bits, sir, on this wall, the healthy bits – gathered up, do they really all fit inside a person?'

'Yes, every person has every one of those.'

'Never!'

'Yes!'

'It cannot be!'

'I tell you it is.'

'We're quite crammed up to the brim, aren't we, sir?'

'Marie, I am trying to work! It used to be quiet in here. Read a

47

book.' Then he seemed to stop, as if in inspiration. 'Better yet, take this charcoal and this piece of paper, go to the corner there, and draw something.'

'Draw what, sir?'

'Draw . . . draw that.'

'What is it?'

'The medulla oblongata, the bulb of the spine.'

'Medulla oblongata. Bulb of the spine. Yes, sir. It looks like a rat with a centre parting.'

'Draw!'

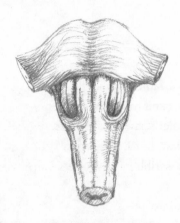

Thus it was that I began to draw. When I was not required at the stove, or passing him his tools, I sat in the corner and drew.

The fourth head Curtius made was that of a hospital governor. Having seen the heads of the surgeon and the hospital chaplain, the governor wanted his own. Here is a truth: people are very fascinated by themselves. He came to Welserstrasse; Curtius was astounded by the attention. The hospital governor put the hospital governor's head in the hospital atrium. He contrived to stand in front of it, often. Soon, people who had nothing to do with the hospital, people who were entirely healthy, perhaps even sprightly, people whose only disease was curiosity, entered through the black gates of the hospital just to see the hospital governor standing beside the hospital governor's head.

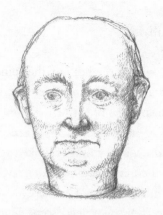

I drew Curtius's father's modelling tools, I drew kidneys and lungs, I drew bones and tumours, the better to know them. I drew Marta, I drew Father's jawplate, I drew myself. I was not good, not at all, not at first, but I was eager.

'Those are just scribblings, Marie,' Curtius said. 'Come with me.'

I followed him into the kitchen. There, he took up a loaf of bread, pulled some white away from the crust, rolled it into a ball, and walked back to the workroom. He took up my drawing – it was a gall bladder, or meant to be – and with the ball of bread rubbed the paper, until what was upon the paper, which had regained most of its former whiteness, was now on the bread ball, which was very black.

'When you make mistakes, and you do make mistakes, go to the kitchen. Bread.'

One afternoon as I was drawing, he asked me, 'What's that?'

'It's one of those,' I said. 'A liver, *hepar*.'

'Is it really?' he asked. 'Look again. Bread.'

Later he said, 'No, not yet, still not yet. Look again, look harder. Bread.'

49

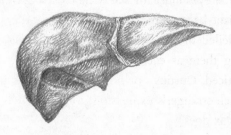

I learned the names of the bones of the body by drawing them, I studied organs of generation and how many bumps there are upon a spine, and I drew everything. I looked at anatomical drawings in his books and copied them in pencil. At night I fell asleep with a pencil in my hand. I drew Curtius.

Thanks to the governor's wax head, some people of Berne began to hear of the name Doctor Curtius and the place Welserstrasse. They began to call. Take my likeness, they said, and Curtius took it. Head of a chandler. Head of a swordsmith. Head of a banker. Head of an officer. People kept coming, one or two a week.

I opened the door to the people of Berne. 'Please to come this way, sir,' I said, and showed each visitor to a seat. Each one stared at the shelves full of Curtius's work. 'Wonderful, aren't they?' I said. 'Wonderful,' the visitors responded nervously. I laid towels around their necks and fronts, gently removed their wigs, washed their faces and pinned back their hair. I asked them to close their eyes and laid some oil over their eyelashes, over their eyebrows, around their chins and at the top of their foreheads. I carefully inserted quills into their nostrils. I was always very gentle. I prepared the heads of Berne for Curtius. 'Berne people no longer come through this door in many pieces,' Curtius happily observed, 'but always and only whole.' The only things missing were women. No woman ever came to Curtius.

Curtius caught every wrinkle and pore, every scar and dimple. For every head, he drew out the region of the eyes, filling sheets of paper with detailed notes and watercolour sketches. When the face is cast, the eyes must for safety be closed up; then, when the heads are finished, they must have open eyes in order to seem alive. Curtius modelled those opened eyes from his drawings and his notes, adding them as each head was finished. With each new person, I noticed, Curtius's own face seemed to shift; he strained to imitate each stranger's expression, to mirror that new face, to creep in as wax does.

Welserstrasse was being discovered by Berne people. Carriages sought it out. But one man was not happy about this new business. Surgeon Hoffmann, seeing all those other wax heads diminishing the effect of his, fearing that the hospital might lose its modeller of anatomy, grew restless and uncertain. What Curtius was engaged in now, he warned, could hardly be called science. Should he continue in this peculiar practice – which must be considered as a sideline and nothing more – he would no longer be supported by Berne Hospital. And soon, indeed, his wages were cut off.

That night, as we sat at table in the kitchen, Curtius delivered an extraordinary speech. Though his head was down as he spoke, as if he addressed his soup, I considered myself his audience, not potato and onion and broth.

'Doctor Hoffmann used to have me model not only for the education of surgeons-to-be,' he began, 'but for the education of the people. Small models of diseases. I should be called to take a casting from one of the hospital wards, to sit beside syphilitic sores about the face of a young boy, to copy a woman's tongue grown rancid or a man brought to nose loss by disease. And each time, after I had made these little models, I was told to take them from street to street and show them to the people of Berne. This here, I was supposed to say, is smallpox: beware. Or this is an example of a siphilide, here is one with alcohol poisoning, here one with opium damage: look out.'

He paused. He slurped. He continued.

'This was my job, and such a job is not good for relationships. Such a job distances you from everyone else. The arrival of such a man on a doorstep with such a job destroys any happiness within. People shunned me! I wept in complaint to Surgeon Hoffmann, and at last I was relieved of any house calls. Then I stayed indoors and saw no one. But I longed for people, and in the end, though he disapproved, Surgeon Hoffmann allowed me my own servants. And you came to me, and your own poor mother left.

'But now I am no longer alone, now I am welcomed. People come to me, they look at me, and though they do not shake my hand, still they look at me. I used to be only, day and night, with death, with dead things, but now life comes to my door, and I say to life: come in, come in, you've been gone so long, welcome, welcome to my house! And I like this new life! But now, Marie, Surgeon Hoffmann has announced that he will not have it! Well, Surgeon Hoffmann does not understand. I shall not go backwards! I shall not do it! A kidney always has another kidney nearby, but I was as singular and as lonely as a vermiform appendix. But no longer. Because of you.'

His soup was over. I took the empty bowl.

'Thank you, sir.'

'Yes,' he said.

He did not see me grinning.

# Chapter Seven

*There is a distant city.*

By the time Curtius's hospital earnings had been cut off, he was making just enough money from the wax heads to carry on. Curtius looked into the store cupboards and confirmed his supply of wax and other necessary materials. He continued to make only heads. Bills were delivered to Curtius: bills for rent, bills for materials, eventually letters demanding that Curtius pay back several months' wages, since in his final months it appeared he had been working not for the hospital but for himself.

One day, Curtius received two foreign visitors. Seeing through the keyhole that they were not from the hospital, I let them in. I said: 'Please to step this way, gentlemen.' Two men dressed in suits, one grey, the other white, both out of breath. The one in white had a notebook and a quill and a travelling bottle of ink with a springed cap; there were blue stains upon his jacket. He was all nose and very little chin.

'We have heard of you,' he said to Curtius in good German, though it was clear he was a foreigner. 'You are not without your local reputation. So. We had time to spare. So. We are here to see for ourselves.'

Curtius invited the men to observe the wax heads upon the shelf waiting to be collected. The man in white looked at the heads very quickly, then sat down uninvited and started rifling through his notebook. The man in grey spent longer with them, his dark eyes close to theirs.

'You are the likenesses of Citizens of Berne,' he said quietly, addressing the heads. 'I know you. I hear you in your small corridors, whispering. It's a hissing sound that you make. A gas of words. I feel your disapproval.'

He turned his back on the heads, stood still for a moment, bent over, and placed his head in his hands, as if he were in some pain, and quietly moaned, 'Where is there a little peace?' He took a withered plant from one of his pockets and proceeded to study it, calming now, murmuring to himself, *'Picris hieracioides,'* words that seemed to soothe him.

The man in white, believing me to be disturbing the man in grey, waved me over. 'Leave him alone, unattractive child; come over to me. He does not understand children. He had children of his own, but he sent them away. But I understand you lot. I can tell, for example, that you're wanting to know what I'm writing in such a furious hurry, aren't you? Of course you are. Well then, since you're insisting, I'll tell you. I'm remembering my walks. A walk has just come back to me. I collect the walks of my life. Some people ask me if I have walked so very far to merit such an activity, but I say to them, it's not about how far you have walked, but how thoroughly. And believe me I *have* walked thoroughly. Of course, now you're wanting to know where it is that I've walked. Aren't you, little boldness' – this he called me, and, very pleased with his own observation, he went on, not caring for a moment how I might take his words – 'little ill-facedness, little minor monster in a child's dress . . . little thing . . . little howl . . . little crumb of protruding flesh . . . little statement on mankind . . . little . . . *little?'* he concluded, not certain in the end of what I was, only that I was little, a little of something.

He scratched his sharp nose and looked down at his shoes and I noticed for the first time that they were both covered in cloth bags that tied up at the ankles, his actual shoes hidden from sight. He undid these bags now and took them off, revealing his shoes: ordinary gentlemen's black leather, worn in places, with silver buckles.

54

'There,' he said, slipping one off and passing it to me. 'Smell it. Smell it with that conk of yours.'

I smelt the shoe. It was rancid.

'Do you know what that smell is?' he asked.

'Is it,' I ventured, for the man had not been kind to me, 'foot rot?'

'Paris,' he said. 'It is Paris.'

That was my first introduction to the city.

'Paris,' I said.

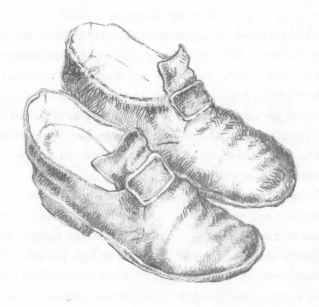

'I have drawn Paris with these shoes of mine,' he continued, 'across the Pont Neuf, along the Rue Saint-Antoine, to the tiny back streets. So many different sentences of streets have my shoes walked me. I write about what I see; I jot it all down. I ignore monuments, great churches, and historic buildings; I speak of people. Delighted people, miserable people, the ones in between: I know them all. I see them in my walks and contain them in my notes. Open any of my notebooks, in any place, and you will smell and hear the great stench and cacophony of Paris. Read any sentence and you'll be walking beside me, amidst it all. With these shoes I have seen them: exhausted encyclopedists, prodigies of chemistry, delegations from the Académie, actors from the Comédie-Française and the Opéra, puppeteers from the boulevards, cobblers of excessive skill, nervous wig-makers, broken street porters, needlessly thorough dentists, wildly inaccurate doctors, rag-and-bone men, midwives, madams, pickpockets, the pock-marked and the powdered, those of royal birth and foundlings; every ingredient in the thick soup of Paris!'

It sounded an extraordinarily busy place.

'We are an inseparable trinity,' the man went on, 'my right shoe, my left shoe and I. We have walked through such horrors, we have trod over such things. Sometimes we slipped, we admit it, but always we got up again.'

He lifted me upon his lap. I was not happy with the perch, it did not suit me, it was not pleasant to feel the man's thighs. Curtius, pretending to be busy at his desk, nearly dropped a large inter-osseous knife for lower-leg surgery.

'Why do you wear those bags, sir?' I asked.

'Because I will never allow my shoes to touch such unworthy streets as the streets of Berne. I am lost anywhere outside of Paris. But in Paris you can blindfold me, you can spin me around and deposit me anywhere, and instantly I'd know which of the sixteen quarters I am in, and not only that but which street too; in fact even the names of the people who live in that street. I have left my city – a terrible thing for me – to visit the man over there whom you disturbed. He's in exile now. His books are banned in Paris and burnt in Geneva.'

I turned to the other man; he was still observing his plant. This, I thought, is a man who writes books? Books that offend people?

'She is my servant,' said Curtius at last. I slid down happily and stood beside my master's desk.

The man in white pointed at the wax heads. 'Altogether, though, you will admit, it does not amount to so very much. There is

56

nothing the matter with the work, that itself is perfectly acceptable. It is the subjects of your work that leave me in doubt. You may just as well have picked up any person from a Berne street and proclaimed him someone worthy of attention, someone who should be queued up to be seen and crowded around, when in truth these people are simply common.'

'I never,' said Curtius, 'distinguish. Not with the body parts; not with the heads.'

'Perhaps you should,' the man said. 'What you need are faces that deserve your gifts, faces that will challenge you. You could carry on here sculpting mediocrities, but consider this: how will you ever progress if the faces are so dull, so petty-minded, so mean-spirited and obscure? You should come to Paris, find a shop there. You'd be far better off. It is a small tragedy to have your talents wasted on Berne. Think of the heads you could have. All the best heads are in Paris, not here. Ah, but I don't suppose you will come, will you? Alas, you do not look the type. Well,' he concluded, 'if you ever change your mind, I'll give you my address.'

Tearing a page from his notebook, he wrote down his name and his address, the word PARIS inscribed with a flourish and many underlines. His name was Louis-Sébastien Mercier.

'And this here, with the plant,' Mercier said, 'we shall call Monsieur Renou. Though it is not his real name. No, we call him Renou to discourage attention. Now, *his*,' he said, pointing to Renou, 'his is quite a head, I'm sure you'll agree. For your information, since you please me, I'll whisper who he is: in your own room, standing just over there, is the author of *Émile* and *Du Contrat Social*. What do you say to that?'

But we had no knowledge of the works or of the celebrated gentleman.

'Should you ever come to Paris,' Monsieur Mercier concluded when we failed to adjust appropriately to his news, 'should you come to where the only pertinent heads are, why not call upon me? I'd like to put you in my notebook – though, alas, coming from Berne as you do, I cannot. But you *are* singular, I'll give you that, with your heads and your rude-faced serving child.'

'All the good heads are in Paris?' asked Curtius, shocked.

'Nowhere else,' said Monsieur Mercier, nodding and smiling. 'Come on, dear Renou – for Renou it is today – on we must go.' Turning back to us, he explained, 'We were being pursued in the city, and finding ourselves near your street, we decided to duck in for a while. But now it is likely safe to venture on. We thank you for your time.'

Curtius showed them to the door, shook the energetic hand of Mercier (whose feet were now fully shod and bagged), and bowed to the distressed author, who in response looked the other way.

I gave the visit barely any significance.

# Chapter Eight

*Which is a worrisome one.*

Surgeon Hoffmann returned at last with final warnings and dark clouds. Very soon, he told Curtius, indeed before the week was out, bailiffs would be coming. Everything he possessed would be claimed by Berne Hospital unless he was somehow capable of immediately paying his considerable debts. He was ruined, the surgeon said; he was drowning in his debts. There was, however, one possibility, one hope that he might be saved: Surgeon Hoffmann, describing himself as a kind man, and as Curtius's only friend, had arranged for him to have a room within Berne Hospital itself, so that he might be kept inside the grounds of that great dark monolith, and be succoured by it. There he could be looked after, he could be watched over, he could work on his anatomical models without any fear of distraction – he could, in short, said Surgeon Hoffmann, be happy.

'Am I in trouble?' asked Curtius. 'Am I in very great trouble?'

'Yes indeed, Philip. I am afraid you are.'

'I don't like to be in trouble. I don't like it at all. I'm worried, Surgeon Hoffmann, worried and also frightened.'

'You should be, Philip,' the surgeon replied, 'and it is not good for you to have so many worries. Let me take them from you. You were not made to battle the commotions of this world; you were made to be looked after. A person of your type always needs protection. Come to the hospital, there's a room for you already assigned. You'll be given your meals every day, everything will be taken care of, there'll be no worries for you any more. You shan't get muddled in your finances again, and since the hospital will provide you with all your comforts, you will have no need for money yourself. I shall see to your well-being myself and I alone shall instruct you on your labour. I shall keep you thoroughly occupied in the spirit of surgery. So, Philip, be sensible, while I can still help you. Should you decline my help, I am very much afraid that people will come for you and put you in prison.'

'Prison!' gasped Curtius.

'For stealing from the hospital. What you have done is not lawful.'

'I did not know! I did not know!'

'But you will be safe, Philip, within the hospital walls. Keep the rest of the world beyond those walls, let it do what it may, but you shall be safe inside.'

'I shall be safe?'

'Indeed yes.'

'Making models?'

'Of course.'

'Not heads?'

'Sometimes, perhaps, heads. The insides of heads.'

'But I don't want the insides any more. They bear down upon me, the insides do, and they turn me,' said Curtius. 'I'm much happier making heads.'

'Philip, are you happy now?'

'No, no, I must admit that I am not.'

'And that is because you've been making heads. It is the only cause of your present unhappiness.'

'And my servant? She will come with me? She and I in that assigned room?'

'That is not really within the laws of the hospital. Besides, you shan't be needing a servant, since everything will be provided for you. You are not really capable in the end of having a servant, are you? But I am here to help. Work can be found for her in the laundries.'

60

'Among so many diseased sheets, in so much sickness?' my master muttered.

'Will you come now, Philip?' asked the surgeon. 'I think that you should.'

'Very well. Yes, the laundries.'

'Sir, sir?' I begged.

'Paris,' whispered Curtius.

'Did you say something?' asked the surgeon.

'Nothing at all,' my master said. 'Surgeon Hoffmann, could I, do you think, be allowed a little time to pack my things alone? I'm such a precise person; I do like to do things exactly and in peace. It will take me a week, I should think.'

'Very good, I shall send porters. In a week. Well done, Philip, you are being sensible. Your father would be very proud.'

With that the surgeon left. I never saw him again.

'I'm very brave now,' Curtius whispered as soon as the door was closed. 'I'm not frightened at all. You can't frighten me, Surgeon Hoffmann – well, well, you can; in fact you do,' he said to the door. 'I'm very frightened, but I'm packing it in with you and Berne. Such a dull, petty-minded place. So mean-spirited and obscure. There are no good heads here, none at all. Not even yours, Surgeon Hoffmann.'

Curtius went into the atelier; he began packing his tools up.

'Can I help, sir?' I asked.

He did not reply.

'Sir,' I asked, 'what is happening?'

'Paris, Marie,' he said, 'Paris.'

He said nothing about my going with him. He said nothing about me at all.

'Am I coming?' I asked. 'I can light the stove. I know the names of most things. I can smooth people's faces down, I can put straws up nostrils. I can do all this. In time, much more. Sir, please, please take me.'

Curtius stopped his business. He lifted me up onto his table top

61

and crouched down, so that our heads were at the same level. 'Something has happened,' he said, tears springing from his eyes. 'Have you not noticed? Something extraordinary. Just as the smaller radius bone is fused to the taller ulna, just as the fibula is to the tibia: we are connected. You and I.'

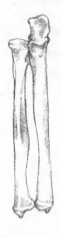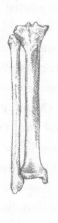

'Sir?'
'I shall not do without you.'
'Thank you, sir! Thank you!'
'No. No. Thank *you*.'
And so then to Paris. Together to Paris. But how was that to be achieved?

To go to Paris, you have to be brave. To be brave, you have to sell some things to gain money. Some of his father's tools, for quite a sum, and two of his books. To be very brave, you must be prepared to say, very often, Paris, Paris, Paris. To be very, very brave, you must get out your papers and fold neatly away the one belonging to a dead mother. To help you be brave, you can hold on to some bones of humans or pieces of sculpted wax.

'Wax helps people in distress,' said my master, passing me a wax epiglottis. 'In certain Catholic countries, it is understood that, should a person or a relative be suffering with acute pains in a part

of his anatomy, that person, or his relative, can purchase, in miniature, in wax, a model of the troubled part – alas, abominably
sculpted, but the principle is there, and the substance undeniable
– which he can then place in the correct chapel in church, so that
God may see where the person is hurting and be moved to cure
him. And thus: wax helps wounded people.'

Slowly Curtius pushed himself, dragged himself out of
Welserstrasse, and went to buy seats for the journey. Afterwards
he was sick, just round the corner, a little on his jacket, but it was
done. Marta, Father's jawplate, and my few clothes were packed
away with other necessary items into my grandfather's trunk. They
did not quite fill it. Curtius packed the wax head of me very carefully. 'We shall need this,' he said, 'to show ourselves off.' What
tools and devices and books he had kept from selling, he packed
up in his father's old tool case, a creased leather thing.

We left the little house in Welserstrasse in the company of two
hospital porters. Curtius gave them the key. He told the porters
that we were going for a walk together, and that afterwards he
would be at the hospital.

'Going for a walk with a trunk?' they asked.

'Oh yes,' said Curtius doubtfully, 'it's very light. To the hospital.'

'We'll take that,' they said; 'put it down.'

'It's no bother,' said Curtius, 'no bother at all. If you may bring
along the furniture, my desk, my bookshelves, that should be an
enormous help.' These, Curtius had told me, would be sufficient
to repay his debts once we were gone. 'The wax pieces, though,'
he mournfully instructed the porters, 'do please be careful. They
are very lovely, and I am sad to leave them . . . if only momen-
tarily!'

We left the house. We had, Curtius supposed, several hours
before our escape would be noticed. We went directly to the hotel
where the coach picked up its passengers. How long the coach took
to arrive; how Curtius kept his head pointed downwards. But at
last the horn sounded, and Mother's trunk and Curtius's leather

bag were taken up. Our seats were on top of the coach. Finally the horses began to pull. Curtius was in tears again.

Half an hour later we left the city gates. Goodbye to my lost mother; I was going like Father before me out into the world, into those uncertain places where, among other possibilities, you could have your jaw taken from you.

Berne went further and further away.

It would never be coming back.

## Book Two

### 1769–1771

# A Dead Tailor's House

*Until I reach ten years of age.*

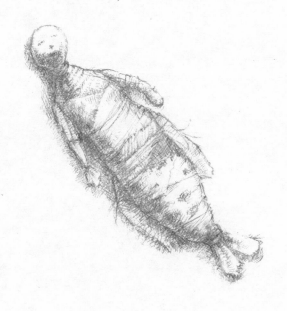

# Chapter Nine

*The newest children.*

Along the way, Doctor Curtius was mostly very silent. He pulled his coat up around him and tried very hard not to look out. At Neuchâtel he changed all his money from Berne thalers to French livres. We swapped coaches before crossing into France. At Dijon we stopped for the night. Since there was one bed in the tiny room Curtius rented, I slept at the end of it. Curtius pulled his knees up to his chest, but often while asleep he involuntarily attempted to straighten himself, and I, awake and anxious, would see the great galleons of his feet rushing towards me, causing waves in the sheets. The following night, at Auxerre, my master called out in his sleep, naming body parts.

The next day we arrived at last.

Paris at first was a smell to me, a stale smell living upon the left shoe of a gentleman called Louis-Sébastien Mercier. Then, as we approached the actual city on top of the coach, Paris was a great mist of dirty yellow seen from a distance: a canker in the sky breaking the winter air, something huge, just out of sight, breathing.

Everything grew darker as Paris drew closer, shades of dirt accumulating in the air. At last we reached the customs gates on the verge of the city proper. Right in front of us was a thirty-foot-high obstruction, a great, forbidding arch. The customs men, unhappy fellows in green coats, appeared. We were instructed gruffly to get down. Cold hands moved about us. All bags and trunks were taken off the coach, opened and searched. Curtius whispered that he would probably be dead any minute. I trembled in fear that we would be separated, for if that happened, how would I ever find him again? Everything was examined. Curtius's wax head of me was passed from one official to another and shaken, until with reluctance the object was proclaimed legal. Our papers were stamped and finally we were waved along. Through the arch the coach went, passing on its way a vast grey block of misery that I would come to learn was the prison fortress known as the Bastille.

As I counted off crooked whitewashed houses, the smell of the city came back to me. I suppose it was the same smell that had resided on Monsieur Mercier's left shoe, only here, at its source, it was far more powerful. I thought I might choke upon it. All around the carriage people darted in and out, locals as muddy as the streets beneath us, yelling at the top of their voices. We arrived finally at a large square. A ladder was banged against the side of the coach for the roof passengers, and Curtius unsteadily descended, his back unable for the moment to straighten, his lower body exceedingly numb. I went down after him. My eight-year-old feet touched the city of Paris for the first time and were, from those very first steps, dirtied by it. I kept very close to him, grasping for a portion of his clothing.

'So,' Curtius said in a whisper when at last he had his breath, 'hello to you, Paris. I'm Curtius, Philip Wilhelm Mathias. I'm here. I'm here.' Looking at me for agreement, he added, 'Here we are, Marie.'

'Paris,' I said.

Paris continued without obvious astonishment. 'This is the address,' he said, taking out Mercier's much-troubled piece of paper.

People knocked into us, a whole gallery of Parisian visages, and none of them kindly. Red noses, yellow eyes, brown teeth, bewigged, shaven-headed, male, female, wrinkled, smooth, and all busy and all finding us inconveniently in their way. Curtius at last managed to show a porter Mercier's address, and the porter, an unhappy youth with a mealy face, took the several coins Curtius proffered, speaking impatiently all the time, though

I understood not a word of it, and filled his barrow quickly with our belongings.

At last, through busy furious streets, we found Mercier's house. Curtius used the knocker such a deal, but there was no answer. The porter was quick enough to leave us there with our luggage. We sat on the doorstep to wait. Two hours or three or four went by, during which Curtius wondered what was happening in Berne now, and whether the hospital was perhaps not such a bad place after all, and that perhaps the laundries were not so miserable, not really if you considered it, and that people working there were not absolutely guaranteed to catch the diseases they scrubbed from the linens. For my part, I wondered what happened to people here if they slept rough upon the streets.

Then at last came the sound of shoes approaching, tapping and clinking, and then they stopped. A voice spoke in French. I looked up and beheld Louis-Sébastien Mercier dressed in shoes no longer concealed in cloth bags but out in the open for all to see, very muddy. Fortunately, he remembered his German.

'Berne, isn't it? What are you doing here? This is my home.'

'You told me,' said Curtius, 'that I should come to Paris. It's a very long way, sir, a long way indeed.'

'Did I? How nice that people listen. And you are visiting for a few days?'

'I've run away, sir,' said Curtius, 'no going back.'

'That's a long time then, isn't it? Do you want me to write about you? What shall you do to make it worthwhile?'

'I do – that is, I did, in Berne – heads.'

'Yes, you did! And you've come here to make heads. Only this time Parisian heads: heads that count. You might, for example, consider mine.'

'I do prefer heads,' said Curtius.

'Any lodgings?' asked Mercier. Curtius shook his head. 'Take my advice, it's best to have lodgings. Money?'

'I make heads. I'm very good at it.'

69

'So you say. And you have brought this child with you, this . . . little bold face, little loud features.'

'Marie, she is called.'

'She's a little exclamation. A little protest. A little insult. In any case, a little something. Yes, I prefer Little. Little is what I name her.'

'She is mine.'

'Is she?'

'Oh yes, certainly!'

'You had better succeed then, because if you don't there shall be two failed starving people, not one.'

'I had to bring her.'

'Did you? An act of kindness, was it?'

'She should have surely perished in the hospital laundries.'

Would I have perished, I wondered, deep in the sheets? And then what new future was this we had bumped into? How long was its rope?

'She would have been fed there, I suppose,' said Mercier. 'There would have been work.'

'You said I should come here. I've nowhere else to go.'

'Yes, there is. There certainly is.'

Mercier told Curtius he was a very careless individual but perhaps quite heroic after all, and that though Paris might seem packed to the brim, it actually had holes in it here and there, many little gaps that were not yet taken up, where a person might live with his servant, perhaps even happily. These places even sometimes drew attention to themselves by little pieces of paper stuck onto exterior doors and walls. Mercier proceeded to list for Curtius places that were available for rent. He could lodge with a tanner just by the river, though the place was somewhat noxious; one tenant had been found a few years back, dead in his sleep and strangely coloured. Curtius did not like the sound of that. Having such a medical background, Mercier ventured, perhaps he might consider the second-floor rooms of a barber-surgeon. No, Curtius insisted, nothing connected in any way to medicine, he was done with that occupation for good and all. For the same reason he refused accommodation with a pill-moulder, a cutler, an elixir wholesaler, and an undertaker. At last Mercier proposed accommodation belonging to a woman, a widow whose husband had been in the tailoring line. There was a son, too, who was being trained in the same business.

'A woman?' asked Curtius.

'There is an abundance of such creatures in Paris.'

'But I have nothing to do with women.'

'What about Little here?'

'I don't think she can be counted, can she? She's just Marie, she's hardly frightening. Sometimes I forget she is even female at all; she seems to have no clear sex really, or one entirely of her own: Male, Female, Marie. She's my Marie.'

I was his; I knew that; nothing else mattered.

'And really,' concluded Curtius, 'after all, that's enough company for me. No, I do not have business with womankind, I do not.'

'Do you want my help?' asked Mercier. 'Or shall I go into my home now and close the door?'

'Yes, yes, please! I need your help. A woman, then, a woman!'

'A tailor's widow.'

'There we are, then. Yes.'

'Good. It is decided. I shall call for a cart.'

'Oh, God.'

'Life,' explained Mercier, 'can be said to start for you now, now that you've found Paris. What passed before doesn't count. Look at you, the newest children in the overstuffed toyshop! I'm sure you don't yet understand the objects, or the playfellows; well, there's plenty of time for that. Come, let us advance.'

Another cart was found, and more money laid out. Mercier rushed us through the crooked streets until at last we reached the place.

Somewhere towards the shrunken middle of the Rue du Petit-Moine in the Faubourg Saint-Marcel was a grim house with a word painted on buckled boards suspended from rusting wires. The word of this house was TAILLEUR. In all the windows greasy black material hung; all was parcelled up in darkness. Here a tailor had died. Mercier reached for the door. As he pushed it open a bell attached to it sounded twice, a loud noise in all that hush. It was a sad sound, two dolorous clangs, that seemed to say, *That. Hurts.* I would come to know that bell, its mottled, calcified clapper like the twin of a kidney stone Curtius had kept in Berne.

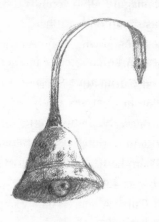

At last someone came to the door. It was a boy with no particular distinguishing features, a pale blank face: here must be the widow's son. Mercier spoke to him, and after a moment his plain face barely nodded and he turned around and went back into the darkness. We followed him into the passageway. Sorrow had choked the house; no sound came, only the quiet whispering of Mercier's clothes as he moved forward, his shoes silent upon the blanketed floor. All was dark and musty. Not only the windows were covered in black material but it seemed every object, all shrouded over, no corner to be found in the whole place. We went through rooms at the back, feeling our way along dark walls, until we arrived in one where a single candle threw meagre light on many bolts of dark cloth. When the son advanced towards one heap of cloth, this heap moved slightly and a hand came out from it and tenderly touched the plain boy and I saw that the plain boy most likely called this heap 'Mother' and that this particular pile of material contained inside it a female human, a widowed one, which now turned around.

Charlotte, the Widow Picot, wore a great black bonnet. Her face was clamped between the surfaces of hard mourning material, though two strands of hair had crept out in rebellion to frame her large cheeks. Her complexion was ruddy; she had sizeable lips and deep dark eyes. There remained about her face the tiniest trace of girl, so that you could just imagine her in younger days, before adulthood had begun to work its stamp on her. She was not unattractive, but it seemed that worry sat upon what handsomeness there was.

Mercier explained to her that we had come to rent a room.

'Heads,' stammered Curtius to Mercier for translation. 'I'm in the business of making heads.'

I was instructed to unwrap the wax head of me and hold it up beside my own. I closed my eyes to increase the effect. There was an unhappy noise. Then the widow exclaimed, and Mercier translated: 'But they are the same!'

'Yes, oh yes,' said Curtius, very proud, clapping.

'How did you do that?' she asked.

'It is my business.'

'And you can do it with anyone,' she demanded, 'or just with her?'

'Anyone, anything,' my master said, 'provided there are surfaces.'

'You earn your money making heads?' said the widow, through Mercier.

'It is to be hoped.'

'She insists,' said Mercier, 'it would not be right to make such things in your bedroom. Rules of the house. You shall rent a working room from her.'

The widow pointed at me. Mercier explained that I was Curtius's assistant. To this she said, 'We used to have a servant. But she had to return to her people in the country.'

'I light the fires,' I volunteered. 'I know all the instruments, I grind colours, I . . .'

'It will be very nice,' the widow interrupted, 'to have a servant again. Paulette always used to sleep in the box room by the kitchen. Would this be agreeable?'

Curtius thought it would. An additional fee would be levied.

'Can she cook?' the widow asked.

Curtius admitted that I cooked for him and even accounted me very good, which made me smile very broadly and keep smiling long after, when they were discussing very different things.

'Welcome to the House of Picot,' the widow said. 'You will find us a very tender people, very feeling, very sore with grief. Do not be rough with us. We hurt very easily. We weep at almost anything, our skins are so thin, my son, Edmond, and me.' I had forgotten about the son; he had been standing there all along, pale and blank. 'Do treat us with kindness.'

'Oh! Certainly!' said Curtius.

Then she put out her hand. I think for a brief moment Curtius was in a panic that he was meant to kiss it, but then Mercier explained: 'Money.' Curtius had come to rent a single room from this woman, and within ten minutes she had him renting three.

'One last thing,' said the widow, 'your papers, please. I shall look after them.'

'My papers?'

'As a guarantee against fleeing should the rent come overdue.'

He handed our papers over. I was not certain that was right. I thought surely they were ours to keep.

The widow took her son aside and a moment later I heard the bell: the quiet boy had gone out. Now she let us into her various chambers. Here were her workbenches, her tools, the spools of thread, her tailor's chalk shaped like flat pebbles. Amidst all these objects, upon the floor, upon the worktables was a tailor's world, a world neat and in its place. Many scissors. Tools for pricking and shearing, tools to scrape cloth, a great variety of needles; there were irons and awls; there were spindles and measures.

'I think I understand,' Curtius whispered. 'I am not unsympathetic.'

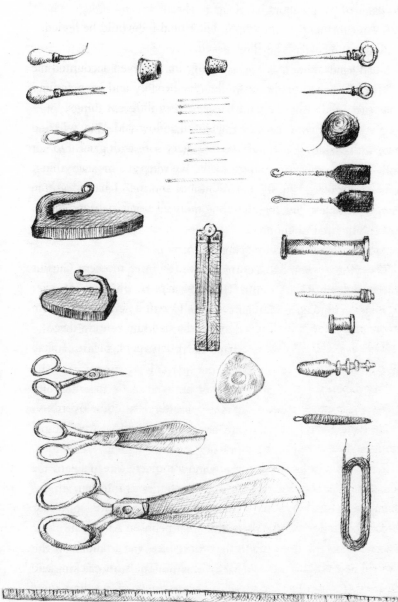

There were four tailor's dummies, which were objects made in the shape of people though lacking any heads or arms or legs. There were three further pretend people, which, unlike the tailor's dummies, had limbs and heads. They had legs that ended in stockinged tapered feet, and hands that on closer inspection were mere flappers roughly in a hand's shape, mittens more than hands. Two were female, one male, each possessing the same bland face, a rough nose, eyes hinted at only by the shadow of the brow, lips that were only thin red lines sewn with thread, that could never open. Not real people, then, but cloth-made people sewn and stuffed with wadding. These were shop dolls, to be placed in shop windows wearing clothes for sale. It seemed possible at first that there was quite a populace in the widow's house, but after a moment it became clear that her workshop contained the most unconvincing companions.

The widow pointed to a corner, where lingered a human-shaped object covered in dark cloth. 'Henri Picot,' she whispered.

'Beneath this cape,' Mercier translated for the widow, 'is a tailor's

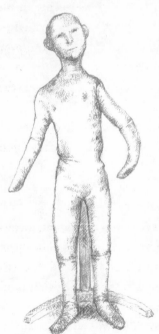

dummy constructed to precisely the shape of this lady's late husband. It was the first tailor's dummy that she and her husband made together, and it is very sacred to her. She insists you are never to touch this. She is most pressing on this matter.' Here, then, the widow's grief was particularly centred, as if the object beneath the covering were the widow's suffering heart.

We were taken to the kitchen at the back. I was motioned to come forward, where I was introduced to the stove and the logs and the coal room, to pots and pans, to cutting boards, to hooks and upon them utensils.

'I shall cook your meals here, sir?'

'I suppose, Marie, yes.'

The widow opened a small door off the kitchen. In the darkness was a room, very small and damp. There was a pallet with a straw mattress. There was no window. Curtius glanced bleakly at the widow, then back at me. 'A room, Marie. Very good. You shall sleep here.'

'Yes, sir. Sir, might I not sleep in your workshop?'

Curtius relayed the question back to the widow. She shook her head.

'I suppose,' said Curtius, 'such things are not the custom in Paris. It is well to do as the Parisians do.'

Curtius's bedroom was upstairs, two windows and a dark bed with a sagging mattress that had surely held many extinguished Picots before Curtius would add his long shallow dent to it.

'I shall be very happy here,' said Curtius, though something in his face seemed full of terror.

The bell rang. The son had returned; he had been sent out for provisions; we were to have a meal together. Mercier agreed to stay. The House of Picot had a very dark dining room, and now the widow and her son, Mercier, and Curtius sat down to some cold meat and cheese. As I prepared to join them, however, the widow broke in loudly.

Servants in Paris, it seemed, do not dine with their masters.

'It is not the Parisian way,' Mercier said. 'Little, I believe you shall be eating in the kitchen.'

I looked at Curtius.

'I have so much to learn,' he said.

'The foreigner,' Mercier agreed, 'is a friendless, ignorant, inconsequential thing, forever asking to be knocked down. Shut up in his rented room, he peers out at the world of Paris and discerns nothing. All foreigners must learn French or be forever shut out.'

'Then I should like to learn French,' announced Curtius.

Mercier agreed to find him a teacher. The widow spoke again, and though I knew little French myself, this time I understood her: 'What is that person still doing here?' I went to the kitchen then and ate as I should always: alone at the kitchen table.

Later on, the blank-faced son showed me where the water was stored and where the bucket of wood ash was for scrubbing, and then I was left to clear away the plates – not only Curtius's but the entire table.

Later still, Curtius came in to see me. 'I shall start French lessons tomorrow. The widow has agreed to help me with my French – a very capable woman she is – for a little remuneration. Mercier will come tomorrow for a sitting. Marie, all is well with you?' But he left no gap for an answer. 'We have arrived. Paris, Marie, Paris.'

My room, with the door closed, was dark and airless. I took out my things, Father's jawplate, Mother's Bible, Marta. When I lay still, I thought I could hear the damp walls weeping.

# Chapter Ten

*Second heads.*

The first head we made in Paris was Louis-Sébastien Mercier's. Mercier explained that there was no real need for him to pay Curtius, since he considered he was doing him a favour, as showing his head around to future clients was the best possible way to explain Curtius's great gift. 'It is all very well,' he said, 'to show off the head of Little, but, you must admit, no matter how lifelike the portrait, no matter how affectionate, still it remains a portrait of an odd-faced child. What you need is a face with some fat upon it, and mine,' he said, pinching his own cheeks, 'is just such a one.' It was indeed a face with fat, that much was true. Mercier insisted that Curtius cast not just his head and neck but a portion of his chest too: a proper bust, he said, as if to suggest that an ordinary man might be compared to the philosophers of antiquity, that man might be contemplated merely for being a man, that we might learn to look better. This change in our work did indeed make the sculpture look more finished, less as if it were missing its body. Moving his hand about his own wax face, Mercier said, 'What a map! What terrain! All the sixteen quarters of my head, and here,' he said, tapping his nose, 'my Notre-Dame.'

Mercier showed Curtius where in the city he might find supplies. I did not go with them. The widow had asked if I might help her, and Curtius said that I might. She pointed to the kitchen floor and the mop, then nodded and smiled and left the room.

'I do like most of all, sir,' I said later, 'to be your assistant.'

'Oh, yes,' he agreed.

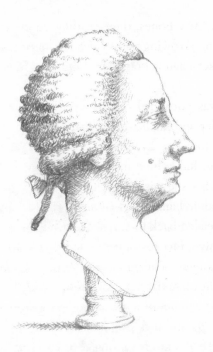

Head of a gossip

'I have been trained, sir, to be your assistant.'

'Yes, of course. But we must help out the poor widowed woman. She is suffering so. Marie, may I tell you a little story? I believe it is like this: once upon a time there was a lonely bone, and it was day after day by itself only. And then suddenly another bone appeared and then another . . .'

'What bones are these that you're talking of, sir?'

'Which particular bones?'

'Yes, sir.'

'Well. Let us see. The spine, perhaps. Ribs. It does not matter.'

'It does not matter which bones, sir? You say that?'

'I cannot tell which, exactly. It is all such fresh territory for me. I never knew any woman before, you see; there never were any. And now perhaps we have newer bones, and it is possible that slowly a creature is being built. What creature it is I cannot say. But these new bones, they fit, they do fit, but it takes some getting used to. Growing pains certainly, one must allow for that, ball and socket chafing together. Bound to hurt a little at first, bound to.'

My day was portioned out between Curtius and the widow, between atelier and kitchen. She wanted me to sweep and polish other rooms too. For as long as possible I pretended I had no understanding, hid behind my German language, allowed her to pantomime what she wished me to do. She pointed to the grimy windows, cloth in hand; I bowed and waited for her to leave, then turned and headed back to Curtius and his tools.

We had only a few customers to start with: friends of Mercier, small businessmen. The first was Mercier's cobbler, to whom Mercier had shown his own portrait bust. Initially Monsieur Orsand could not see the point of a wax bust – he was all about the lowest ends of the body and had little interest in the top – but he agreed to have his likeness taken so long as it cost him very little. With the head in the window, he soon found, he was noticed above other cobblers; he stood out; he was different. People felt they could trust that head with their feet.

After that, our bell began to sound. Mercier brought more businessmen to the workshop. I laid tools ready on the table, lit the fire, ground the pigments. Last of all, the wax was taken out – always Curtius's business – and with the wax in his hands he was home and happy and himself. With wax he could begin to make sense of Paris.

Soon the bell made far more noise for Curtius than the widow, as if she had fallen out of favour with the thing. With my cleaning duties came a necessary freedom of the house, so I wandered from room to room downstairs, familiarising myself with everything. When I was confident in being alone I opened drawers and cupboards, finding mostly empty spaces or mouse droppings. But I had to be careful as I entered a room, for sometimes, after I'd been looking about, I would find that Edmond, the widow's son,

81

had been there all along, standing in a corner or sitting still, his blank face fixed upon me. Most often he appeared in the room beside the dummy of his dead father, which prevented me from looking underneath the covering.

Once my eyes had become accustomed to the dimness of the house, I could move about in the dark and learn where everything was, and I began to see more clearly. Under the grief, I could see now, something else was hiding. The grief could disguise this other thing if you were making a short visit, or if your eyesight was poor, or if you only entered certain rooms, such as the dining room or the front room, where the shop dolls were wearing the widow's tailored clothes. And yet this other thing was surely there: it had gnawed at the curtains, had chipped the pottery, had cracked the windows, had worn away the sheets; it would not light candles in the darkness and left the cupboards bare. This other thing was poverty. The widow's business was failing. Edmond had been sent out to get food that first evening we arrived because there was no food in the house; only after Curtius had paid them did they have money.

Upon a certain evening, I found myself staring at the black cloth that covered the dead tailor Henri Picot's shape. No one else was in the room, I made quite certain. The forbidden object was directly in front of me. I was going to have a very quick look. I lifted the cloth away. Here was the shape of a paunchy human male; old wood and wilting canvas were the substance of the widow's dead husband. The fabric of the dummy's chest was no longer tightly tacked around its frame but sagged inwards, its woodwork chipped and worn. I imagined Henri Picot, when he was substantial, to have been a faint gentleman of impeccable manners, a middle-aged tailor who married a young plump woman and stitched her dresses and must have known his way around female tailoring, for shortly afterwards, before his life was suddenly halted, he fathered her a son. I understood that the man called Henri Picot had factually existed, but I could picture him only as the elderly dummy before me that evening, only as a slightly more complete version of that dummy, with a cloth head and a body of grey faded material and loose stitching, with pale buttons perhaps for eyes, a little moth-eaten man.

I was about to return the black cloth when suddenly there was noise. The widow was there. She had crept into the room, her movements muffled by her mourning weeds.

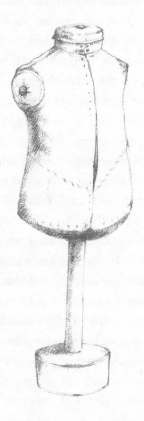

What fury, what rapping of the head, and screams, hers and mine. As if I'd exhumed her poor husband. As if I'd stared upon the actual private corpse.

Curtius came rushing in. 'Marie, my fault,' he said when he understood the disaster. 'Marie, I am to blame. I should have beaten you, I suppose. I should probably have beaten you once a week. I was often beaten. My father and his exactness, you see. I said to myself when the surgeon left you with me in Berne, I said children must be disciplined – I remembered that much – and yet I did nothing about it.'

The red-faced widow nodded energetically, but when Curtius finished his dreadful words she must have thought them insufficient, for she approached me again and slapped me hard across the face.

What noise that contact had; what sound sprang from the violence of her skin as it visited itself briefly and with considerable impact upon mine. I was shocked and hurt, hurt and furious, and I waited for Curtius to strike her back on my behalf. To scream at the widow, to rage and anger at her.

But he did nothing.

'Sir,' I cried. 'Sir!'

He looked surprised and unhappy, but he did nothing other than to whisper, 'Ah. Marie. Please, dear widow, not to?'

But that was nothing at all and followed only by my master biting his own knuckles. Which was also nothing. It was a most terrible nothing, an abominable nothing, for in that nothing the widow understood that she had complete power over me.

The cloth was returned to the private dummy; Henri Picot could sleep his dead sleep once more. I was hurriedly returned to my room; the door closed upon me with no candle; I heard the door of the workshop opening and Curtius and the widow going inside. I was left alone with my swollen cheek.

# Chapter Eleven

*A terrible progress.*

There had never been a woman in Curtius's life before. His mother had died in childbirth; his arrival had meant her departure. But now there was a woman, and he was most struck by her presence. He allowed her very quickly to make decisions for him. He stood still as she picked crumbs from his jacket.

Yet Curtius was ascendant. His workshop was very quickly the greatest room in the house. People came and found sociability and conversation and Mercier laughing. The room held Curtius and his wax; it boasted colours. Happiness was only in that one small district of the house. Who could resist such a place? Not the widow: she found herself visiting the workshop often, watching Curtius, studying his methods, sometimes bringing him wine though he had not asked for it and sitting beside him to study the heads being made. When she left, I noticed, she often left behind one or two hairs in the atelier. I thought of those hairs as spies; whenever I found them I picked them up and put them in the fire. The widow and I were fighting over Curtius; she wished for his complete attention, and I was in her way, and she meant to put me out.

Sometimes, when I returned to the atelier from the kitchen, I discovered that the widow had moved in during my absence. Soon she started to bring glasses of wine for Curtius's customers. After the wine she brought small things for the customers to eat. Curtius did nothing to stop her; he was flattered by it all – worse, he thanked her – and all the while crumbs fell upon the floor, crunching underfoot when stepped upon, and had to be removed by fingernails or with a knife. But most of all it was she who troubled: a woman and her mourning cloth, her smells and hairs and little ways of doing things, smacking her lips together, smoothing down her dress at the knees with her hands, sitting there, uninvited. A woman.

She sat there and watched Curtius and his business; she watched wax busts. And then, at last, she made her move. One afternoon, the widow suddenly stood up and marched out of the atelier. A short while later, she came back with a jacket from her store. She held up the jacket, shook it in front of Curtius's face, and pointed to a bust, which was that of a chandler. Curtius, horrified, said nothing. Then she took hold of the bust and proceeded to dress it. The bust was hollow, and in the hollow she stuffed the back of the jacket, the part that was not necessary for display. Then she set it upright, so that the shoulders of the jacket formed the shoulders of a man. The chandler was dressed.

Silence.

Curtius's chest hunched; I thought he was toppling forward. Then he drew his long arms inwards and there was a very small, and completely silent, joining of hands together, twice. To the uninitiated it may have appeared that he was secretly squashing something small, a fly perhaps, a frog, a snail, a kitten, whereas actually he was clapping.

View a person without clothes, and that person could be anyone from any time, great or insignificant. The human body has changed very little over hundreds of years; no matter what you put over it, underneath it still looks the same. Clothe that person, however, and you pin him down. Curtius smiled at the clothed bust. When he smiled, people often looked the other way, for it was a rather unnerving smile, an enormous dear smile that showed entirely his bad teeth which had gaps between them; it was a smile unlike any other. Most people have many different examples of smiles on which to base their own, but Curtius's smile was grown up in isolation, practised in Welserstrasse to an audience of wax body parts. How should the widow react to such a display? She watched

86

it without looking away, and, forming a conclusion, she nodded. Then she held out her hand.

She wanted paying.

He paid her.

That was only the beginning of it. As if it were not enough that there was a woman with us in the atelier, her son placed his chair in a corner and took up residence. Curtius said nothing. In his corner Edmond would take buttons out and study them very carefully, both sides, then line them up upon his thighs, his face barely changing expression.

'Don't touch anything in here,' I told the boy, though he could not understand my foreigner's tongue. 'He mustn't touch anything, sir. You should tell him.'

'He's just sitting there, Marie.'

'Hasn't he his own business?'

'Will you light the fire now?'

'How do you say "Don't touch" in French?'

Curtius told me, and I repeated it many times. Each time I looked up from work, the pale boy was seated in his corner with his buttons, looking at me, not Curtius, and I would tell him again not to touch. Only when his mother came in did my instructions cease.

That night, when I went to bed, I discovered something terrible.

I had left my doll Marta upon the chair in my room, sitting up, but when I returned she was lying down. Marta is capable of a great many things, she is loyal and always very welcoming, but if she is sitting she stays sitting. She does not lie down; she waits for me to lie her down. Someone had been in my room. I could see no hairs on my bed or on the floor, and so I concluded it was the son who had been here. I held Marta so close. I took her apart and wiped every single piece of her before putting her together again.

It was the first in a series of disasters.

When I came to the atelier the next morning, I found Curtius in the doorway. I told him what had happened and he was sorry for me, but he reminded me that I had recently been reprimanded for a similar act, and also that we lived in Widow Picot's house and that every room was in fact hers.

'Our objects are vulnerable,' I said. 'There are people who yearn for them.'

Curtius muttered a little about things in Paris being so different from those in Berne, which should have alarmed me, should have prepared me. And then it came: he asked me to cook not just for himself but for the widow and her son. The workshop door opened fully; the widow had been seated inside all along.

'It is not right,' Curtius told me, 'for such a lady to be always in the kitchen. Have you seen her hands? They are delicate but punished.'

'I am familiar with them,' I said. 'One of them struck me.'

'She showed them to me. They are very painful hands.'

'That is certain, sir.'

'In fact, I should not mind casting them. She has been so good, I should like to be good in return. Everything is so strange in Paris, and she sets me on the right path. I do need guidance sometimes. I easily turn and get lost.'

'I cook for you, sir. I work for you.'

'Yes, Marie, and you are essential and in every way a blessing. But now when you cook for me, for us, just make a little more.'

'But I am your assistant.'

'That is right.'

'And not hers.'

'But I am asking you. And what I ask you should do.'

'Yes, sir.'

'You mustn't look so upset, no tears; you mustn't; it hurts me here.' He pressed his hand over his chest and its vital muscle.

'Yes, sir.'

So I had less time in the atelier, less time with Doctor Curtius – who seemed not to notice, for the less time I passed in the atelier the more time the Picots were there. The widow began to bring her tailoring work in, and Edmond did likewise.

88

In the kitchen, one day, I chose a plate, a very nice glazed one with a delft blue pattern – I picked it out particularly – then lifted it high and let it go. An accident, I said.

'Be more careful,' Curtius said. He could never abide carelessness with objects.

'Shall I not draw for you, sir? What shall I draw?'

'Don't draw just now; sweep up the pieces. Marie, the widow says if you break anything more you shall be beaten.'

I slipped further and further into the role of household servant. The widow came to me, walking about me with downturned lips, and with her plump digits and a wooden ruler she measured me. The reason for this I soon discovered: she had taken out her former servant Paulette's clothing, cut into it with her large tailoring scissors, and like a butcher severed off pieces of material until what was left assumed my shape. I was to wear a prickly black dress and also a second-hand white bonnet, with someone else's greasy hairs still attached. She told me to change. I went into my room and closed the door.

All the household was there to see the transformation when I emerged, dressed as a serving girl. The widow nodded, her equivalent of Curtius's clap. Edmond looked but revealed nothing.

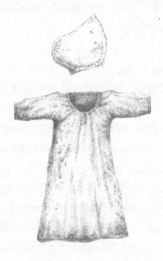

'The widow says you are very lucky to have such clothes,' Curtius told me. 'How beautifully she has made them for you. Say thank you.'

'I am very lucky, sir? These clothes itch – may I take them off?'

I may not. They rubbed at my skin, wearing sore patches into my neck and shoulders. They were made of mourning; the widow's gloom had dyed them. I breathed less well in them, and in them I was inclined to melancholy thoughts. I wondered if she hadn't used her own hairs to stitch them up; if I was wearing widow now. I tried to make my master understand how wrong all this was, but when he looked at me he saw only the widow. The whole city was widow for him now.

Doctor Curtius, out of sorts with dispossession and gratitude, had failed to grasp the significance of my metamorphosis. He had not seen that what had just happened was a shifting of ownership, a possession changing hands. I was rendered a household servant, learning words that were useful to servants, such small vocabulary, and Curtius did nothing to stop it. Adults, I understood, have many faults, they are not perfect – even though they have lived longer, even though they offer themselves as examples to children. They are larger, that is certain, and size has an unearned authority. But they are easily influenced, and they can be easily swayed. He was already lost to her by then. Some hair of the widow, I thought, some fraction of her, had found its way into his lungs.

She cajoled him to be washed, the dirty man, and made him new clothes and burnt the old ones. How he stroked these new coverings. She had him shaved, his hair cut away, and then she wigged him. She was making him acceptable, in her eyes. And how did my poor master react to these assaults? I spied him in his room, crop-skulled and shivering in new underclothes, but holding a wig upon his fingertips, commenting, not without pride: 'I'd recognise you anywhere. You're Doctor Curtius's short-tail bag-wig.'

With this new wig he could be just anyone, any Parisian. To me, it seemed like all the Curtius was being pulled out of him.

\*

Curtius was being managed by the widow, now, just as he had been managed before by the surgeon Hoffmann. Only the surgeon had allowed him far more freedom, had never had him stripped and shaved. Still he grinned all the while at the widow, the dear man.

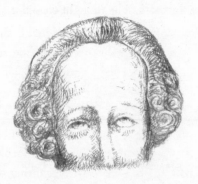

My studies with Curtius grew limited, then all but dwindled out. Before, when I asked him to tell me about the body, he would sit me down and explain at great length. Now he said only, 'Later, Marie, later.' Might I draw? I asked. 'There's no time,' he said. If I drew, I asked him, would he look at my drawings? 'Marie,' he said, 'you are making too much noise; the widow as you can see is napping in the chair there; please don't wake her.'

So I took paper from the widow's rooms – sheets of old yellowing paper she wasn't using – and practised my drawing. I found her pencils, too, and took them for my own. I drew every day without fail. I would remember what I had seen during the day, store it in my head, and relive it on paper at night. I would not stop; I would draw everything. Each drawing I made, each line, was a little proof of me.

Doctor Curtius went out often with the widow, who was eager to show him Paris, but Paris to me was only a dead tailor's house; it was only the market nearby, and the well, and the laundry-women coming once a month. One day, as I was coming back from the market, I saw a mound in a ditch, some heap of rubbish, but when I came closer I saw hair upon one end. A head, a female human head, grey and fallen in, a body lying dead in the street and all the people walking by it and paying it no heed. A person all stopped, collapsed and ignored; a person of indeterminate age that had once dressed itself and been among us. This is Paris, I thought: dead people punctuating the streets, and no one to care for them. The thought chased me home.

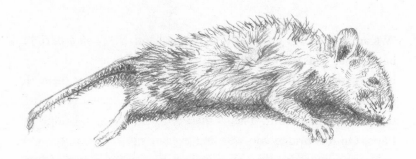

I have substituted a dead rat for the dead woman.

The body was gone next time I went by, a strange horrid little patch where she had been. What were the rules of Paris? Were there any?

On those brief occasions when Monsieur Mercier came in to talk to me, I received some schooling in the subject.

'I do love Paris so,' Mercier told me, 'but in truth, Little, I fear for it terribly. It is getting too, too big. It can't be stopped.'

Each time he came, I asked him to tell me where he had walked, and he would. I listened carefully and imagined myself busy about the streets. Seeing me concentrate so intently, he spent more time with me, took me on longer walks as we sat in the kitchen. I held his hand, I closed my eyes, and together we went travelling.

# Chapter Twelve

*Paris: a tour given by Louis-Sébastien Mercier.*

'We are at the river now, Little. Are you here? Yes, you are, right beside me. This crowded bridge is Paris's vital organ, the very heart of the city. It pumps not blood but people. Pumps them all around the city. Throws them off the bridge with more energy than they came onto it. This is the Pont Neuf, biggest bridge of Paris. On this bridge you will find everything: the beautiful, the ugly, the young, the old, the wretched, murderers, saints, givers, takers, geniuses, charlatans, babies, and skeletons all mixed up together. Here creatures are born and taken away; here life-saving operations are carried out, and life-taking ones too. On this bridge, throughout the day, are the ever-changing tides of song pedlars. Many of these singers are somewhat lacking in something: eyesight, limbs, sense, for example. They take their place and sing out, bawdy songs, slow songs, songs to make you cry, songs to whip you up into a dance, songs to give you peace, songs to take you to war. These song sellers are all around Paris, it is a singing city, but the Pont Neuf is their capital. They control the volume of the bridge, and the bridge controls the volume of the city.

'On we go through the Place Dauphine. Bear right now, Little, around the sad buildings of the Palais de la Cité; there's the top of Sainte-Chapelle in their midst, the great glass jewel case. Now, eyes front, Notre-Dame looms up ahead, but come with me this way. Into these unhappy structures, past a portal of misery. This is our next stop. Come in. Do.

'Welcome to the shame of Paris. Officially termed: Hôtel-Dieu,

93

the House of God. Also known as Death Hole. Here priests and nuns run about, ordering diseases from one bed to the next, marshalling illnesses incorrectly, spreading infections as they attempt to spread God. This is what the poor of Paris fear: these damp walls. This is what the poor of the city say to each other: I shall end in the hospital, just like my father. The Hôtel-Dieu will not turn them away. This is where poor people come to die. Despair, despair, despair, and follow me. There are generally six thousand patients here, though it varies with the season of course; there are dying seasons in Paris. Six thousand patients but only one thousand two hundred beds. No matter what your ailment, you will be thrown into a bed with someone who has a far different and possibly very infectious illness: your bedfellow most likely will kill you. They carry out the dead in carts at the earliest hint of the morning or in the darkest minutes of the night, so that no one can see the daily harvest. Buildings of the Sunken Spirit! Do not breathe too deep, for the air around these buildings has an evil, angry nature, made worse by the river, which makes everything heavy and damp. There's not a corner of dryness in this entire hospital. Forgive me now, for this building needs to be kicked. I kick it every time I pass with these beloved shoes; they're quite used to it by now. It scuffs the leather a little and bruises my toes, but even so this building must be kicked. There are many such buildings across Paris that need kicking.

'Come, there's something else you should see. Here in this small courtyard, where the air you breathe has been long forgotten by everywhere else, you see flush against a dripping, moss-covered wall a small hut. A sty, perhaps, something fit for a pig. Or a kennel for an unloved dog. This is what I found on one of my walks. Please be quiet. Look in. Now I must whisper. Inside this tiny wooden cage is one of this place's patients. A boy wrapped in a soiled rag, shivering, mumbling away to himself. A child with a massive head. The child, you see, is so thin, but that great head pushes the eyes apart, the cheeks two globes in themselves, the whole a great dome of swelling. A hydrocephalic child, stagnating in the dark, nibbling eagerly on a bone long picked clean of nourishment. See the sign around his neck: DO NOT FEED. You must forgive me now, for being overcome with allegory. I call this child *France*. His real name, I believe, has been lost. France, you understand, is a rickety child whose every nourishment goes only to the head, leaving the body weak and emaciated. Each time he eats only his head grows, never his body. And he can't stop eating. He's always so very hungry. France's head grows and starves his body. How long, do you think, can he live? How long do you think our country will survive? Sssh now, come away. It's time to move on. Don't linger there. There's nothing you can do for him. He's only excited because he thinks you might feed him. He doesn't care for people, only for food. Come; from this dark and cramped hovel, we'll climb up into the air, climb as high as we can go. I'll make you two hundred and seven feet taller, and then, when we've no higher to climb, we'll look down on it all.

'So. Notre-Dame. Here is time, Little, carved in stone. Greatest monument of our city, most famous of edifices. Wisest and most complicated of buildings. Or, do you not think, with her flying buttresses coming out from her sides and behind like so many arched legs, that she resembles a great spider athwart this thick and complicated web of Paris, fed by her visitors who leave small coins of charity? She is, after all, the first object worthy of note in this monstrous mess. Let us ascend the spiral stairs of this monolith. I shall go ahead, I shall advance before you around each corner.

'Can you hear my voice echoing now, Little? Sometimes closer, sometimes further away? The stairs here grow narrower, round and round, up and up, to such a height. You can catch glimpses of the city through slit windows, diminishing, growing further away, as we climb. Can you hear my breathing now, my beloved shoes clacking against the stone steps? And the steps turn grudgingly now; they have built up a rhythm and want to go on ascending

95

forever, but one last twist and we have reached the top of the North Tower.

'So. Here it is. Paris, as it looks from the top of the tower. What can I tell you? This: Paris is situated in the middle of the Île-de-France, on the banks of the Seine. It is forty-eight degrees and a half and three minutes north latitude, east of London. Two miles in breadth, six miles in circumference. You will observe that the city is near perfectly round. Have a look, do please, there it is. Paris, formerly called Lutetia – which means, you will be unsurprised to learn, the City of Mud. Or, we might call it, Subterranean Town. Or perhaps: Labyrinth of Shadows. Or even: the Universe Abridged. It's all there, look at it, alive and moving. You can see palaces – there's the Palais des Tuileries. You can see hospitals – there's the Dôme des Invalides. You can see theatres – there's the Comédie-Française. You can see prisons – behind us the monstrous oblong of the Bastille.

'But what do they all mean? How can you ever learn it, how can you ever read it, this great mess of roofs, this great confusion of buildings and of people, this melting pot, this great sink down which everything is poured, eight hundred and ten streets, twenty-three thousand houses, home to seven hundred thousand people? All kept inside the city by lock and key – you can't get out without permission – and all of them, or most of them, trying to live, wanting the best for themselves in this home, this world of Paris!

'And yet! Alas! Listen to me carefully, Little. I have come to understand the awful truth: Paris is suffocating. It can't go on, it can't breathe, it gasps but no air reaches its bloody lungs. You want to ask a question, Little, I can see you do. Everyone does. You want to know how anyone can endure this place, this vile home, capital of misery. You want to know how people can breathe this poison air each day. Why people dwell in such urinous pools, why people choose such an excrementious location, why people whose eyes can still register light lock themselves voluntarily in this darkest of abysses. Well, I'll tell you, it's very simple: habit. The Parisian connects himself to all these evils, because this place, putrid and corrupt, is the hell we call home. And we would never leave it, for despite everything we love it. We love it. I love it.

'Here ends my tour. Now I slip off a shoe and pass it around. All gratuities gratefully received. You have no money, Little? Then give me a kiss, odd child of Paris that you are.'

And I would kiss him on the cheek, and off he would go, leaving me behind in the kitchen, eyes closed, imagining myself floating about the city.

# Chapter Thirteen

*I am shut out.*

I drew the heads in the evening of the fish I had bought in the day. Everything was to be drawn, and my piles of yellowing paper dwindled. The drawings themselves I rolled up and hid at the back of a kitchen drawer. At night I would creep into the atelier and draw Curtius's heads of Paris. By now my own head, modelled in Berne, had been taken off the shelf, wrapped in cloth and tucked away in a cupboard. I sat with those new wax personalities, and I felt they were very happy to have me there. They longed to speak, I thought, but were not quite able. There is a melancholy to wax heads: they were never born, they capture life, but life shrugs away from them. In the quietest moments, I whispered to these half-personalities: 'I'll sit with you,' I said. 'Are you frightened of the dark? Don't be.'

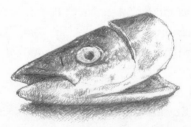

Living inside the dead tailor's house in those days, you could just hear it, barely audible at first: the sound of a distant ticking, of cogs creaking, the noises of a great machine beginning to live. And you would have to have great faith to hear those sounds, for all there was then was a widow and her measuring son, a thin foreign doctor and his little servant girl, and a house in mourning. It was a small business then, nothing likely to attract attention, very unassuming. People find such varied ways of getting on. There were many thousands of private concerns operating throughout the city. On the Rue des Chiens, so I learned from Mercier, a father and son blew glass eyes; Curtius began to use these for his wax heads. On the Quai des Morfondus, a man dealt in second-hand wigs; Curtius bought these for his wax heads. On the Rue Censier, there was a small school for making artificial flowers, founded by a matron from Toulouse; the widow used these to decorate Curtius's atelier, now rechristened the Sitting Room. And on the Rue du Petit-Moine, a small private business Rue consisted of making busts of small-time Parisian businessmen out of wax. People find such varied ways of getting on.

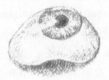

Months passed. The widow worked on clothes for the busts. Once, when I was polishing the tools, I saw the widow take up a bust while she was talking. After a while she set it down again, but not with precision, so that it rocked back and forth a little. Curtius looked at the bobbing head and shouted – *O marvellous noise!*—

'To hand it so! As if it were a butcher's thing!'

That's Doctor Curtius, I thought, there he is again! But instantly he looked appalled at himself. The widow was silent; she did not understand him, but she had heard his anger, and then, suddenly, she was in tears. At the sight of this Curtius teared too, until the room was filled with a general wailing. What sorrow on her face, what a choking up, the son immediately to her side. The tailor had been dead mere weeks, I reminded myself; it was a very fresh grief and it held her still very hard. She never showed herself again like that, but in that moment there it was: a human being, trying to survive.

Then, as she dabbed her face with her handkerchief, the widow looked around and caught me observing her, and in that instant she knew I understood what I'd just seen. The mouth turned down a little, in a look of absolute recognition, and I knew I'd made myself a greater enemy. I'd comprehended her vulnerability.

Afterwards, the widow never handled a head with indifference. At first she just moved more carefully, but as time went on, I admit, her work began to show some tenderness. She seemed to register how Curtius cared, how concerned he was for all the chins and ears, how he sympathised with every fold of flesh. Curtius was in love with eyelids and lips; he would swoon over an eyebrow, fidget in excitement at a mole or dimple. If a subject had two or three small hairs beneath his nose missed by the barber, Curtius would ensure that they were a part of the finished head. It did not matter if the head he was making had burst corpuscles around the nose, or pores so large they could be seen several paces off; it didn't matter if the head was wall-eyed, or the skin was so shiny that the wax must be varnished to suggest patches of sweat: whoever came to him, Curtius loved. And of all the faces it was the widow's that he saw most, and in that familiarity grew an interest.

All of this, the widow watched and learned.

And as she learned, I regret to report, possessions got very muddled. Returning to the workshop whenever I could, I discovered new and terrible progressions. Her tools, for one, had joined his upon the table. To begin with they kept to one side, but later I saw those different tools, his and hers, moving closer and becoming acquainted. Once I saw the widow reach out and take a hold of Doctor Curtius's trocar, the trocar with straight shank, which was designed to penetrate the skin to evacuate deep abscesses, but was used very successfully by Curtius for making passages in wax ears. The widow took this object up and used it to penetrate calico. But that was not all: incredibly, Curtius sometimes borrowed the widow's narrow buttonhole hooks and used them to draw out nostrils. And so, it will be understood, I had to take action before it was too late.

Only I could return order to the household. Only I could help them. I was supposed to keep things in their right place; that was one of my functions. And that is what I did. I took up all those tailoring things and lined them up neatly in the tailor's workshop, where they should always have been. And did I get thanks for my great carefulness? I did not. How they complained, both of them. How they moaned, how they protested that they could no longer find anything. I was bad, they said, very bad. The widow said I should be discharged, sent back to Berne, returned to where I came from, for moving other people's property; that I should be expelled from France, where I was neither wanted nor welcome. To whom would I be returned, I wondered. But my master would not dismiss me, though my actions must be addressed.

I was to be punished for my sins, it was announced. I prepared myself for a beating, wondering who should beat me, Curtius or the widow. But I was not beaten. I wish I had been, for the punishment I received was worse than any beating: I was forbidden access to the workshop. I must never go in again. Life, out of bounds. I pleaded with my master, but he simply tapped me, fondly, on the top of my head, my servant's cap, and repeated that the decision had been made. And that was a sort of goodbye. Thereafter I saw him for only a few minutes each day, and these were mostly observed by the widow.

Curtius had shown me so many things. He had shown me such affection, too. Perhaps, I thought, he should never have done it. Perhaps if he hadn't I should have been quiet; I should have been an excellent servant; I would not have had so many thoughts. But he gave me a taste for it – for work, for thinking, for wax – and I could not get that taste out of my mouth. I clung to it. Every night, when they were sleeping upstairs, I went into the workshop and the wax heads there told me of everything that had gone on

101

during the day. And I drew. I took out his anatomical books and I studied and I drew. How I longed to see him, but he never came into the kitchen to see me any more; only Mercier would call in, now and then, to pinch my cheeks with his inky fingers before rushing out to wander over his city.

And so, on that particular day, I was delighted at first when the kitchen door was knocked upon and my master entered.

'Marie,' he said, but then these words followed: 'The widow is missing many sheets of tailor's patterns. Have you seen them?'

'Tailor's patterns, sir? I promise I don't know what you are talking about.'

The widow was livid. Those yellowing sheets of paper I'd lifted: these were patterns belonging to her late husband. Now she accused me of burning them. I was called an evil foreign child who would never learn her place.

'Marie,' Curtius said, and his eyes were wet, 'you shall be beaten now.'

'No, sir, no!'

But then the blank son said something. Just three words, which Curtius had taught me: 'I' and 'took' and 'them'. And then was silent again.

But that was not right. He had not taken them. I had. Why should he lie? Why should he speak those words, which made all silent in the kitchen? The widow marched her son from the room.

'She should apologise to me, sir,' I said, hardly believing my reprieve, but hoping to make the most from it. 'She should apologise.'

'Marie,' he said, 'I must apologise to you. I was sure you had taken them. For that I am very sorry.' These words hardly made me feel better.

But why had the boy lied? Why had he? I was told nothing.

One evening, climbing the stairs to lay out Curtius's bedclothes, I discovered a terrible thing. When I happened to peer into an open door, I noticed that the widow had removed her bonnet, revealing an incredible mass of hair. Moving around the hairy

102

greatness went Edmond, diligent with a comb. The widow's bug eyes were closed; she was peaceful. I kept there in the darkness, watching Edmond bother out tangles, up to his arm it seemed to me in his mother's head growth. Here was all the widow's softness, kept sealed up during the day, but pulled out and gently managed by the son in the evening. He tended to his mother's gentleness before gathering up all that affection and plaiting it into great hair intestines, which he coiled and pinned neatly around her head before tucking them out of sight beneath a large black cloth cap. The widow herself tied the bow around her fleshy underchin, and with the hair out of sight hard-heartedness returned. The widow's eyes opened, turned suddenly, and glimpsed me through the door. I rushed onwards. All that hair recalled to me one of Mother's people from her Bible, Mary Magdalene, out in the wilderness.

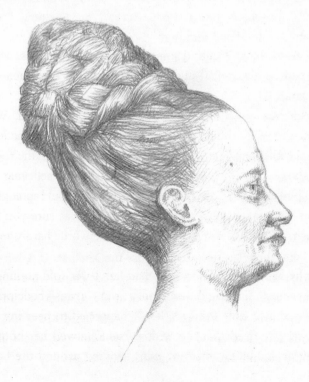

The reward for my spying upon the widow in her bedroom – 'spying' was her word – was that I was no longer to come upstairs in the evening. 'Please, Marie, do not upset her,' Curtius pleaded. I was no longer, in fact, to clean my master's bedroom at all; this the widow would see to herself. I had become little more than a kitchen maid. Sitting in the kitchen, how I seethed. I seethed until I could bear it no longer and went into the workshop without knocking.

'If I am a servant, I should be paid. Apprentices don't get paid but I'm certain servants do.'

'Marie, what are you doing in here?'

But Curtius spoke to the widow. I understood by their gestures that they were discussing money. I put my hand out. The widow laughed.

'No money?' I asked.

'Well, you see,' said my master, 'I do want to pay you. I shall pay you one day. Only now we do not have so much money. Later, there will surely be money and pay. But not yet. For now, Little, you are paid in food and lodging.'

'I should be paid,' I said. 'I'm almost sure of it.'

'Well, yes, you may be right. I do not know the ways of Paris. All will be well.'

'Will it?'

'Oh, yes.'

The widow said something. Curtius smiled weakly.

'Ah, Marie . . . I think you should go now.'

'Is that what you think, sir?'

'Ah . . . yes, Marie, it is.'

'I'll leave then.'

And I had nowhere else to go. Just the kitchen. If I left the house, what should happen to me? There seemed no other option but to stay there; it was my one chance at life. Otherwise I might fail, like the dead woman on the street. And besides, I could not flee my master. How could he manage without me? The widow would quite eat him up. She'd digest him.

104

# Chapter Fourteen

*Edmonds, in the kitchen.*

I was standing on a stool in the kitchen skinning a rabbit, and I must have been concentrating very hard, for suddenly I was aware of a faint rustling sound. I was not alone. The widow's son was beside me. He looked at me for a long time, and I looked back. 'No touching,' I told him in his language. And then, after a while, 'Thank you.' His ears, I saw, immediately reddened. He had, I may say this now, the most eloquent ears of anyone I have ever met. His face remained pale, he did not tremble, but his ears flushed. At last the boy nodded faintly, as if he had been considering something quite seriously and had finally reached a conclusion. He dug about in his pocket and pulled out a very scrawny doll made of cloth.

'Edmond,' he said, indicating the doll.

'Edmond?' I asked, pointing at the doll.

'Edmond,' he said.

'Edmond? Edmond and Edmond?'

He nodded. The boy had named his doll after himself. This doll, I saw instantly, was a relative of the tailor's dummy in the shape of the dead tailor. Here, in this grim home, family shapes were duplicated. There was the family in the flesh and then there was a second family, the family of cloth. You may not see this cloth populace at first; the cloth people mostly kept themselves to themselves, a sullen, sulky tribe; but after a time their coarse material made its presence known through their vaguely human shapes, in their almost imperceptible sighing. They took up space.

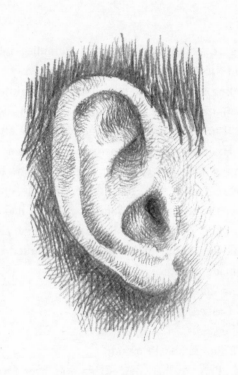

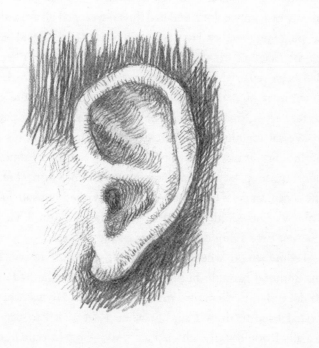

Human feelings made from scraps, hoping in the half-light. Here was a representation of Edmond, a son to the tailor's dummy. I observed the thing.

After some silence and consideration, I washed my hands and carefully took her out. 'Marta,' I said. Edmond had met her before but he did not know her name.

I lay Marta on the table. He carefully lowered Edmond. Edmond the doll was fashioned of ten or twelve different pieces of cloth, mostly of a grey colour, and had thread wrapped all around the body keeping him together. He was a mess of torn and clipped bits; I could not be exactly sure where his limbs were supposed to be. The doll had been repaired with thread, over and over it seemed, and with new pieces of material sewn on by Edmond. Miniature cloth boy, secret keeper, small person to be worried over and whispered to.

We sat together at the kitchen table, I looking at his Edmond, he looking at my Marta, until Edmond returned Edmond to his pocket, got up, bowed, and left without another word. I understood the significance of the meeting. He'd revealed himself fully, in the only way he could: through slightly damp cloth. That was only the first time Edmond visited me in the kitchen.

From then on, whenever his mother went out, the pale boy came in. Edmond brought buttons with him so that he had something to do, ordering them into rows on his knees. He was very quiet at first. I tried to draw him, but when I set pencil to paper, where usually I would start with a person's nose, now I would be confused, for the nose did not seem very much of a nose, nor did the eyes really, or the mouth; only the ears were helpful when they reddened. At first I feared that the cloth representation had more personality than the true boy. The more I focused upon him, though, the more he began to appear, like a deathwatch beetle that comes out only after all others have gone to bed, and you've stayed up all night to keep a corpse company. Once I had found him, once I had him in pencil before me, I saw him clearly thereafter – as if he were a puzzle and I'd solved him.

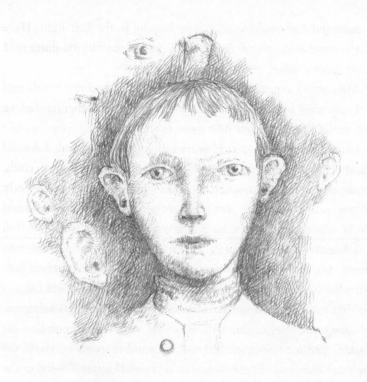

He had plump lips; green eyes; his nostrils were not quite even; he had some freckles around the bridge of his nose; there was a small mole on the back of his neck. I drew him several times, until he became quite accustomed to it. After a time, when I did not draw him, he seemed rather put out.

In those days I existed in that foreigner's fog, as Monsieur Mercier called it, which meant that I did not fully exist. I could comprehend little beyond the few words drummed into me by the widow. But later on, when she went out with my master, I had a tutor too. When Edmond came in the kitchen, I decided that he must do more than take out his doll and buttons. I picked up a rag – a word taught me by the widow – and showed it to him.

'Rag,' I said. 'Rag. Rag.'

Edmond said nothing.

I pointed to the window. 'Window,' I said. I pointed to a chicken hanging in the kitchen. 'Chicken,' I said, 'chicken.'

Edmond said nothing.

I pointed to the button in his hand. I pointed to it. I pointed to it. At last he asked, 'Button?' in his language.

'But-ton,' I repeated, 'but-ton.'

Only after *shirt* and *collar* and *hair* did he understand that he was to teach me French. We went to the tailoring rooms, which, neglected by his mother, had become his province. I pointed to an object and he told me its name, and that I must remember that name, that he should test me on it next time. He was very serious. When I was wrong, the blank face shook a little, but the voice was never raised. It was always quiet and gentle.

I learned French through the language of tailors. Just as my master had shown me his particular knowledge, so Edmond told me what he knew of the world. My first words were not *cat* and *rat*, but rather *thread* and *scissors* and *bobbin*. I knew *gusset* before I knew *good night*, *hessian* before *how do you do*, *calico* before *hello*, *thimble* before *hymnal*. I learned *croquet* and *poinçon*, knew my *marquoir* and *poussoir*, my *mesure de collet* and *mesure de veste*. I was immersed in this world of words.

Edmond's most essential object, besides the cloth Edmond, was his tape measure, a long strip of thin leather with small and large markings drawn along its side. There were many other measures, long wooden rods with numbers down their sides, but the tape measure was Edmond's own, tied around his waist when it was not in use. Edmond measured me. After months of our clandestine lessons, it was no longer sufficient for me to say to him 'My name is Marie'; now I must say 'My name is Marie, my shoulders are two and a quarter inches, my neck seven and an eighth, my arms from pit to cuff fifteen and a third, my legs sixteen and a seventh, my waist seven and a third.' By the time I had learned my figures with Edmond, I could comprehend most of what Edmond had to say.

After a time, I demanded more from Edmond. I wanted books, primers to help me learn. I wanted to know more than just tailor's words. With Edmond as my tutor, my language progressed. I began to catch up with my distant master and, after a while, even to overtake him, for the widow would sometimes stop me and ask, 'How did you know that word? I never taught it you.'

Standing before the tailor's dolls in the front room, Edmond asked in his quiet, precise manner, 'May I show you our shop dolls properly? We sell them to some shops on the Rue Saint-Honoré, perhaps five a year now. Some are male, some are female; here they are. They have the same faces and the same expressions, you see, all of them do, regardless of sex. They vary only inasmuch as some of them sit and some of them stand, and some have breasts and are slightly wider at the hips. There are more that stand rather than sit. They are based on me, did you not notice? Male and female, I am the general measurement for the shop dolls. It was Mother's idea; she likes to have me up and down the Rue Saint-Honoré wearing such things. They are, I suppose, my brothers and sisters.'

How many Edmonds were there in the world?

'Thank you, Edmond, thank you for showing me.'

'Welcome.'

'You are so talkative today.'

I thought of Edmond when he was away; he was my company. As our afternoons progressed, I learned more things. I learned the words for bits of the body: arms, legs, head, ears, eyes; that was easy. But it wasn't enough.

'I need to learn more,' I said. 'I need to see things. I've such a hunger, Edmond.'

'Do you? This is the kitchen. There is food. I'm hungry myself.'

'It's not that sort of hunger I have.'

'No, Marie, you say not?'

'No, I want to know things, I want to know everything. Even here in this house there is so much to learn. I think I have seen it all, looked in every cupboard, lifted every curtain, explored shelves from top to bottom. But then, just when I'm certain there's nothing else, when I think at last I've looked everywhere there is to look, suddenly I see something else.'

111

'Marie, have you been nosing around again?'

'There's you.'

'There's me?'

'You are someone.'

'I am, I do think so.'

'I don't know what you look like,' I said, 'under your clothes. That's a drawer I haven't opened. Take off your shirt, I would like to draw you.'

'You must not!'

'Oh come, don't be fussy. I've seen so many bodies. In Berne I did. I've seen *inside* bodies. Come along, Edmond, let me take a look.'

'What are you doing?'

'I am undoing you.'

'Oh no!'

'I am going to remove your shirt.'

'Oh! Please!'

'I know all about bodies. Doctor Curtius taught me.'

'Oh dear!'

'Yes! See how I unbutton you!'

'I do see it. I feel it.'

'I am going to learn you, Edmond Picot. Every section of you.'

'Mother! Mother might come in.'

'She's gone out.'

'She may be back.'

'There's time, you know there is.'

'I'm cold.'

'Then move to the fire.'

'How you look at me!'

'I want to see you.'

'How you stare!'

'Can I touch?'

'I should go.'

'I see your little frame, your ribs, the life under you moving! Edmond with the human skin! You're lovely!'

112

'Marie! Marie! Stop!'

'I want to look. Take your hands away, Edmond, I want to look!'

'I can't! I cannot! It's too much to have you staring so.'

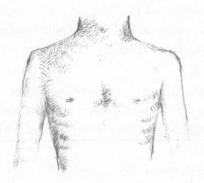

The bell sounded. The widow and Curtius were home. Edmond rushed his shirt back over him, in such a panicking.

'Edmond!' called the widow. 'Edmond, where are you?'

His hands were shaking terribly as he fled to her. He did not return for several days. When he did, on a pretence, he was still clearly uncomfortable.

'Oh, you are here! I did not know you should be . . .'

'It's where I generally am, the kitchen.'

'Yes, yes, for now. And perhaps you may remain thus situated, until the end of the month. Perhaps.'

'Why a month?'

'I do not think you shall stay much longer than a month. Mother does not like you, and Mother is used to having her way.'

'Oh, Edmond, please, Edmond, will you help me with your mother? I don't want to leave. There's nowhere else for me to go.'

'You must do everything she asks.'

'Yes, I shall. I shall do my very best.'

'You must not break things or move them about.'

'I will do my best.'

'She says you are always lurking.'

'I do not mean to. They should pay me, Edmond. I haven't yet been paid.'

'Do not ask it, Marie. Do not anger them in any way.'

'I will try. It is not always easy.'

'You must not take off my shirt.'

'I shan't, Edmond; I shall never again.'

'You are a servant.'

I said nothing.

'You are a servant, and I am the young master of this house.'

I said nothing.

'One day I shall be a tailor!'

Nothing.

'One day a great tailor. You a servant.'

'Will you help me?' I asked.

'Yes. I shall try.'

'I do want to stay.'

'Then you must behave.'

I worked. I was a servant, the best servant I could ever be.

I put myself away. I came up with the great vanishing system, in which I could retreat so deep within myself that, though I may appear still the same creature, actually I was very different. I thrust all thoughts and feelings in the depths of me, where they were safe, but in an outward way I became something like an automaton. I was wound up by their orders and performed them mechanically but perfectly. I muted myself and put on the role of servant so that I might have a chance at living. But when I was alone, when they were elsewhere, I recalled myself to me, then I was all about Marie again. Still there.

# Chapter Fifteen

*The citizen of the year 2440.*

I must talk for a moment of larger things, things of French significance. For suddenly it happened that I knew someone very famous.

While wax busts were made and clothed, another world away, so it seemed to me, the Dauphin of France was married to Marie Antoinette of Austria. In Paris, during a mass celebration for the wedding, some prematurely ignited fireworks started a panic in which one hundred and thirty-three Parisians were crushed to death, among them many women and children. After the fatal stampede, Louis-Sébastien Mercier was in such a temper that he found it quite impossible to calm himself. Collecting all his notebooks, he saw a terrible theme running through his work, and the theme was suffering. For a few days he found it impossible to walk out in his familiar streets.

'I hate this place now, Little, this abattoir, this cesspool. What casual monsters we are. What calamities we are capable of.'

Having talked to my master and the widow until she barked him away, he came to me. I sat him down, gave him a glass of wine from the widow's decanter.

'Tell me,' I said. 'Tell me all. Quickly before they call you back.'

So he told me of crushed bodies and screams and blood. And that the king had done nothing about it. He took his shoes off and put them on the kitchen table.

'My shoes are insulted,' he said.

'I have just scrubbed the table,' I said.

'Perhaps you are right to stay shut up inside.'

'No, don't say that.'

'What a world it is. I want none of it.'

'Is it? Won't you tell me?'

'If I could but walk the land of this wooden surface, washed and fresh, a new land, an undiscovered land. Yes, if only . . . but . . . well, why ever not? Yes, that's it! A new home! Yes, clean! Yes, Little, with your scrubbing brush, make it shine!'

He tore his shoes from the table and bolted from the house.

Yearning to promenade in a happier place, Mercier set himself down to write a guidebook to a Paris in the future, a problem-less, harmonious metropolis, a utopia. He would call his new book *Paris in the Year 2440*. He brought pages with him when he came to visit, and read them to me in the kitchen.

'"No children are ever crushed by coaches in the city of Paris in the year 2440. The king himself frequently wanders about on foot, obeying the traffic laws wherever he goes. There is no mud on the streets. The poor receive medical attention for free. In the year 2440, on the place formerly occupied by that hideous castle, the Bastille Saint-Antoine, a Temple to Clemency has been erected."'

And eventually the book was finished and it was published.

In the year 1770, many Parisians began to read Mercier's book, to discover exactly what their city would be like in six hundred and seventy years' time. Written in fury, it made its readers furious. Suddenly they found themselves living in Paris in the wrong year: they resented 1770, they preferred 2440. And so Mercier became famous.

The widow placed Mercier's bust in the window, with a placard reading CITIZEN OF THE YEAR 2440, for passers-by to marvel at. And it was the sight of people gathered in front of the window, day after day, that gave the widow her enormous idea.

One afternoon, the widow took Curtius and his black bag out with her on a visit to Mercier. Later that day they came back with Mercier, and also with a new plaster mould. The head in that mould was soon labelled JEAN-JACQUES ROUSSEAU. I recognised this head: it was Renou, the fellow in grey who had visited us with Mercier in Berne. He'd been in hiding, but he had since returned to Paris, and now he looked very ill. The next week, the three went out again and came back with another head, this one very energetic and friendly; they labelled it DENIS DIDEROT. Afterwards came a very unhappy head called JEAN LE ROND D'ALEMBERT. These people were no doubt very well known in the world; I knew not what they had done, only that their heads were to be celebrated.

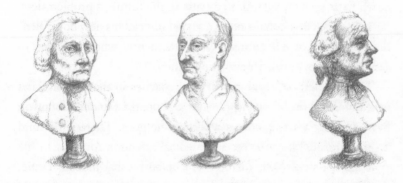

Three old men variously contemplating death.

The widow had a huge sign made announcing whose busts were inside, and many more people came to see them. The widow nodded a great deal. My master clapped. The widow went out again, this time on her own. She was very busy.

Then, late one evening, Edmond came to the kitchen and said that I was to go upstairs to his mother's room and to bring wine and two glasses. He helped me to ready the tray.

My master was seated in the widow's own bedroom. I poured out the wine. The widow untied her bonnet, and all her great brown-russet-chestnut hair tumbled out. Curtius swallowed several times.

'Edmond,' said the widow, 'you may begin to comb me now. Henri used to comb me every night; when he died that duty fell

117

to Edmond. Now, Doctor Curtius, please attend very carefully. I want you to understand. I want to tell you a history. Little, get out.'

I did get out, but, feeling the tremendous import of the evening, I stayed just beyond the door, and heard all.

'Attend me, please. I, Charlotte, widowed piece of womanhood that I am, mean to educate you, Doctor Curtius. We are known to each other now, we have business in common, and so I shall let myself a little down.'

'We are known, yes! To each other!'

'Edmond, comb, comb away. I reveal myself to you, sir, through the biography of a business. I shall talk to you of my husband.'

'Oh, yes?' was the doleful response.

'My Henri Picot's parents dealt in second-hand clothes. That was the beginning. They had a little shop here in the Faubourg Saint-Marcel. That is the essential beginning.

'Comb, Edmond, harder.

'The first thing you learn about a second-hand clothes shop is that it must be kept very dark inside. It is essential that the customers can't quite see what's there. It's amazing what poor light can do for a bit of old clothing. You won't see the stains or the loose threads, you won't see the patchwork. His parents did not like me at first, but I stood outside and pulled people in, and on Mondays at the big second-hand clothes market on the Place de Grève, I shouted hard and loud and the parents watched me and approved.

'But comb, Edmond, do!

'We sold undershirts that people had died in, panniers from prostitutes, old greasy bonnets belonging to shrunken widows who'd finally given up the ghost. Stockings very mended. Old clothes that had been used, that other bodies had pushed themselves into. There's a shirt we had in the shop, came back to us seven times, seven different Parisian owners. Our coverings go on and on without us.

'At our shop, we'd see people trying to climb up the slippery

118

ladder of Paris. A market girl would put on the lace cap of a dead lawyer's wife. Young women would strip almost to nakedness in the shop and fight each other over a petticoat. Sometimes, at night, when his parents were snoring, Henri and I would go into the store and try things on ourselves. He would dress me up as a lady.

'Plait, Edmond, tight! Tight!

'After a time, Henri wanted only the finer stuff. The sight of an old linen cap would upset him. He sat dreaming of gowns for rich people, of silks and satins. His parents didn't understand; they shook him and struck him and told me to wake him up. But in the following seasons they died – one by tripping on a slick paving stone one February morning, the other in May through an infected cut got from some old clasp – and their demise laid open the possibilities, and a tailor he became. Yet this business, unlike the second-hand clothing business, was never profitable.

'Now listen, to this, Doctor, attend particularly. Some businesses have no future and should never have been launched. Others must be prodded at the right time, or they will stagnate. We have work making busts. You are very skilled, Doctor Curtius, everyone can see that, and the work is increasing, and we might work somewhere better, particularly now we have our famous heads – not down some quiet passage, but, shall we say, upon a boulevard. We might find more heads, particular heads of great worth. Here we are at the crossroads, you and I. Picot made the change and it killed him. And now we try it on. We attempt to take two steps up society's great ladder. And my question is this: will you come with me?'

'Yes, yes, I will!' There was no pause.

'Will you hold tight and not let go?'

'I will, I will by all means. But how, tell me, do we go about it?'

'In short, dear Doctor, I have found somewhere. It is a bigger property than perhaps we have need of, but got for a bargain. Rent for the term paid down in advance. The building is a little used, but it is sturdy enough. A business has gone under, and it makes way for us. Let us not follow it. So, Doctor Curtius, float or drown.'

'Float! Float!'

'Edmond, you may return my bonnet.'

As glasses were clinked, I crept back downstairs. Where would we go, and what would happen in such new territory? Then, suddenly, I took to wondering: would I be going too? What was to become of me? No one had mentioned me going, but then no one had said I should not, and I feared so to ask them. And so I helped with the packing up and was very useful.

On the day the carts came, I followed them, trembling in fear of dismissal.

The widow and my master went first.

Followed by Edmond.

And then I a step behind him. I *was* coming too. Curtius turned to look at me, a slight nod of his head, then back widow-wards. But the widow was focused elsewhere.

'This street was not good for us, Henri,' she said to her husband's shape upon the cart. 'We're moving on, and we'll never look back.'

## Book Three

### 1771–1778

# The Monkey House

*Ten years of age until seventeen.*

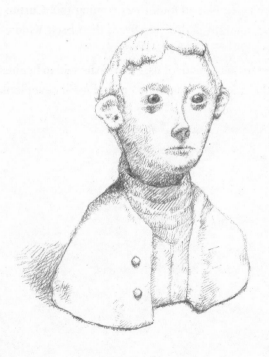

# Chapter Sixteen

*The hairy man.*

Number Twenty Boulevard du Temple was a wooden building that stood hard by the city wall, with a deep ditch along one side. In rather gaunt letters, it boasted of its purpose: HOUSE OF THE WORLD-FAMOUS PASCAL, THE PHILOSOPHER PRIMATE – ALIVE! – AND OF HIS MANY BROTHERS and above this HÔTEL SINGE, which meant TOWN HOUSE OF MONKEYS.

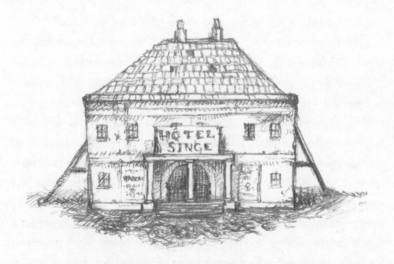

It looked something like a square temple, with three columns in front and a double-door entrance. Look around the back, though, and you would discover that the entire structure was held in place by two great wooden supports – crutches, as it were. This was to be our new home.

Outside the Hôtel Singe, furniture had been stacked on several carts: everything from cages to boiling pans, from chairs to peculiar, unfamiliar skeletons. And on top of them all, in the cages, were three living things, with staring black eyes, cramped in their homes, with sores on their skin, and large patches of their fur missing. These were monkeys. As we drew closer to the propped-up house, they started screaming.

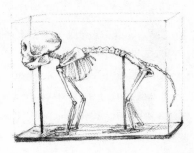

Curtius marvelled at them. 'So long! So thin! So hairy!'

One monkey let out a terrifying, very sorrowful, very human howl. We were each of us shaken by it, even the widow.

'Good day to you,' said Curtius to the monkeys, lifting his tricorn.

Into the wooden house we went.

The ground floor was dominated by a wide hall, so empty it echoed – almost empty, I should say, for sitting on a footstool to one side was a fat man dressed peculiarly in a kind of bear costume, his whole body, except for head and hands, covered in furs patched together. Here was the bankrupt monkey-keeper Bertrand le Velu, which meant Bertrand the Hairy. A black-suited official stood a step away from him; le Velu, it seemed, was being taken to prison for debt. In his lap was a small heap of darker fur, which was in fact Pascal the philosopher primate, dead. Orbiting Bertrand le Velu and Pascal, moving about the room taking pieces of property and stacking them near the entrance, were other men in suits.

'These other black animals,' the widow said, 'are bailiffs. They bite.'

As the widow signed papers with the bailiffs and a notary, the monkey-keeper signalled to me, waving insistently until I approached him. He seemed most eager to talk, and he scratched himself as he chatted, on the crown of his head, under his armpits, around his behind, all in a peculiar fashion which I began to suspect he had caught from the monkeys.

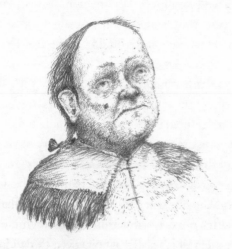

'I've been on and off in the monkey business since I was twelve, I don't mind telling you. My father was a wealthy man, a merchant dealing in cinnamon and cumin, in nutmeg and in vanilla. He would bring back creatures as well as spices from his long absences. The very first was a pan troglodyte, a chimp, that I called Florence. Florence bit my finger off here,' he said, brandishing a stump.

'But I loved her, and I could not stop wondering at what creatures there are upon the earth. And so I collected them to me, and spent all my father's wealth upon them. They were bought from so many different traders. I could never have enough. I've worked with many apes; I used to count a baboon among my friends. I prefer monkeys to humans. They're more honest. You know where you stand with them. I've been marked by the monkey business. I had a snub-nose monkey once, but it didn't last. He was all the way from the tropics, and no bigger than that,' he said, indicating

125

a length of about four inches. 'Tiny little thing. Such a lovely littleness. That I called Emmanuel. That's Emmanuel's frame over there. I boiled him down myself. This is his.'

He touched a patch of fur on his shoulder.

'He cost two hundred livres. People loved him for his tininess – he was ill, I think, when I purchased him. But there was no one so good as Pascal, was there, my love? No one approaching you. They're saying I killed you. Why would I kill you when I love you? When it's you who made me famous? You do believe me. Don't you?'

'I am trying to, sir,' I said.

'You quite resemble a monkey yourself, little girl. With a nose like that, with such thin arms. Such a proboscis. Given your look, perhaps you'll understand how it was: this whole house was a place of monkeys. At one time there were over twenty of us here in this house, and only three of us human. Each had his own cage. You went from cage to cage, seeing the Hôtel about its business, seeing the inhabitants asleep on their beds or combing their hair or putting on wigs or beauty spots. I had a chimp in livery delivering food on trays. What a Hôtel it was! How people crowded in, how they learned about themselves by watching the monkeys. A spider monkey chewing a cigar – they'd remember that the rest of their lives. A capuchin brushing his hair with a rhinestone-studded comb? A baboon sipping wine from a decanter? What a Hôtel! But it didn't last. Some of the residents, though well fed, well cared for, died entangled in their silk sheets.'

He pointed to a patch of his left elbow.

'A baby rhesus monkey was found drowned in a porcelain potty.'

He rubbed a portion of his chest.

'A Barbary ape hung himself from a bell cord. I couldn't sustain it; I had to let my staff go. One day the chandelier fell down, singeing the fur of the liveried chimp and cutting into him.'

He touched the fur of his right arm.

'The monkeys began to riot. They wouldn't calm. But still then I had Pascal. Greatest of primates. You should have seen him in

126

his smoking jacket, wearing his little cap with the gold tassel. I couldn't always control them; sometimes they got the better of me. Such a Hôtel, my Hôtel, not a full Hôtel for sure. Admittedly, the upstairs meaner rooms were empty by then.'

He smoothed the fur on several portions of his body.

'People would still come to see Pascal sipping cognac. But things got muddier. Muddier and muddier still. They said they could hear me every night shouting at you, Pascal – that every night they were disturbed by my shouting and your screaming. And now you don't make a sound. They've taken everyone away. They say I hit you! I never hit you. Why should I hit you when I love you? And then on Wednesday I go to the cage and there you are in the corner, all lonely and still.'

He was silent then, stroking the monkey's corpse.

After a while I said, 'Thank you very much, sir, for telling me.'

He stroked on.

'Excuse me, sir?' I said. 'May I touch him?'

'You want to?'

'Yes. Please.'

'Then you shall, spirit, and free of charge.'

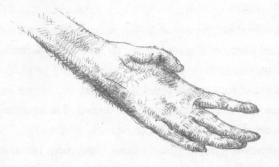

I took Pascal's right hand. It was very elongated and black, with sharp claws, longer than mine, but thinner and cold and very stiff.

'I'm sorry he died,' I said.

'Yes,' he said, 'such sorrow.'

'Sir!' I called to Curtius in our own language, breaking out of myself. 'Sir, shall we draw him together?'

'What an idea,' my master replied. He was smiling; I could see his teeth.

'In French,' the widow said, 'in French please. Doctor Curtius, we should understand each other, don't you think?'

'Yes, certainly, Widow Picot.'

'Then let us, from this moment, always and only speak in French.'

My master said, merely, 'French.'

'Pascal was a genius,' Bertrand whispered to me. 'I'll never see his like again. What am I going to do now?' he asked, taking hold of my free hand, the other still holding on to Pascal's. 'What's going to happen to me? What shall we do, my love, my little man? I'm stuck.'

He looked at the widow, then asked me, 'Is she in charge?'

'She thinks she is,' I whispered.

'Excuse me, Madame,' he said with great urgency. 'Do you have any animals? I'm very good with animals.'

The widow turned to the bailiffs. 'This house is ours now. You must vacate. Little, come away before you catch something that further impedes your usefulness. How typical of you to seek such company.'

'Can I help you with any animals you have?' Bertrand called. 'I'm gentle. I'm very, very gentle, I'm . . .' and here Bertrand le Velu could contain himself no longer. He let go of my hand, and I let go of Pascal's, and he brought the dead monkey to his face and sobbed into his fur. As he was escorted out, he called, 'I wear all my memories, so I never forget a thing. I'm dressed in memory. I'm dressed in all my friends. They're always close. They keep me warm. What a fine hat you'll be, Pascal, a very fine hat, and how I'll love you always.'

The shrieks began again outside and slowly died away and we were left alone.

128

# Chapter Seventeen

*The Monkey House.*

What an emptiness it was. I didn't think it suited us at all; I thought the widow must have been terribly mistaken. She had struck out too far. There were only four of us to fill this space, us four and traces of what lived there before. It may once have been a celebrated attraction, a highly visited place, but disease and death had soured this house of natural miracles. People had apparently lost their taste for monkeys, as if they'd collectively made up their minds that they no longer believed in them. But the monkeys, though absent, would never be forgotten to us.

It was not just the leaflets littering the floors that boasted LES SINGES À PARIS. Up and down the narrow stairs, along the bumpy passageways, the walls were marked by scratches and rips. The stairs themselves had been gnawed. It was, all in all, a partially eaten place, a nibbled house, a very chewed residence.

'This is our new home?' Edmond asked nervously.

'A monkey house, that's what it is,' my master said. 'Monkey House,' no matter that it had once been a small hotel and before that a café with gambling tables, no matter that it was to be a house of wax personages, the Monkey House is what it was always called.

'Little,' said the widow, 'be useful, unpack. Get to it.'

I carried our boxes and sacks upstairs. Painted on the doors of the first-floor cage-rooms — a few of their metal bars remaining — were the names of the former occupants: MARIE-CLAUDE, FRÉDÉRIQUE, CATHERINE ET SIMON, DOMINIQUE,

129

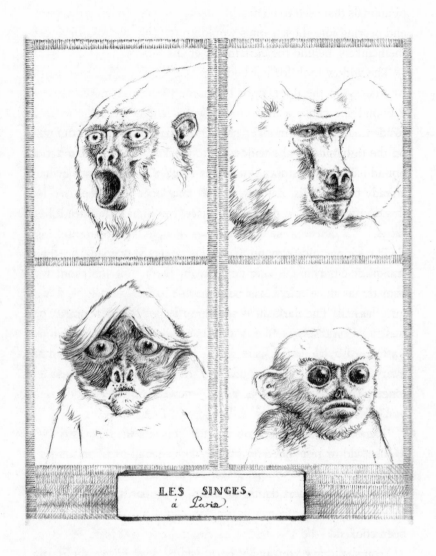

LES SINGES,
à Paris.

LAZARE, AUGUSTINE, AUGUSTIN, NICOLAS ET MARIE-ANGE, CLAUDIA ET ARNAUD, GRAND JEAN, PAULINE, HÉLOÏSE ET ABÉLARD. By each of the names was a small drawing of the animal or animals that used to be nearby, so that people climbing the stairs and peering into those rooms would know what to look for under the blankets, behind the curtains, over the lintels.

The widow took for her bedroom a chamber with CATHERINE ET SIMON on the door, once the home of howler monkeys. For Edmond she chose a little room to the left of hers, the former residence of a spider monkey named PAULINE. Curtius's room was on the right side of the widow's, the former home of a hundred-pound baboon called LAZARE from eastern Africa, captured when already mature. His obituary, written by Bertrand, was posted by this door: Lazare had died at thirty-five, after swallowing a silver rattle.

The widow told Edmond to carry his father's shape up the stairs and place him on the landing just outside her door, facing the banister, as if he might wish to lean over and have a look down into the hall. The dark sheet was removed; in this new house, he was to be on display.

'Here you are, Henri,' she said. 'From here you can see almost everything. We are very proud. We do so well. I shall hide you no longer; I want you to see how we come along. Indeed, I declare you!'

'Excuse me, sir,' I asked my master, 'where am I to sleep?'

The widow responded by marching me back down the stairs.

'Kitchen,' said the widow. 'In the kitchen. Out of the public eye.'

It was a black and damaged room, floorboards scraped, walls scorched by flames from the fireplace, as if the room itself had been cooked.

'You shall have your pallet here, and be most comfortable. It's at the back of the house, closest to the boulevard ditch. It should fit you very well.'

'It is a very unhappy room, I think.'

'No doubt it is you that makes it so.'

'Yes, Madame.'

'You'll be in here, mostly, not out there. We shall have a very new public, and when the public is present in the great hall, then shall you keep yourself shut up in here.'

'Yes, Madame.'

'But now you must tidy this place, this mansion of ours.'

'Yes, Madame.'

'So get along!'

Well, then, the broom.

'We shall call the business the Cabinet of Doctor Curtius,' announced the widow in the hall. 'The words *Widow* and *Picot* shall not draw people; they have an everyday ring about them. But *Doctor* and *Curtius* have a certain sound.'

'Do they?' said my master. 'A certain sound!'

'And should our venture fail, I shall need to find another employment and we need not both be condemned for our failure. I am a widow, you are a man.'

'I see. Yes. A widow, a man. Yes, that is how it is.'

'But most of all,' she added, not without unhappiness, 'a woman's name does not encourage. Women are not supposed to have businesses. Of course, Doctor, we shall not fail.'

The house needed such a deal of cleaning that all four of us went about it at first, mopping and sweeping. After several hours it looked really very little better, but Curtius was coughing uncontrollably and had to be taken out. The widow and her son would promenade with him; I should stay behind and carry on the work.

'Hello,' I quietly said to it after they left. The response was creaks and scratching. I closed my eyes and felt them moving, then – all the unhappy spirits of dead monkeys, running at me, swinging for me, curling up their lips, showing me their teeth.

'I'm not frightened.'

The house clicked. Something fell within the walls.

'You're a very grand place, I know.'

Something upstairs groaned.

'I'm going to live here. I've come to live here.'

Dust seemed to gather up and whirl about me.

'Do your worst, why don't you? I've nowhere else to go. I'm staying. I mean to work you, house, until we are friendly.'

A crack then, a crack that started small but grew in noise until it was a long shriek. It was the crutches, I thought, the crutches outside adjusting to the new weight of me.

'Please,' I said, 'let us come to an understanding.'

A scurry upstairs as if someone or something were running along the landing, though when I went up nobody was there. It wasn't right, I thought, to leave me alone in such a place, with all those afternoon spirits itching to attack.

'Very well then!' I called to the house. 'Do go ahead and crush a child. Here I stand. Go on, I'll not fight you!'

A door swung open. No one came out. No one was there.

'I know you're unhappy, but come, let's talk to one another and feel at home together. So it's true, you have swallowed me! And I mean, O big house, to nurture you, to be wholesome to your great insides. To fill you up! Even me, your supper! Little chitterling that I am, small beer. I'll tell you everything. I give myself to you.'

I cannot say whether it was my fanciful thinking or not, but the house seemed to breathe a little then, and let me touch it without unhappiness and learn its every corner. This was where I lived now, inside the beast, and I would make it the best of all possible beasts.

As I swept, as I spoke to the place and told it who I was and what I had learned and how much I wished to work with my master again and how good was his work and how Edmond had shown me his doll, and that though he might seem a very quiet fellow, still he was company and that the house should be good to him, for though he could be self-important he was actually not unpleasant, with his freckles about his nose, and his white chest. The mother, though, I told the house, do feel free to trip her feet, to gnaw at her in her sleep, and make her as miserable as such a fine and glorious abode can.

As I spilled all to the large place, as I felt less frightened and more at home, there came a dull murmur, a storm approaching from a distance. I thought at first it was a great colony of the dead monkey-folk come to visit me, but then I understood these were new sounds, not from the nervous house but from beyond. From the boulevard outside.

It was the noise of shutters opening. Of door bolts being pulled across. Of wooden planks being laid down in the mud. A flame whooshing into life. Then a sound like the clearing of a hundred throats, and a murmuring of a hundred voices slowly rising in volume, as if the Boulevard du Temple itself were being wound up by those voices, stoked into life, until there was no quiet any more, no pause to interrupt the great noise that spread over everything and was amplified alarmingly inside the empty container of the Monkey House. The Boulevard du Temple, the entertainment district of Paris, a living and painted creature, was waking up.

I ran upstairs. From a window I watched the boulevard swelling with people, from the repairer of broken china to the rat-catcher, from the water carrier to the sedan-chair carrier, from the feather merchant to the brick maker, people of Paris were coming in. Here opposites mixed: flour-covered wig-maker's assistants walked beside coal carriers thick with black dust. And among them were the boulevard people, shouting: itinerant musicians, men with puppets, toy sellers, actors in bright costumes, a man walking a great bear, blind men playing fiddles, children singing, old men dancing, flame swallowers, sword swallowers, a great circus of extraordinary people. Oh, here was living!

The noise of the boulevard echoed so loud inside the Monkey House that I did not hear the doors open below, nor the widow enter the building until she was upon me. I was roughly instructed to return to the main hall and there to keep brushing until the hideous animal smell was gone. But that smell would never entirely leave us.

When it was time to sleep, the widow, summoning monkey shadows all around her, took the light upstairs and with it Edmond and my master. In the darkness I heard shouting and weeping and laughter coming from the boulevard. Many of the noises seemed to originate from the house directly opposite, labelled THE CELESTIAL BED and in slightly smaller letters DOCTOR JAMES GRAHAM (*LATE OF LONDON*). Peeping through a shutter, I saw people arrive there late into the night: sometimes couples, sometimes single men.

Twice in the night, the doors of the Monkey House were noisily rattled from the outside by unseen hands. I tried very hard not to sleep, for my fear was up again and I was not certain it was altogether safe to surrender to sleep in such a place, but eventually, exhausted, I closed my eyes. I dreamed of a monkey sitting on a kitchen chair, rocking back and forth, staring at me with huge eyes. As I sat up in bed, in terror, I saw that someone indeed was there. It was Edmond.

# Chapter Eighteen

*Voices in the night.*

'Mother's asleep,' he said.

'Yes.'

'The doctor's asleep.'

'Yes, I suppose it is very late, Edmond, or very early.'

'He calls out in his sleep, Curtius does.'

'Yes, I know that well enough.'

'I can't sleep.'

'No.'

'Can you sleep?'

'Yes.'

'I thought perhaps I might come here to see how you are.'

'Well, here I am.'

'In truth, I was frightened. Mother would hardly let me go into her room for comfort. She'd call me childish. And I wouldn't want to go into the doctor's. I was scared, you see, of the house, of what's beyond it. Mostly of the house. I miss home. I don't think this place can ever be home; I can't see how it could be. I fear this house could be the death of me. Are there ghosts, do you think?'

'Any number of them,' I said.

'I thought there were. I could hear them scratching.'

'I know them very well – they came to me, you see. I have seen them moving about in the darkness; I have heard them whispering. Just this afternoon when you went outside and left me here alone, they came upon me – and in a rush!'

'No!'

'Oh yes! And they nibbled at me and stroked me and were about to eat me whole when—'

'When?'

'—when I talked to them and gave them harsh words and I think we are friends now.'

'May I be friends with them too?'

'They might not have you.'

'Why not?'

'They are very moody.'

'I am moody too.'

'Not like them.'

'Are they very furious?'

'You will have to be brave.'

'Yes. I will be.'

'Very brave!'

'I will.'

'Then perhaps, in time, I may introduce them to you.'

'I think I should much rather they left me alone.'

'Don't say that – don't ever say that. You shall make them *mad*.'

'I'm sorry, I didn't mean . . .'

'See that?'

'What?'

'There was one just now! He stood just before you, with long teeth and claws, but, seeing me, he darted off again.'

'Truly? I didn't see him.'

'Yet he was there.'

'You're trying to frighten me.'

'I am not.'

'I'm going back to bed,' he said sullenly.

'Edmond, wait, you do not have to.'

'I think I'd better. Mother might hear us. She wouldn't like it.'

'You'll be all on your own.'

'Yes, but if Mother heard us.'

'Of course you must always do what your mother says.'

'No, that's not true. But I feel less scared now. Having seen you, though you tried to fright me. Still. May I come, Little . . .'

'Marie!'

'Yes, sorry, may I come again, Marie? If I have such a terror upon me, may I come to you?'

'Always.'

And up he went, with the ghost upon the stairs shouting at him with every step he took. And I on my pallet could hardly sleep for happiness.

# Chapter Nineteen

*Third heads.*

Bees secrete wax through glands in their bodies; with this secreted wax they build their many-celled homes, their cities made of wax; within small wax walls their young are raised, their honey stored, great passages and halls, homes for thousands. Wax is essential to their lives. Without wax they would have no home; their offspring would have no roof above their heads.

People take the wax away from the bees and render it to remove impurities. Then wax is made into candles. Wax gives us light; without wax we would live in the darkness. How much of our lives have we seen because of wax? How would we illuminate theatres and ballrooms without it? How would the little boy with monsters under his bed dispel them without wax? How would the old woman in her darkling terror know that she still lived without a little candle-light to cling to? We strike a match and burn a candle and a little bit of daylight is restored to us, because of wax.

In the Monkey House, a future was built from wax. My master sliced it and heated it in his great copper bowl, to a temperature between sixty-two and sixty-four degrees. Out of wax he grew Parisian heads. The widow fixed up Henri Picot's bell by the door. She put the famous heads in the hall; they took up so little of it.

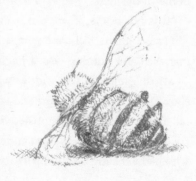

Two days after our arrival at the Monkey House, I heard them together in the hall. They were speaking of me.

'Why must you be so strict with her?'

'Because she offends me.'

'She is just a child, Widow. And she has much improved, you must admit.'

'So common. So foreign. Such a face. I cannot help it, it unnerves me. As if she's dead already and yet still living. A face from a nightmare somehow let slip into the everyday.'

'Is it no more than that? You do not like the look of her?'

'Is that not enough? Such a bad-luck face!'

'How you imagine, Widow Picot!'

'It's how I feel. A woman may have feelings.'

'Yes, yes, a woman may.'

I lost some of their conversation but caught more a little later.

'I am so grateful to you,' said my master.

'Yes.'

'I wish you to understand my gratitude, my affection.'

'We are partners in business, Doctor.'

'May I be so bold? Could there be a greater partnership?'

'I am deep in grief and not available.'

'But one day?'

'I cannot say. Do not press me. The business must be first, there is no space for foolishness. Foolishness killed my husband.'

'Yes, I see, the business! First the business. And here we are at home in business, Widow Picot, you and I. Home, home!'

'It is our home, if we can manage it right.'

Home, home. If I can manage *her* right. The business was what mattered and nothing else; I begged it to remain that way.

My master and the widow went to visit the most successful showmen of the boulevard and soon had them in wax. There was tall and scowling Jean-Baptiste Nicolet, who had a theatre of tight-rope walkers; there was short and swollen Nicolas-Médard Audinot, who had a theatre of child performers; there was smiling, freckled,

140

auburn-headed Doctor James Graham of the Celestial Bed, who entertained adults in his establishment.

Nicolet and Audinot owned the only two brick properties upon the boulevard; all the others were made of wood. When the wind rose upon the boulevard, how the wooden places groaned and shrieked. The Monkey House creaked particularly. The attic space, the most vulnerable part of the house, complained all night long; it had loud conversations with itself, all full of misery and recriminations. One day, while she was exploring that space, the widow slipped and fell and a whole widow leg came through the ceiling on the first floor. From then on, she proclaimed the place too dangerous to enter, and the attic door was kept closed. But the attic would not be forgotten. It called to us, it muttered and chattered and implored us to remember it.

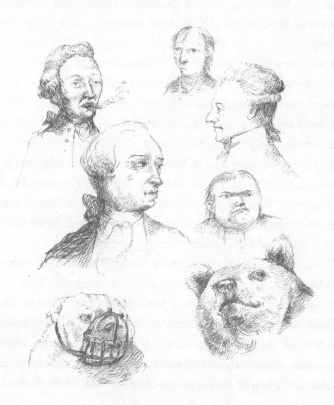

The atelier in the Monkey House was upstairs in a large chamber formerly occupied by a pair of piebald chimpanzees and so I, in the kitchen downstairs, was kept far away from it. Exploring it at night involved climbing the main staircase – and, so doing, letting off barks and whoops from the wooden steps – so I had mostly to wait until everyone had gone out to look.

When I could, I watched all the boulevard business. Our neighbouring building to the right was a small chess café; to the left was THE LITTLE WORLD THEATRE of MARCEL MONTON. The residents of these two establishments did not, I think, welcome us between them. When Doctor Curtius bowed to them, they looked the other way. When I could, I watched the people of the boulevard in their leisure hours. I saw a man without legs, progressing up and down in his cart, overtaking many. Another walking a pack of muzzled bulldogs. One taking his four dwarfs for a stroll; one out with his lumbering bear. I saw the redhead Doctor Graham again, flamboyantly attired, smoking a cigar, always accompanied by a different beautiful lady. What strange and varied life there was here! I should never have seen all these things, never have imagined them, if I had stayed in the village of my birth.

Amidst the characters upon the boulevard, I soon became aware of a certain conspicuous, ugly bully of a child, a vagrant whose principal friends appeared to be feral dogs. I saw him playing with them, snapping at them, howling with them, searching for food beside them. When I pointed the boy out to my master he was astonished; he stared with wonder at the boy's broken skin, his matted hair, and filthy clothes.

'This, even this, Marie, though brought so low, this too is a Parisian.'

I knew he would find the filthy boy interesting. I knew the sort of head that would move my master. The widow was always telling him that we must concern ourselves with noble heads, heads of distinction, but my master saw nobility in gutter folk. If he had a passion for a certain head, it was hard for him to shake it. I saw him several times looking at this wild boy, his hands moving hurriedly in the air as if modelling his face. In my turn, in the night, for the briefest moment, I put my own hand out and touched Edmond's face.

'Ow! Do not do that.'

He had come down to me again. He came sometimes twice a week, learning to be so soft on the stairs. He was so unhappy in the new place he needed someone to talk to. That was when Edmond slowly, tentatively, made sound. He lived his life working around his mother's louder volume, hushed under her daily clamour. We spoke in whispers, and in those hushed sounds, in that delicate noise, he let more of himself out.

'Am I so quiet, am I, Marie? I don't think I always was. I used to run around at school and be very loud; I had many friends, but when Father grew ill I stopped school to help him with his work. I suppose I was quieter then, as Father grew louder and made noises in his illness; they were not happy sounds. Mother insisted I be quiet, so that I should not disturb him. And so I learned my quietness, until I spoke only in whisper. I don't mind whispering; in fact I prefer it, everyone else being so loud.'

'What more, Edmond? What more can you tell me?'

'Nothing, nothing at all.'

'What do you hope for?'

'One day to be a very fine tailor.'

'That is your mother speaking.'

'No, no, it is my deepest wish.'

'And I, Edmond? What shall I be, I wonder?'

'A servant, I suppose. Whatever else?'

'I know how to draw. I can mix colours, prepare faces, ready the wax.'

'Not that again, Marie. Mother will never have it. You must learn your place.'

'But what if I don't like my place?'

'Mother will toss you out with barely a thought.'

143

'She'll have to pay me first.'

'Be good, Marie.'

'Though I hate it.'

'You are fed. You have shelter.'

'I'm glad you come to me. I should forget myself if you didn't.'

'I don't mind coming down sometimes.'

'I look forward to it.'

'But you shouldn't expect things, Marie. It's not your place.'

'You'll come again?'

'I may. But you shouldn't expect it.'

# Chapter Twenty

*Sounds of the outside falling in.*

One afternoon, when the wild feral boy of the boulevard was sleeping nearby, propped up against a poplar tree, my master stepped out to have a better look at him.

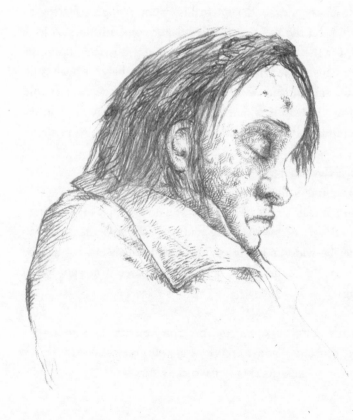

There was no harm in that, perhaps, but then the boy opened his eyes and those open eyes watched my master. Curtius quickly began to walk back towards the Monkey House. When he turned round, after a few steps, the boy was no longer there at the tree. When he stepped into the Monkey House, he saw the boy had been following him, was sitting across the way now by Doctor Graham's establishment. The boy pulled a sausage from his pocket, wiped it with his grimy hands, took a good-sized bite, and aggressively began to chew. When I checked later, at my master's request, the boy was still there. He lingered near the Monkey House all evening. Once he had seen Curtius, had seen how thin and fragile he was, I believe he began to consider what a vulnerable place the Monkey House was. Unnerved by the wild boy's closeness, Edmond kept to his room at night, fearing to disturb him on the steps, and I dared not come upstairs to look for him, for the one time I had tried, the noise I made upon the fifth stair caused the widow to shout, 'Who's there? I hear you!' My master and the widow were likewise not themselves. The wild boy followed Curtius whenever he went out, always just a few steps behind. It was as if our house and our lives were under siege.

'He's always there,' Curtius moaned.

'Ignore him,' said the widow. 'If you do, he'll go away.'

'I begin to fear, Widow Picot, that you do not know everything.'

Edmond was dressed smartly and sent out into the streets to distribute the widow's newly commissioned bill sheets. He handed them to people in the parks, on the better streets, in appropriate gatherings.

FAMOUS FOREIGN SCULPTOR, DOCTOR CURTIUS, GENIUS OF WAX, GREATEST PORTRAITIST IN PARIS, LIKENESSES TRULY REMARKABLE. CUSTOMERS AMAZED!

SCULPTOR OF ROUSSEAU, DIDEROT, D'ALEMBERT &C. DARE
TO SEE YOURSELF, YOUR LOVED ONES, WIVES, DAUGHTERS,
SONS, GRANDSONS, AS IF FOR THE FIRST TIME.
*(For a reasonable fee.)*

In response came not only boulevard heroes and celebrated philosophers, but also something new: women. Women to be talked to, women to be modelled. They entered the hall and were seated upon our chairs. Such women! Paris women. With women's skin, soft, wrinkled, windswept, tough, blistered, greasy, clean, sweet-smelling, rancid, stinking of onions and of flour and of chocolate and of strawberries. Curtius touched them all. And as his digits descended onto female flesh, he hesitated and his eyes flooded, but sometimes, so very close to a customer's female face, his hands met together in a silent clap. Surrounded by so much femininity, I considered, perhaps my master's widowish affection might fall away. In one such rare moment, he came to tell me.

'Oh, the nose! These noses! Oh freckles on foreheads. Oh creases on lips, so perfect, so chapped, so wine-marked. Oh curls of eyelashes! Oh dimples! Oh cheekbones! Such moles, such redness, such whiteness and greenness. Oh pinks, oh reds, oh you blues and yellows! I am moved! Necks! How I have cried over the napes of necks! Lips! Lips, again!' he said in wonder. 'Happy! Oh, happy! Alive!'

Curtius made skin. The widow covered it up. Edmond sewed buttons. I scrubbed floors.

The rough boy slept on the steps.

On the second week of the wild boy's proximity, Edmond at last came down again. I heard him upon the stairs, making such slow progress. I listened out: it was certainly him, for I could just hear the widow's heavy slumber and also my master in his sleep-muttering. Edmond's small footsteps, coming with such

147

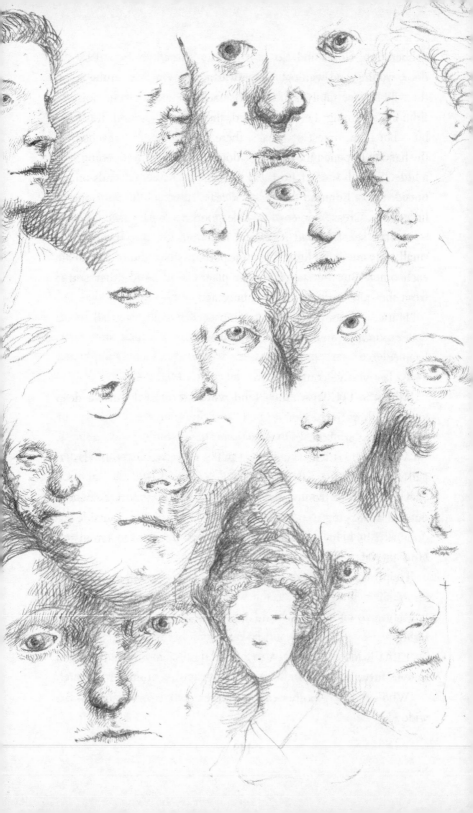

deliberation, closer and closer. I got out of bed and stood by the door, waiting and waiting. There was a noise outside on the steps: the wild boy, certainly, shifting. I listened out again for the noise of Edmond's coming; he had stopped, there was no sound, not for a bit – but then, tiniest of creaks, there he was again. I reached for the handle; I opened the door; the door pronounced its opening, just a little. The advance of Edmond paused. There were sounds on the outside steps. Edmond continued. Creak. I pushed the door open a little more. Creak. Someone outside stood upon the steps. Crack.

I could see Edmond now, and he could see me, through the small early-morning light. We were perhaps just twenty yards from each other. But we stayed in our places. Crack. Another sound from the steps outside. Then silence again.

'Marie,' Edmond whispered, almost no sound to it at all.

'Edmond,' came my smallest answer.

Silence.

'At last you've come,' I said.

'WHO'S THERE?' Such loud words suddenly! Such a deep voice! Calling from outside.

We kept very still.

'WHO'S THERE, I SAY? WHAT'S INSIDE? WHAT HAVE YOU GOT IN THERE? UNLOCK YOURSELF!'

And then the front door was knocked and shaken. Someone outside was trying to get in. Then a roar of fury from outside the door, as if by being so lawlessly out of bed we'd awoken a monster. How the door was hammered then!

'Help!' whispered Edmond. 'The whole house will come down upon us.'

He ran to me then and I held on to him, my arms around him tight.

'LEAVE ME BE! UNHAND ME!' the voice outside bellowed now in fury.

'Who's there?' Another call, a different call, from upstairs – the widow!

149

'Mother?' cried Edmond.

'Edmond!' she snapped back. 'What's going on? Why are you up? Who's there with you?'

'The sounds, Mother. It was the sounds.'

'Little? Little!' she cried. 'What are you doing?'

I let go then.

'Do you not hear it, Madame?' I whispered. 'There is something beyond.'

Another noise outside, the door being smashed upon, and then an enormous scream. And as that scream, a hurt beast's yell, so shocked us from outside, so it was echoed inside, for the widow screamed, a low mounting call like something bovine in distress. Edmond's cry followed – his own much higher, like a rabbit in a trap – and then it was picked up and followed on by another, this from my master at the top of the stairs, a horse's whinny, and the house screamed and chattered, yelped and growled like a great menagerie of all beasts at once. In that noise, I could not help but insert my own small sound among the others, a small mouse wail, a shrew's.

But suddenly the hammering and thumping ceased, leaving just a whimpering and a scuttling, as of someone hurrying away. We stood all four of us, each his own island, not daring to make sound, until at last from our entrance steps came a deep snoring, as of some great mastiff. Then, shaken and pale, we returned in muffled terror to our sleepless beds, in hope that the morning and the sun would bleach away our agony.

# Chapter Twenty-One

*In which the Cabinet gets its guard dog.*

With daylight came an explanation. Someone, it seemed – some drunk fellow – had been snooping about the Monkey House, hoping to upset us by rattling the door, when he had accidentally trodden upon the wild boy. He had had no reward but pain for his mischief, nor would two of his teeth ever grow back.

My master stood at the window and watched the bully still asleep upon the third step. 'I think,' he said, 'I think we must thank him.' I watched by the kitchen door as he opened the front door and cleared his throat.

'I don't suppose you slept very well,' he said. 'None of us did.' We all came a little closer, then, to see what happened next.

The wild boy slowly sat up, curled his lip, but Curtius did not come back indoors. The boy moved up a step, but Curtius stayed where he was. The boy climbed to the top step, and so Curtius did the only thing left for him to do: he put his hand in his waist-coat pocket and tugged out a coin. The wild boy took it. And, having taken it, he ceased his growling at once. My master looked very brave then, brave in front of the widow. She, unused to such a turnabout, stammered and huffed but could find no obvious path.

'This creature is the lowest of the low,' the widow said. 'He's not to come inside.'

'You're a good fellow,' said this new Curtius. 'I like you, but you are rough. And inside are some delicate things. So keep outside, bellow and thump there by all means, for you're made for the

151

outdoors, aren't you? You're not to be limited by architecture. But, no, don't come in.'

'In fact,' said the widow, 'keep out.'

Turning about in her exasperation, finding me too close for comfort, she recalled something else from the shadows the night before.

'Last night, Edmond, I saw you!'

'Yes, Mother, and I you. What a fright we have all had.'

'You were in the closest proximity with the servant.'

'I . . . I . . .'

'Do you deny it?'

'No, Mother, I cannot.'

'You cannot lie to your mother!'

'No, Mother. I never could.'

'Why then such communication?'

'I was frightened, Mother. She was . . . near.'

'Edmond! Learn your place; it is not, it never was, with the kitchen rat.'

'Yes, Mother.'

'You seek comfort? Come to me, I'll comfort you.'

'Yes, Mother.'

'And you, Little, scum, boil, dropping, touch my son and you shall find yourself in the gutter!'

'Yes, Madame. Certainly, Madame.'

I long for you to die in agonies, I thought, and I could almost picture it. Why was she always so cruel, I wondered, even after I had worked so hard for her? Perhaps she needed someone beneath her to know for certain that she was not on the bottom rung. Perhaps being cruel was proof of her success.

I was certain that with this latest proclamation there would be no more creak upon the stairs. That I should remain alone in the kitchen, and be taken over by that place.

'It disgusts me!' she concluded. 'Just because this vagrant makes a little row on our steps, it is no cause for all society to be overturned.

We must hope that that breathing rubbish shall tire of us very soon and then all shall be returned as it was before.'

But that was not what happened.

Once the wild boy had conquered the Monkey House steps, neither he nor my master could be stopped. Not only did the boy spend his nights upon the steps, but he remained during the day, and soon he began to serve my master's Cabinet on various small errands.

The rough boy did not merely attach himself to Curtius. He sent out messengers of his personality in the form of fleas. There were small pimples on Edmond's forearms; I saw him through the kitchen door, scratching them. The widow discovered a tick upon the back of her neck. How Curtius respected that tick, made its removal into a great drama. I was summoned – such was the trauma – to bring a basin of hot water.

'Why must you see my shoulders?' the widow squawked. 'The creature is on my neck. No, I shall not loosen my jacket!'

These medical attentions of Curtius must also be put down to the advent of the rough boy, for my master should never have dared touch the widow's neck without the help of the rough boy's tick, and here he was pinching and squeezing it. Curtius would keep that dead tick in a little box, resting on red velvet, upon the mantelpiece in his bedroom. I saw it when I came to empty the chamber pots.

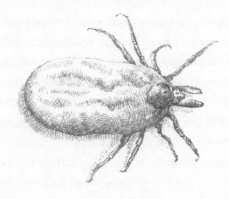

Some people will leave their dogs outside in the cold; others will have them indoors on their laps or on their beds. You can tell a person's character by how he treats his dogs. Here is an indication of my master's character: Curtius not only insisted on letting the boy sleep on the steps, as if he could stop him, he even gave him a rug from his own bed.

Finally, Curtius asked the boy his name. In response, the boy forced a sound out from deep within, more a bark than a name.

'What was that?' Curtius asked. 'Try again. Once more.'

This time, I seemed to hear words: *Jacques*, that much I felt confident about. Of the second word, I could make nothing.

'Visage? Oh – Beauvisage!' exclaimed the widow.

Beauvisage? *Pretty face?*

'Jacques Beauvisage,' he growled and nodded.

And Curtius, those syllables splattered upon his face, was enraptured. Such a name for such a creature! Rather than laugh at the beast, Curtius just smiled. 'Indeed, so you are, Beauvisage.'

With the coming of bad weather, Curtius's character showed itself again. After much behind-doors negotiation with the stunned widow, he invited Jacques to sleep inside, curled up by the door. Now I was certain Edmond would never come down again. In desperation, I passed him a note. It said only,

HALLO, EDMOND! *From Marie.*

He looked shocked to receive such a thing, and scrunched it up very quickly, but his ears, I noted, had gone their reddest.

Jacques Beauvisage was instructed to remain by the front door and ordered never to touch the wax heads. But it was already too late by then: once you let a dog sleep inside, you cannot expect to turn it out again. You must never bring the wild things into your homes. His old friends, the boulevard's stray dogs, came to the steps, whining for him, but in the end they slunk off, confused. And the wild child was left friendless in the Monkey House.

I was to look after him.

# Chapter Twenty-Two

*I become a teacher.*

I, the kitchen thing, creature of grease and soot, spirit of steam and flame, I, dirty thing with the black, stained fingers: I was the one. I was to look after this new man. There were rules to be learned. He must not be in the great hall during business hours. He, like me, belonged to the back rooms. And so my days became occupied with a wonderful parenthood. My child, my difficult charge, took all my patience and care and love. I spoiled him perhaps, fed him sweetmeats, but I was stern with him also. I raised my voice, I wagged my finger. He lashed out, but I took breath and went straight back into the battle. How Edmond fussed over my scratches! I saw him once in the distant hall, looking into the kitchen, putting his hand to his mouth in horror.

I was domesticating a wild thing, and it kept me busy. Jacques must urinate and defecate in the chamber pot; it took him months to learn. There'd be a smell, I'd find a puddle and a stool, and, howling, Jacques would rush out of doors.

Perhaps I overdid it a little. Perhaps, overflowing with parenthood, I could not see clearly; perhaps I made him out more feral than he really was. He knew how to talk, of course; he did not have to be taught words, though I sometimes forgot this, and in his misery as I groomed and broke him in, he would call out names of people. He might howl *Yves Sicre*, for example; he might lessen his discomfiture by snapping *Jean-Paul Clémonçon*; he might thump the ground repeating the name *Anne-Jérôme de Marciac-Lanville*. And just uttering these names – names of people he'd heard upon the boulevard, I presumed – did seem to hush him a little. He learned not to whine and grow quite so agitated whenever a female customer entered the Monkey House. But he must, the widow instructed, he must protect everything that belonged to the Monkey House.

Jacques's face perfectly described his thoughts: sad, angry, frightened, happy, all would show openly upon his face. He was, unlike wax, the poorest of actors; he could be no one but himself; he was stuck with himself, and that was at times a very desperate and troubling state to inhabit.

After Jacques began to sleep inside, I think he came to be frightened of the outside. It didn't happen immediately; it crept up upon him. He grew a little fatter, grew accustomed to the warmth of indoors. As we sat together in the kitchen, I told him of my mother and father, of my life before I came to Paris; if I didn't tell him, I had begun to wonder, how could I ever be sure it had all happened? If I didn't tell the story it might dry up and I would be left short and grimy of the kitchen. Slowly he breathed it all in. And one afternoon, his mouth opened and the words came out.

Jacques Beauvisage had stories of his own.

'Bernard Balliac cut his wife. Into pieces. Fed them to a dog!'

I heard these words, these clear signs of intelligence. I leaned forward, listening attentively. After a long while he spoke again.

'Butcher Olivier axed up his family. His wife. His children, two. Sold them for pig food. Pig food was too rich for pigs, pigs took sick. Law called.'

I kept very quiet. He went on. Small blurted words, his messages of thanks to me.

'Isabelle Torisset and Pascal Fissot lay together in bed. But someone was with them there already. Her husband, Maurice! Maurice was a cripple. Three's a crowd, so they do say. They took him to the top of the house where there were birds on the flat roof in a big cage, a building downriver, nearby the granaries. They put the husband in the cage. And the husband was pecked apart

156

by birds but found, months after. Alive! Bony! Unlike the lovers! They were soon dead! Hanged on Place de Grève! Public! I saw it!'

What a breakthrough that was! How my teaching and instincts were confirmed that night! For then, as if all victories had come at once, he started to share with me his own passion, which before he had kept only to himself. Jacques, I discovered, was a great memoriser of Parisian crimes and murders. We sat in the kitchen together and Jacques in his growl let out small, bloody, miserable tales of unfortunate people leaving life in a hurry. One after the other I heard them, deep into the night, delivered with increasing confidence. Tell us another story, Jacques, tell us another. I couldn't go to sleep without one. Under his tutelage I became very knowledgeable of appalling acts.

He told me of his life too. I begged it out of him: 'Jacques, tell me. Do!'

# Chapter Twenty-Three

*Jacques Beauvisage, an account of himself.*

'I seen hangings, but not murders. I should like to grow up one day to see a good murder. A bloody one. I missed a throat-cutting on the boulevard by only a few minutes. Saw the blood, even the bleeding, but not the cutting itself.'

'How old are you, Jacques?' I asked.

'I don't know. What d'you think?'

'I think perhaps something like twenty? I don't know. Even thirty? I can't say.'

'Well and what then?'

'Where were you born?'

'Here. Paris.'

'Who was your father?'

'Don't know.'

'Your mother?'

'No, don't know.'

'What do you know then, my pet?' I gently persisted.

'You sound like an old granny.'

'Tell me, what happened to you?'

'I was left at the foundling hospital, Rue Saint-Honoré. That's sure. There they named me, nuns did. I was never pretty, so they say; I am big of face, and been made bigger no doubt by my living. Called me Jacques, which I go by, and Beauvisage on account of my good looks.'

'What was it like? At the hospital?'

'I lived. I ate. There wasn't much food, so I took some from

158

others who weren't strong enough to fight for it. So then maybe they starved; that's how it was. I was loud and did hit and was not always to be ordered. I hit one nun, and I hurt another with my shouting; she went deaf, they say. Children died, 'specially in winter. I didn't. Couldn't kill me. Haven't yet, least. Was ill one winter, thought I'd gone, lay in the ditch by the wall day after day, buried in filth. Came back though, sat up, ate some, shat some, up again. Better and better.'

'And after the orphanage?'

'I was taken. Audinot, the theatre manager, he always comes and takes some, four or five a year, to be on the stage in his Ambigu-Comique.'

'Yes, I know him. We have his head here!'

Jacques spat. 'All the performers there are children and are took from orphanages because they're cheap; he doesn't have to pay for them – he's paid to take them away. I played there mostly wild animals. I was well known, people came just to see me, but they didn't like to come in the front seats when I was on, on account of I might come down off the stage and hit them. I have a temper, better now a bit, but then I'd hit a person just because I could, and Audinot would scream at me, and he feared very much I might have at him too. I had a good girl at the Ambigu, that was Henriette Peret, and we knew each other a lot and she was the first for me. But she got ill on me, and they she died on me, and I got so angry I hit about everything and threatened to kill Audinot and so he got his heavy men on me and they broke me all over and shoved me out. That was when I was in the ditch and thought that was my last resting. But at last I got up again. So then. I hung around with dogs mainly and they kept by me and were company, but we fight so. And do frighten. Been with them can't say how long, seasons on seasons. I nearly become a dog, I think. But then comes Curtius and you, who is an old woman and a child both at once, who makes me talk again. And so here I am again. Among the people, or a single person, small and busy. I'm every day on the boulevard

159

except when there's a hanging; then I do go to the Place de Grève. Those are the good days. I like me a good hanging, very good for me.'

After he had begun telling me his own tale, I cleaned Jacques with a kinder touch. I convinced him to sit in the tin bath, and there I made him look more and more like a person every day. There was a man under that grime, a rough-looking one with appalling teeth, who laughed at the most inappropriate things; a clumsy youth, a thuggish one, but one who, in the midst of his miserable tales, had a certain beauty about him. There were so many scars upon his skin from burns, from rips, from being cut, from self-scratching. I asked about the marks, one after another, and sitting in the bathtub, he nonchalantly told me one by one. 'That from the theatre, Master Audinot with a spike. I was littler – he shouldn't try it later. That one from Black Dog. That one I did, to test a knife, I stole it, very good knife. Very.' Under the widow's instruction, Edmond made him a woollen suit of double weave so that it might last longer, each seam stitched four times, but Jacques tore it soon enough and so a new tougher outfit was made for him of leather.

Jacques's tales were so good that they could not be kept in the kitchen; they very soon spread themselves about the house. Like those monkey phantasms, they began to make their presence known in the upstairs room. Though the widow and my master had not listened to them exactly, still those stories began to enter them, finding a way through their nostrils in their sleep. Why else could my master be heard in the night walking back and forth in his room? Why else did the widow always wake in such black moods?

He was such a very different creature from me, Jacques was, that I was like some innocent learning the world. The pupil became the teacher, telling me, in his way, what it was to be alive and how many ways there were to die. It was as if I had had almost no real contact with life before he came along to me, as if I'd heard only rumours, small whisperings of what human beings could do. I was a toy doll from a nursery, being instructed by a rat. Afterwards, when Jacques dozed after a telling, I would visit the wax populace in the hall, still a child no matter what he called me, but shedding that childhood as I walked among the counterfeit humans.

One early evening, I was clearing away the plates in the dining room before the visitors were let in when I observed Edmond sitting there, avoiding my looks. He'd been so distant since Jacques's coming.

'Jacques knows such stories,' I spouted at him.

'What?' asked the widow. 'Did you speak?'

'Jacques Beauvisage knows such wonderful stories. You should hear them.'

'Get out,' said the widow.

'Stories?' my master said. 'What stories?'

'They are Paris stories, sir, all of them.' I cleared my throat. 'Of murders, of killings. He knows them all. They are very extraordinary, sir. They must belong to heads we don't know. Certainly I've never seen the faces of men and women that have done such things.'

To my delight, Curtius asked me to send him up. My master and the widow would listen to these stories. I expected to hear my master clapping very soon, but what I heard was shouting from the widow. She boxed his ears; Jacques came down miserable.

When I went upstairs, the widow scolded me. 'You bring such ugliness into my house. This is a place of fine faces, of beauty and accomplishment, not the dirt you know. You'd have us in the gutter. Don't get too comfortable here.' She glanced down at the floor, spotted a speck of dirt. 'Look out there – mud!'

Later, my master tried to scold Jacques. 'Bad boy, my own bad boy.' But his face did not seem to fit his words. To me he said only, 'What wonderful work, Marie, how he thrives! What excellent care you take of him. I do thank you.'

# Chapter Twenty-Four

*Which contains an outing of great significance.*

'What news, what news I have, Curtius, dear widow,' said Mercier to my master and the widow as he burst into the Monkey House, full of joy.

'News, no doubt,' said the widow, 'that shall involve the drinking of our wine to ease its telling.'

'I shall not say no!' cooed Mercier.

'You never do,' said the widow and nodded to me.

I brought the wine as fast as I could.

'Well, then,' said the widow, 'if you are sufficiently primed.'

'The year 1774 began with headaches,' Mercier began.

'God save us,' groaned the lady, 'we know the date.'

'As January progressed,' continued Mercier, undeterred, 'so came body pains and fever. February arrived with a rash. In March the red spots called and wouldn't leave; they began to spread themselves everywhere about. By April the smell was undeniable; by mid-April the spots became lesions that soon filled with watery pus; by the end of April the lesions had crusty scabs. On the eighth of May the lesions began to haemorrhage, on the ninth the holy men were crammed in, on the tenth of May 1774, Louis XV, King of France by the Grace of God, has died of smallpox. Better times are here, Doctor Curtius, Widow Picot! Little too! Even your new hound! France is great again. Long live the new king, and long live the new queen! In Versailles, Parliament has been recalled! Now may Paris be saved!'

'The king is dead,' said the widow, clearly shocked.

'Dead and rotting,' replied Mercier. 'It is younger bodies that concern us now.'

But after all the talk of newness came restlessness. Soon Mercier came back, rushing around the Monkey House in agony, shaking his head. The city had changed its ruler, but his presence was impossible to detect. When nothing new was apparent, when all was business as usual, spirits broke; there was rioting on the streets; people were killed. Shrieking crowds passed by outside, shaking the Monkey House. Jacques wanted to go out, but the widow would not let him, so he spent his days whining at the door. The riot was contained, arrests were made, punishments decided. Jacques screamed hideously that he needed to watch the punishments, and kept screaming until Curtius promised to take him early next morning. The widow refused to let my master out alone, so would accompany him, and Edmond, she instructed, would accompany her. To a hanging. I was to stay behind and watch the house.

They were such different people, the ones going out of the Monkey House, from the ones coming back. Jacques brought me a souvenir. It was a doll, not particularly well made, roughly in the shape of a man but without arms, only dangling legs. It wore no clothes and had no face drawn onto its head; no hair either. It was made of simple cloth in a single colour, stuffed with dried corn. It came with a piece of looped string tied around the neck. Jacques told me that dolls like this one were always sold at the hangings, for people to hold and dangle in the direction of the scaffold. When the body fell and twitched and writhed, its move- ments matched those of the dolls held by strings in people's hands; the legs of the dying man, like the cloth legs of the hanging dolls, kicked and pitched, desperately seeking land.

'Charles Lesquillier!' proclaimed Jacques. 'Stole bread!'

Curtius was crying as I took his coat. 'Stopped! Right before me. As I watched.'

The widow was in a haze of reminiscence. 'I have not seen a

hanging since I went with Henri. We used to go together. In happier days.'

Edmond was shaking, and even paler than usual. He stumbled rather in the hall, and then dropped down to the ground. The widow screamed. Jacques carried him upstairs; a doctor was called for. When I, barefoot, braved the stairs that night, the widow was asleep in a chair by his bed, but Edmond was awake and looking at me. I saw he was crying. But I could not speak to him, only, fearfully, return kitchenwards.

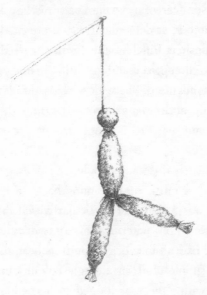

# Chapter Twenty-Five

*Our first murderer.*

The dispossessed were everywhere about Paris. They were daily growing in number, said Mercier, with no one to help them. Our neighbour, Monsieur Pillet of the chess café, lost his job and his house and his chess pieces. Many others followed. The widow wrote down the names of casualties, a list of those that had failed, and pinned it up in the workshop.

| PERSON | BUSINESS | OUTCOME |
|---|---|---|
| Marchand, Pierre | café for Latin-speakers only | bailiffs, prison |
| Roland, Michel | pies | burnt, hospital, death |
| Arlin, Georgette | silhouettes | beggary, madhouse |
| Dixmier, Alain, Hortense | conjurors | suicide, first him then her |
| Pillet, Alain | chess café | bailiffs, prison |

As Edmond recovered from the hanging, he was not allowed downstairs but kept in his room around soft objects. I think that, having seen that death, he had felt a little of it enter into him, a crumb of it somehow inhaled, and knew he must thoroughly fight it off. I had horrible notions he would die too.

One murder followed upon another. It was as if we had picked up a new language to which we'd previously been deaf. Now that we spoke murder, we heard it everywhere. And there, as if conjured by our conversations, was suddenly an enormous new one, a black new history with so much marrow in its bone. In our house it was of course Jacques who let this story in: the unpleasant history of Antoine-François Desrues.

'He poisoned with arsenic!' crowed Jacques. 'Arsenic in hot chocolate! First a mother drank it, down she goes! Bang on the floor! He pulled her old body into a trunk and buried her in a rented cellar. What a fellow! What days we live in! And that's not it yet. For then the mother's son comes calling and out comes the hot chocolate again and down goes the son. Bang on the floor! And this time he's put in the type of trunk they call a coffin and buried in a false grave. And then? The father comes and guess, guess?'

'Hot chocolate? Bang on the floor?'

'No, no, Marie, no I'm sorry, but no. When the father comes he brings the police too, and it must be that Desrues did not have enough hot chocolate for all of them, and they, suspicious, sent out posters all over the walls of Paris, and the landlady of the rented cellar recognised Desrues's likeness, and she screamed and she screamed. And then they dug up the cellar, and what do you think, Marie?'

A body, decomposing.

Hearing the noise, Doctor Curtius came in, and Jacques told the story again, and he called in the widow, and she, all disgust, listened too. I heard them later, raised voices in the workshop.

'You never discriminate,' the widow was saying. 'We cannot have just any head.'

'But I am very interested in this head. I should so like to see it. There must be something new about it – something I've never seen before.'

'Please, Doctor, let me decide which heads we cast.'

'I wish it! Widow Picot, just this once. I must have this head.'

'We do the fine people, the beautiful and the brilliant.'

'Just this once.'

The next day, Curtius and the widow left together. I counted to one hundred and rushed up the stairs. Edmond was in his room, his body under the covers, his head resting on the pillows. I thought

166

he was asleep at first, but then I saw his eyes were open and his mouth too. He was keeping very still.

'Edmond,' I whispered.

He just lay there, so pale.

'Edmond!' I said.

Edmond blinked.

'He's dead,' Edmond whispered. 'I saw him die. It was such a shock. The poor hanging man. I can't get him out of my head. I close my eyes and there he is.'

'You mustn't think of it.'

'I think of nothing else.'

I kissed him on the cheek. I felt I should do it. It was not something I had planned upon, but it just happened, and then in a rush I was back to my duties. He was looking better, I thought, a little colour in his cheeks after the kiss, no longer the pale calico of before.

My master and the widow walked to the Conciergerie, where the murderer Desrues was being held, and they returned with permission, for a fee, to visit Desrues in his cell, to make a cast of him.

'But can it be right?' the widow asked.

'We see so many businesses going down,' my master said. 'Think how many will come.'

'But it is as if we celebrate what he did.'

'No, no, we are shocked by it. More than anyone else. We are the ones who are most outraged by it! That is why we must look it in the face, dear Widow. I feel we must.'

'But does a murderer belong with our other heads? It's as if we are saying there's no difference between them.'

'He'll look different.'

'How?'

Curtius paused. Then stirred. Looked away and back again.

'The great men in our hall, Widow – politicians, writers, philosophers – they are men of the mind. We show their heads. Desrues is a murderer. His mind lost control, allowed his body to murder. So here is what I propose: we'll do *all* of him! Every bit of him, full length, not a bust but the whole vicious man. This time we say, this is exactly how he looked, and how he walked among us!'

The widow said nothing. I went back to sweeping. But early that evening, they all went out again. I was to stay behind again to guard the house. Even Edmond was to go, to give him courage, to toughen him up. The widow insisted he was not like his father, really, not so vulnerable. It was only this once, she said. How thin he was, how uncertain upon his feet.

'Don't take him,' I said. 'He looks ill.'

'And when do servants make orders?' asked the widow.

'I just thought.'

'Don't think. Your thoughts are not necessary.'

When they came back, Jacques was almost dancing with wonder. My master went directly to the workshop, the widow, shaking and sweating, to her bed, and Edmond, white and miserable, came to the kitchen to tell me what had happened.

'He was in tears when we saw him. He cried the entire time, which caused problems with the plaster mould. He kept saying, "They're going to kill me, they're going to kill me." Jacques pinned him still so that Doctor Curtius could place the plaster over his face. When Curtius took the dried plaster away, he said, "Will it be like that? Will everything suddenly go dark?" When we left his cell, he said, "Our Father, which art in heaven. Oh God! Oh God! Oh God!" Oh God, Marie, I measured him! Oh God, Marie, there is death everywhere!'

I kissed him again on the cheek. He stood very still. He did not run away. I put his hand in mine. His ears reddened just for a moment and then paled once more. He could not shake Desrues from his mind. His mother called out to him – as if she always knew when he was near me – and away he went. But there is something else. Before he retreated, he leaned forward, and I felt a moth flutter by my face and go away again. Edmond had kissed me. I held my cheek afterwards, till Jacques laughed at me; in the night I thought of it over and over. No one had done that to me before.

I did not see our Desrues until he had been cast, not until Curtius had finished and called us all to come and witness. Antoine-François Desrues was a puny man, with a pale, uneven face. It was not an exceptional face after all. It was an everyday sort, such as would not be out of place on any Parisian street. But then, after a while, it did seem a murdering head after all, a very terrible physiognomy.

'This could lead,' my master mused, 'to a greater understanding of people! At the very least, it will prove forever that such a man could exist. We'll trap barbarity in wax!'

The real Antoine-François Desrues was placed in a white robe, given a white hat like a bishop's, and a crucifix. His limbs were smashed with a sledgehammer and then what was left of the sorry man was burnt alive. Jacques went, and when he returned he told me all about it.

The wax Desrues was the first full-length wax figure that was made. He was presented standing up, bent slightly forward, offering in his hands a porcelain cup and saucer. Word of his arrival brought many people. People who were not interested in Rousseau and Diderot came to see Desrues; to them he seemed wonderfully horrible.

In this manner, the House of Curtius went into the business of murderers. The widow nailed a length of rope to the floor, dividing the hall in two. She kept the better visages to one side, and sequestered Desrues on the other. Once the business had started with murderers, it was very hard for it to stop. Jacques spoke ceaselessly of bodies found incomplete down back streets. Edmond screamed in the night, until the widow went in to comfort him.

One morning, as I laid out their breakfast, the widow wondered aloud: 'If we invite murderers into our home, what does that make us?'

'Brave?' offered my master.

'It is a terrible hunger, yours, Doctor Curtius.'

'I do thank you for allowing Desrues. You do note how our business progresses? You are a very fine woman, you see,' said Curtius and in a rare, rash gesture he touched her arm.

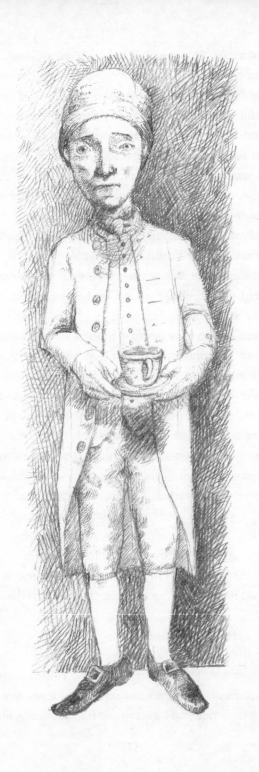

'I am a widow in mourning,' she reminded him. 'That's my husband atop the stairs.'

Desrues increased the profit of the Cabinet, it could not be denied. The widow, scratching her bonnet, herself reluctantly nodded, but she turned the dummy of her dead husband to face away from the ground floor, where the murderers were. For once Desrues's earning potential was proven, indeed other villains joined him. Curtius was taken with his murderers: he had cast the body parts of hanged men back in Berne, but he had never had such a comprehension of personalities before. They affected him greatly; he rubbed and rubbed his neck until his skin was raw. He studied the ways these people had killed; sometimes, he told me, he felt as though he'd not only died all those deaths but also committed them. They were too strong, perhaps, those murderous heads – they led him into the insides of people. He was like a child at a well, holding on to the rim of the neck of a vast decapitated body, looking down into the depths, terrified but yearning to see more, craning ever further forward into the bloody depths, at risk of losing his balance and tumbling inside. If he should fall in, he might never get out again.

In the early mornings I mingled with the late murderers in the hall, sweeping around them, getting them ready for the next viewing. The very latest people.

# Chapter Twenty-Six

*On itching.*

By the time the third murderer was cast, other people had been modelled besides, people who delighted the widow: two aeronautical gentlemen of genius called Montgolfier, who could, they said – though I never saw it – rise up in the sky in great silken balloons. A pockmarked composer called Gluck. Another, his rival, lean and handsome Piccinni. What people I kept company with!

Jacques helped with a few basic tasks in the workshop, hauling the sacks of plaster dust, sawing wood for armatures, but he was never allowed close to the models. He was clumsy, he was too rough, he upset things. Objects were terrified of Jacques. Without meaning to, he would shatter glass and porcelain; he didn't mean anything by it; there was nothing to be done about it. He made people cry. But Jacques wanted to get closer to his murderers. One night I awoke to terrible screams and moans – not a monkey, but a similar horrifying sound, as if those noises were echoing years later. We found Jacques upstairs in the workshop with his feet in a large pail of plaster. Hoping to prove his ingeniousness to Curtius by casting his own feet, he had mixed the plaster himself, but when he slipped his feet into a great iron bucket of the stuff, it had trapped them. Plaster on living flesh must be used in small layers; place a foot into a deep container, and it will hold your foot prisoner till it scorches and cooks it. Jacques couldn't get his feet out, and neither could I, or my master, or even the widow, and all Edmond could do was cry, 'Do something! Do something!' The pain was terrible, the widow gave him brandy, I held his hands, he screamed and screamed. By the time Curtius had chipped away and freed his feet, the plaster was growing cold. Jacques would never allow the wounds to heal properly, picking at them and scratching them. He would hobble for the rest of his life.

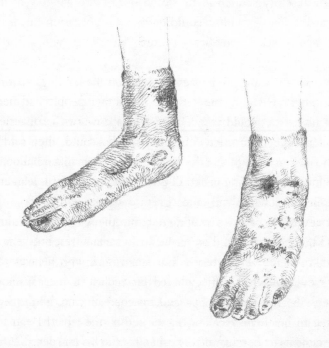

'Plaster,' said Curtius to Jacques in his pain (what music it was to me to hear his lessons again!), 'knows nothing about life. It is a dead substance. When light shines upon it, all it knows is sterility. It reveals facts without personality. It can show pores, it can show wrinkles, it can copy – but never with character. When mixed with water, the plaster powder becomes gypsum, and for a moment the combination of water and plaster make heat, but there is no passion in this heat. It is hot, yes, but a hot *nothing*. There's no comprehension of flesh with it. Wax, on the other hand, is fleshy. Wax *is* skin.'

The Monkey House up and down suffered from itches. Jacques's feet itched, but that was barely the start of it. An itch racked

Curtius's whole body, and he scratched at it, he clawed at his skin, bruising and cutting at it, blaming the exquisite agony on so many murderers. When Jacques itched, we all knew about it; he could not be controlled. He would sit on the floor and rock back and forth, or absently scratch as he stared out of the window at the boulevard. Even the widow could be found on occasion furiously patting at her head, sometimes rubbing hard at it with a butter knife.

Sometimes I heard my master at night, on the landing, visiting the dummy of Henri Picot. Perhaps once a month, in those clandestine hours, he would take a pair of small scissors, of the type called *découseur*, from the widow's tools, and sever a stitch on the dummy, seldom enough that the widow never noticed. After a while the back came away, the neck fell down, and beneath the object a small pile of sawdust and chips grew, augmented by droppings from a slew of tiny slashes, waiting to be swept up. One day Widow Picot, who had not looked at her husband's shape since turning it around, suddenly remembered him again, and with a heave of passion and renewed grief, gathered his replica in her capacious embrace. She repaired her husband, patched him up, bound him tightly with her love, recalling as she did so the troughs and the small gradients of her dear dead husband. After several days he was back at his station, more Henri than ever. And my master miserable.

And other itches were afoot. I itched. And Edmond did too, I knew he did.

'You are a certain age now, Edmond,' the widow observed one morning at the breakfast table. 'Seventeen. Beyond childhood. New things will happen to you. New beginnings. Different people, new measurements.'

'What new people, Mother?'

'I want you, Edmond, to grow up. And there's something else you might think about, that someone of your age and quality should consider.'

'What, Mother?'

'The getting of a wife,' she said, pausing to marvel. 'Edmond with the women!'

But at present it was Edmond without the women, for when he was marshalled into proximity with his opposite sex, with the single exception of myself, Edmond became a dead shop doll. Like me, he had his very own vanishing system. In such circumstances, he magicked his insides into sawdust and hemp waste, until the only blood left in him was concentrated in his ears; he made himself over into nobody at all. Movement only resurfaced after the woman had gone away, after several minutes of standing quite alone waiting for life to return, blood flowing slowly from his ears back into his body, soaking all that hemp waste until it became lungs and livers, bladder and bowels once more.

The first of Edmond's potential wives was the daughter of a cotton wholesaler. A ruddy-faced thing, she had tiny eyes like swine and visible white eyelashes and smelt of urine. Her father was a huffing puffing sort of oink, her mother a pot-bellied sow. Their sty was doing well, and the mother wished to combine business with pigness. The girl sat beside Edmond as directed and looked hard at him, but Edmond never moved. The parents spoke to Edmond, but he never made a sound, so they got a little puffy about that, and the girl began to look unhappy, her almost-white hair growing greasy before my eyes. Finally she took hold of Edmond's hand. As she held it, though, her white face went whiter and a little whiter, she whined a bit, and then she gave the hand back. They never returned.

That night there was a quiet knocking on the door.

'Hello, Marie.'

'Who's there?'

'It's me. It's Edmond. May I be with you a little?'

'Come in, close the door.'

'Thank you.'

'Edmond, you were wonderful today with the visitors.'

'I was?'

'Certainly.'

'Marie, I don't want to be married.'

'No, you mustn't be. You must stay here with me.'

He stayed a whole half-hour. He showed me his doll Edmond, quite distressed now in his trauma. I wished he would put it away; it was as if it were another person come between us, stopping our privacy. When at last he did pocket the beloved thing, though, it was only to get up and leave.

The visit from the cotton wholesaler was only the first of several horrors that Edmond was put through. There was the daughter of a dressmaker who found Edmond 'ridiculous', and the child of a barber-surgeon who wondered if 'he was quite right in the head'. None found him desirable, but rather strangely absent and unappealing. They were blind and foolish and undeserving people, and I was giddy with gratitude and relief for it. So they left him there. But his mother was not finished upon the hunt yet.

Edmond and I were an essential part of the great itching house, its engine perhaps. We came together that last summer as if we knew that our time was running out, that we must discover while it was still possible. Nightly there was a creaking on the stairs. The night was ours, and we were to be found in it.

He would arrive at night, while Jacques was sleeping.

'Look at you,' I said. 'What a sight!'

'Here I am.'

We would look, and we would talk.

'I'm five foot five inches and an eighth of an inch,' he said.

'My head's about at your heart, isn't it? Let's have a listen! There! That's the sound of Edmond. What noise you make.' We talked, we held hands, then he left again.

The house itself itched. With the great progress in business, the widow and my master were able to purchase the Monkey House for themselves. And once purchased they set about redecorating it. The walls of the ground floor were covered in crimson paper.

'Each time I come home,' Curtius said, 'I feel I am entering the vast body of some titan, that the red walls are the walls of the chambers of a colossal human trunk.'

Curtius and the widow bought objects to decorate the hall, purchased from a theatrical-prop maker. There was a great clock which was actually only a piece of wood shaped like a clock, with a clock's face painted upon it, so that it always told the same time. There were matching elaborate chests of drawers made of painted board; these had not one functioning drawer between them, but they *looked* real enough. There were wooden plinths painted to look marble. At night, when Jacques was snoring, Edmond and I would go into the hall and drift together from new object to new object, pretending we were wealthy Paris people, that we had come into our own kingdom. In the large room you felt you were in a magnificent palace, though the windows looked out not on elegant gardens, but on the mud of the boulevard, and Doctor Graham's house across the way.

'Thomas-Charles Ticre of the print-works,' said the widow to Edmond at breakfast, 'has a daughter. Cornélie. We might think about that. What a future that would be. What a solid future.'

# Chapter Twenty-Seven

*Our latest great heads.*

We acquired two more doctors. The Place Louis-le-Grand, a place I had never visited, was where Doctor Franz Anton Mesmer, recently fled from Vienna, set up his clinic in February 1778. He soon had many patients. He cured, a leaflet delivered to me from Edmond explained, everything from paralysis to constipation, from impotence to the vapours, from bunions to herpes, from sties to cataracts, from gallstones to gangrene, from epilepsy to dropsy, from hysteria to hiccups, from sterility to incontinence. He was a miracle man; he placed his hands on people's bodies and they felt a strange power coming over them. I came to know Doctor Mesmer, not in person, but in wax. He had a very flat face with almost no profile at all, as if it had been grown face down in a frying pan.

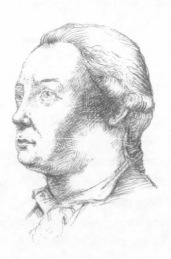

The second doctor was the Commissioner for the Free America, Doctor Benjamin Franklin. I never saw this man either, not the actual man himself – though my master and the widow were given audience – but even so I have cause to remember him particularly. I am most grateful to Doctor Franklin for his long grey hair, for that is what got me admitted properly back into the workshop – as a worker. There was a great shortage of time in those days; there were so many heads to complete that my master needed more help, and so at last I was remembered. The most tedious and time-consuming job was putting hair into wax heads; usually a wig would simply be placed on a head, as nearly everyone of significance, male or female, wore some other person's, or some horse's, hair. But this American doctor wore his own.

'That instrument,' I said, 'is a ring-handled, long-necked needle with polyp tip, sir.'

'Yes, it is, Little. How did you know that?'

'You taught me, sir, in Berne.'

'Did I? Indeed, I believe I did. I had forgot. I shan't again. Do you know what it is for?'

'It is for the propping up of tissues during operations, but you use it for threading hairs, one by one, into wax scalps.'

'Well, yes, yes, that is exactly right.'

'Must she?' asked the widow.

'For the sake of getting things done, Widow Picot. We are so overstretched.'

'But no talking, Little. Sit in silence.'

'Yes, Madame.'

'As if you are not really there at all.'

'Yes, Madame.'

And so I made my triumphant return. I studied Benjamin Franklin very closely. The head was like some massive tuber, a potato of a man. There was a deal of rather wrinkled double chin at the bottom of the face, great hams of cheeks going upwards, a sizeable forehead. In the centre of the face a bulbous nose grew,

179

flanked by two droopy grey heavy-lidded eyes; his mouth was bracketed by considerable folds.

'This personage,' I said, 'has come all the way from America.'

'Yes, Little,' nodded my master.

'It's as if we're learning the world, isn't it?'

'You may say that, indeed.'

'No call for noise!' snapped the widow.

Hair by hair, I made Franklin look like Franklin. I threaded in the long grey hairs, cropped by the widow from an old chestnut seller on the Pont Neuf who needed the money. With the rounded tip of the needle I pushed one end of the hair into the wax; when I took the needle away, the hair remained. This I did several thousand times, and with portraits of the new doctor before me. Cheap images of his face were to be found all over Paris: on prints, on a snuffbox, a matchbox, a fan, even on a chamber pot, over the inscription *'He wrested lightning from the gods and the sceptre from tyrants.'*

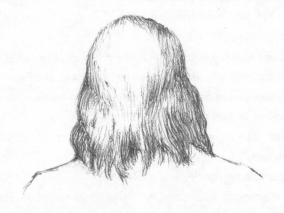

'Perhaps now at last,' I ventured, standing to admire the hair, 'you shall pay me.'

'You are to be quiet in here,' said the widow. 'You are not to be heard at all.'

'We shall look into it, Marie,' said my master. 'We certainly shall. Do be patient.'

I smiled as I worked on the doctor's remaining hair. Perhaps I was finally becoming a true part of the family. Perhaps, if my work was good enough, I might even be permitted to marry into it.

Many people came to see the wax Mesmer and Franklin. Some even called during the day to visit Curtius and the widow in the workshop upstairs. And so I, now a part of the workshop business, witnessed new people every day. One such man was Jean-Antoine Houdon, a very famous sculptor. If I had not learned that, I should have called him only Another Little Bald Man.

'Your name, of course, is not unfamiliar to me,' said Houdon. 'You do thieves and murderers. You rob everyone of grace. There's no dignity, no elevation of the human form, only degradation. You are a cynic, you have no love for your fellow creature, you are incapable of music.'

'I love the heads,' said my master, softly. 'I do love the heads.'

'Your business is good for the streets, perhaps. Your material is cheap and easily obtained, commonplace. There's nothing subtle about it. No wit. No brilliance.'

'Wax is . . . flesh!' Curtius said.

'Then marble the soul.'

'I've made my life of wax.'

'Keep to the murderers,' said Houdon. 'They deserve you. But this head' – he pointed at Franklin – 'is demeaned by you. You dishonour it.'

In February of 1778, as I became an official part of the workshop, an ailing and toothless eighty-three-year-old man, François-Marie Arouet, known to the world as Voltaire, returned to Paris from exile in Switzerland after nearly thirty years. Paris went wild for him. They hurled honours at his shaky frame. Voltaire, in response, haemorrhaged.

In his convalescence he was shut up in the house of the Marquis de Villette on the banks of the Seine. A worried crowd lingered outside the house, hoping for a glimpse, but only the most esteemed visitors were allowed in, among them Doctor Franklin. On two

181

occasions, the small and bald sculptor Jean-Antoine Houdon was admitted for sittings. Then he rushed back to his studio, where he locked the door and didn't come out again for a week and a half. Houdon was determined: this would be the greatest work of his life. Day and night he tap-tapped against his marble. Slowly he found the protruding lower jaw, the thin grinning lips. His thoughts took shape in sunken cheekbones, bald ancient heads, wrinkled chicken necks.

At the marquis's house by the river, there was an old man who daily looked less and less like Voltaire. Now, to see the true Voltaire, you took yourself and your family to Houdon's studio. That's where he was, keeping regular hours, never disappointing. From eleven in the morning to seven o'clock in the evening, every day, grinning without cease.

My master visited it. 'No colour! No life,' he said, but he bit his knuckles.

'If we could only have Voltaire,' the widow said, 'think who would come.'

'I do want Voltaire's head,' said Curtius. 'I want it so much that I hurt.'

My master and the widow joined the dwindling crowd in front of that house by the river every day. Every day they were not permitted entrance. And every day Edmond and I sat together in the workshop. We chatted as we worked and I began to think that this is how it could be if we were married. Every day they went out, the widow knocking fruitlessly on the door, my master holding his father's great leather bag filled with stopped bottles of water, pomade, and plaster dust. Not until the thirtieth of May, after the old man had been moved into a servant's lodge behind the house, and after they had passed money to a servant – an amount my master and the widow referred to only as 'the certain sum' – were they invited inside. Because, by then, it was all over. Voltaire had died. My master took his death mask.

The model of Voltaire had to be ready as soon as possible, but the face my master had taken in plaster was collapsed, slumped, lacking in life.

'I know he's dead,' said Edmond. 'That's a dead face. You've been at his grave, Mother!'

'Not his grave,' she said. 'Doctor Curtius has made it clear to me, Edmond, it is perfectly reasonable to take a death mask of a great man. Death masks have been taken of kings. It is quite acceptable.'

'The murderers were alive when you saw them! This man was dead. A dead thing!'

'Edmond, Edmond,' she said, wiping a tear from his eye, 'you are entirely too sensitive. Do please find a way to bury your nerves.'

My master adjusted the philosopher, stroking and shifting his features, and from the wax death mask he made in clay a plumper face, with open eyes, grinning. My master studied Houdon's head, studied many prints of the philosopher. I watched him shifting his own face until it took on Voltaire's expressions. Then he tamed the clay and the wax until it became Voltaire. It was a marvellous thing to behold. Only four exhausting days after his death, Voltaire was resurrected on the Boulevard du Temple.

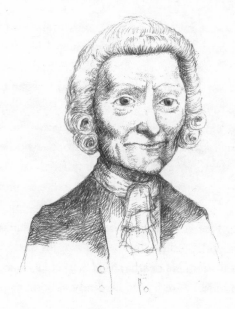

This Voltaire, so lively that he appeared on the very verge of speaking, brought many people. 'At Curtius's,' they said, 'Voltaire still lives.'

'A famous head,' said the widow, 'a glowing head.'

People came in such numbers that the Monkey House grew and grew and someone else came to be employed inside its doors. Florence Biblot was a large, shiny-faced woman who already provided meals for several other of the boulevard businesses. Sometimes she cooked in the house; more often, she brought the food to us. She was not a great talker, Florence wasn't. When she was complimented she said nothing, only gave a little laugh that revealed her tongue bouncing north and south and small, ground-down teeth. She did this every time, without fail.

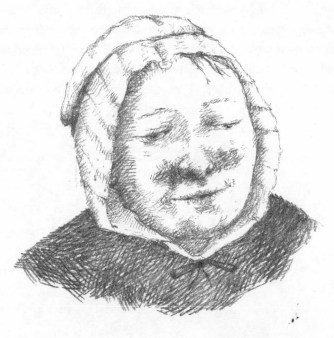

'Thank you, Florence, that was a lovely stew,' said my master.
'Ddddd, ddddd.'

'At long last we remember what food tastes like,' said the widow.
'Ddddd, ddddd.'

I taught her how to make the Swiss dishes that my master so liked. *Rösti*, grated potatoes cooked in fat, and *Fleischkäse*, which is made by combining various meats together with onions and baking in a bread pan.

'Dddddd,' she laughed, putting a liver through the grinder.

More people came, so many that the widow took Edmond on a visit to Monsieur Ticre's print-works.

# Chapter Twenty-Eight

*New clothes.*

With prosperity came bricks. With bricks came builders, who surrounded our walls with brick atop brick, up and up and up, until the old wooden Monkey House was dressed in a smart brick suit. Four brick buttresses were added to help the wooden crutches. 'It's not in the correct spirit,' said Mercier in the workshop. 'No good shall come of it. There shouldn't be bricks on the boulevard. They'll hate you for it. One day they'll take revenge on you for those bricks.'

'And who are you to say such things?' demanded the widow.

'I am Mercier himself.'

'And of what account is that?'

'I am your old friend. Have you forgotten it was I who introduced you to Curtius? Look downstairs: there I am, made by his own fine hands.'

'Yes indeed, I thank you for the remembrance. I am so familiar with our works that sometimes I forget what is before me. I meant to have that one removed months ago. Jacques, do take that head away. Do not worry how you handle it, we shall melt it down.'

'But I am Mercier!'

'Yes, I know, such a shame. Couldn't you be someone else?'

'I wrote the book *Paris in the Year*—'

'Yes, yes, but you see it no longer signifies. You'll have to do something new, won't you? And let us know when you have. Make sure, this time, that it's something that will last.'

'Please, dear lady. Don't take my likeness down.'

186

'It is done. We are not running a charity.'

'I do so like to see it there,' he said, crestfallen.

'We accept only the very best and very worst heads. And yours, like the great multitude's, lies somewhere in between. You do understand, don't you?'

How quietly Mercier left.

He was right, at first, about the bricks. Neighbours would shake their heads and fists as they passed us on the street; some would spit; on occasion, in the dead of night when Jacques was asleep, some would empty their swill buckets on the steps. Of all the buildings upon the boulevard, only three were made of something more solid than wood: Nicolet's Grands Danseurs de Corde, Audinot's Ambigu-Comique, and now the Cabinet du Docteur Curtius.

As it settled, now, the Monkey House made new, strange noises, as of a very large mouth grinding its teeth. The attic creaked in agony, louder than ever before. There was a gradual drop of two inches in some of the upstairs rooms. Once, as the widow was walking along the landing, a floorboard un-nailed itself and sprang up, nearly smacking her in the face.

Newly dressed, the Monkey House provoked a revolution in everyone's clothes. It began, as it must, with the widow. To her customary black she added shades now, some trimmings of purple, a little dark blue to her cuffs; her bonnet was lined with purple silk. She purchased for herself a gentleman's Malacca cane with an ornate silver guilloche handle, never again to be seen without it. There seemed to me a fresh outbreak of moles upon her skin, little bumps and dots that had not been there before, and might never have been, but for the bricks. These growths and pimplings were like medals upon a soldier, smart decorations, each a further proof of her enormous progress.

To my master the bricks brought only a stiffness, as if the building were longing to turn him into a caryatid. The widow announced her disapproval of his cotton suit: that suit, she said, was a personality that had no understanding of bricks. Edmond measured him, and a new personality was created, this in black velvet, which gave my master back pains and strange throbbings down his thighs, but caused him to utter more proclamations of how fond he was of the Widow Picot and what she had done for us all.

Some people cannot be contained within clothes, some people are too full of life, some people are all motion and upheaval; such energetic bipeds and quadrupeds are the enemy of thread. Jacques Beauvisage wasn't made for clothes. He tried very hard, but it was hopeless. Even in finery, he still upset everything around him. One evening, in his clumsiness, he knocked over a murderer; the head shattered. While Curtius sadly sorted through the remains, the widow flew into action. She blew the bugle of her voice: *Scissors! Hot water! Razor!* She was going to cut the animal out of him. In those days of silk, she proclaimed an end to fur. She, who would keep her own enormous hair hidden beneath her cap, now forbade my poor miserable Jacques his matted topper-most. She chopped off his great mane, then shaved the stubble crop that remained. His hair was dismissed like Curtius's old suit; it fell onto an old sheet that had been laid on the floor to receive the gentle tumble of Jacques's wildness and with it a great nation of lice, which I consigned to the fire. If the widow's intention had been to create a neat gentle-looking person, she failed utterly, for shorn of his hair he looked more terrible than ever. I sat with him as he sadly stroked his stubble-head, a chipped cannonball.

Even I could not escape the wardrobe upheaval, this war of cloth, this famous defeat of new over old. From the widow I received dark dresses, very plain, very workmanlike, five modest sisters and a new cap. Of good, though not exceptional, material. Still, here I was, part of the family. I thanked her for it, very much. She grimaced.

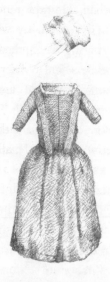

Even the dummy of Henri Picot was seen shining upon the landing, in a new white lace shirt with mother-of-pearl buttons.

Edmond was robbed of calico, which was his material, and put in silk. What whines from him, of uncharacteristic volume. From his room, from the widow's, came loud noises of a family in dispute. 'Please, Mother, no, I don't want to.'

'I won't have this, Edmond, I won't have it!'

'It must not happen, I tell you, Mother, a terrible error!'

'You tell me? Nonsense! What's this new boldness? Where's it from? Put this on now! If I have to strip you myself, you will put this on!'

Edmond in a crisp white silk suit was almost an albino; only his ears were a different colour from the rest of him. There's Edmond, I remember thinking, quick, watch him in that suit of his. Most people did not think much of him, most people did not spend emotion upon him of any sort, and he was left forgotten; I used to think that fitted him well enough and I was very grateful for it. But I saw him in his white suit, exposed as never before; there were blue veins at the sides of his temples. Delicate aquamarine rivers flowing through the Country of Edmond. How to chart such territory? Where could suitable explorers be found? I saw him in that white suit, certainly I saw him, very early one morning, when he would usually be wearing his nightshirt. He came in to me wearing that horrible white suit. He did not say anything. Instead Edmond's blank face came closer and closer to mine, so very close that my lips touched something that felt like cotton but was in fact the lips of Edmond Picot. And then a deeper kiss than ever before, his mouth opened, there was Edmond beneath the cloth, the within of him. But he stopped so soon.

'Sorry,' he said. 'I'm sorry.'

'Why are you sorry, Edmond?'

He said, 'I find you pretty.'

'Edmond? Edmond? Do you? Do you!'

'I don't want to go. I'm sorry.'

'Edmond?'

'I'm so sorry.'

But he didn't say why he was sorry. As I put my fingers to my lips, that white suit went out of sight. The widow had proclaimed the availability of her son. As if she had nailed a bill on an external wall of the Monkey House, and the bill had grown very old, had seen every weather, had been doused by rain which turned to ice, dripped dry, curled and yellowed in the sun, had lost its whiteness and was now almost impossible to read – and yet, incredibly, suddenly, someone had seen it there. Someone read the message carefully, and understood it, and even read the final small words, APPLY WITHIN. And did.

# Chapter Twenty-Nine

PUBLIC NOTICE:
THE NUPTIALS OF CORNÉLIE TICRE.

I have been a little dishonest perhaps. I may have mixed bricks with clothing. I forgot to mention the clothing was for an event, or that the event was the marriage of Edmond Henri Picot to Cornélie Adrienne Françoise Ticre, of the print-works on the Rue Saint-Louis.

The Ticre print-works was responsible for advertisements all across Paris. They printed not only the bills for the Cabinet of Doctor Curtius – ALL THE BEST AND ALL THE WORST PEOPLE OF PARIS – INSIDE! – but also the sheets for the Comédie-Française, for RACINE'S ANDROMAQUE, and they didn't stop there. The print-works went on through day and night, and all day Sunday too; they never stopped; they were hot as all the talking heads of Paris. The presses slammed back and forth, churning out thousands upon thousands of words, until it made your head pound: letters on small metal or wood blocks, positioned in order back to front, rolled with ink, then thumped onto the paper, causing the paper a jolt of agony. Oh, those people, they'd print anything. They'd alert Parisians to the latest book, the latest medicine, the most shocking notices of bankruptcy, the grave importance of elastic stockings, the most advanced varnish for teeth. How many walls in all Paris, I wondered, were covered by the outpourings of the Ticre press alone? All those words revealing all those lives, all those businesses, all those hopes, all those futures, all those little pieces of the human mass.

191

It was the Ticre press that printed out broadsheets for the hangings, for church services and puppet shows, for things missing: a poodle, a turtle, a walking stick, a snuffbox. LOST: A MUFF. LOST: SILVER ASPARAGUS TONGS. LOST: AN ELABORATE CANDLE SNUFFER. LOST: A SILK UMBRELLA. LOST: A DOUBLE-FACED TIMEPIECE. LOST: A TOUCAN. LOST: A BELOVED DOG. LOST: A CHILD.

Lost, lost. Lost to Cornélie Adrienne Françoise Ticre. Lost: Edmond Henri Picot, the model for shop dolls. My chance. Lost forever. I sat, lost, in the kitchen. No one ever thought to ask me. No one came to me to wonder if Edmond should be married off. No one thought I cared; no one thought of me in any way connected to him. So they did not see my grief, or even hear me weeping in the night. Even Jacques slouched away. A miserable servant is no massive concern.

The widow had finally found a buyer. When poor Edmond was lost, in his white silk suit, two strong businesses were combined. Several thousand livres came into the Monkey House with that marriage. The pale boy went to live at the Ticre print-works, where he was expected to learn a new and profitable profession and one day to govern it himself. The widow did not trust the Cabinet alone; she was shoring up greater security with a more certain business.

There was more money in printing than tailoring, even than in wax. The widow went to visit him often, but I never saw him. In my quiet moments, when I was alone, I closed my eyes and cut the widow open – slit Cornélie from her mouth to her anus – sitting all the while in the kitchen, waiting for no one to come.

I could not sleep in those lonely nights – and so instead I stole from Curtius and the widow. Bent over stolen candles, I stole Edmond from Cornélie, or tried to. I stole wax and clay, I stole paper and pencils and wire for armatures. I made a small wax head of Edmond about the size of a heart or a fist: they are the same size. So hard to recall his face, so hard to bring it back; I'd look at the shop

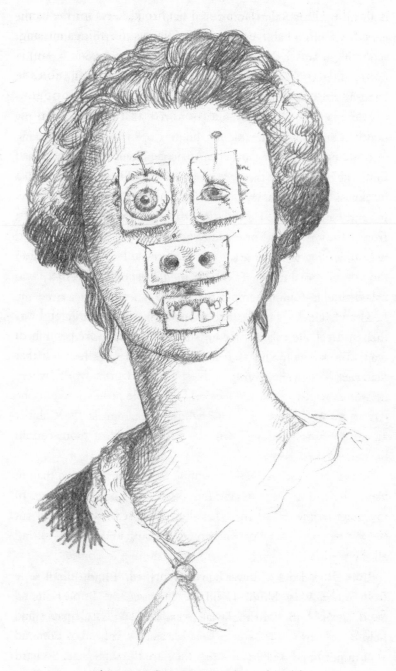

The new Madame Picot, not drawn from life.

dolls on the Rue Saint-Honoré for help and always start with the ears. It became a habit, the stealing of things, to crouch and squint in the night and make my small heads. Always Edmond; no other head mattered. Even if I could never quite find him, still I thought I might yet, one day, if I kept at it.

Perhaps it was my eyes, always so red, that finally alerted my master. I am worried, he told me, holding open my lids and looking into my eyes. As if my eyes were the problem! But he thought I might have a disease there. Most people would muddle on with a weakness such as mine, but my master had my small problem instantly attended to. He took me to a man who put glass discs in front of my eyes and proclaimed me 'weakling'. What I needed was something to help me see things close to. Things further away did not matter so much. The medicine I must take, externally, was called double-folding-temple spectacles. The man measured my head and said he would make temple arms of no more than six inches. Steel, he asked, or coin silver? Curtius looked at me. 'I want coin silver for her, but for now I fear it must be steel.' My facewear cost twenty livres.

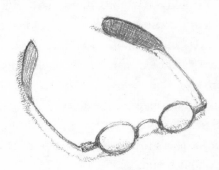

'Blind?' said the widow when we returned. 'Blind. Blind!'

'Not blind! Not blind!' I said.

'If she's blind, Curtius, what use is she? We shall need more help.'

'I'm not blind, sir!'

'What a noise she makes!' said the widow. 'And not only in front

194

of us, also crying in the kitchen. The other day I saw her thumping her own head. And such slovenliness. You may say nothing, Curtius, but I have noticed how poor her work has become. And now how she scowls!'

'And, Little,' asked my master, 'are you eating?'

Jacques Beauvisage was upset by my spectacles. He thought they signified something wrong with me, as if I myself were made of glass. He feared I might shatter.

'I am just the same, Jacques, as ever I was. I just see everything much clearer, sharper, and closer. As if I'm seeing you properly for the first time.'

'How you look at me!' he cried. 'What do you see now? What is different?'

'Look for yourself. Here they are.'

'No! Shan't! Won't! Must not!'

I saw better, saw them all well, now, at last. I saw all the holes in human skin, I saw film over eyes, I saw hair on tips of noses. I saw all the little wonderful truths of the human face that before I'd never known. Was it good to see so much? Was it happy-making? Not if I could not see him. I only wanted him to look at, and here was everyone else save him. I could not at first find a use for such sharp eyes. But I could not stop looking. Even children had creases; that I had not known before. Everything was as it had been, only more so.

'Florence Biblot has small teeth marks on her lips,' I observed.

'Has she, Marie, there's a thing!' said my master.

'The scar on Jacques's forehead turns slightly blue or green or red depending on his mood.'

'Does it? Ha ha!'

'The Widow Picot has a small dot on her left nostril.'

'No, no, she doesn't.'

'She does indeed.'

'No one knows her better than I.'

Even so my master went to look.

'She does! Never had I seen it before. The smallest mole.'

And the fact of it brought him to tears.

Those were the days when the removal of the spectacles from my face left an impression of the spectacles' clip upon the bridge of my nose. There I was in the shadows, hall-creeper, dish-washer, little lost woman of hair. Before the red sore could grow into a callus, a very different visitor arrived and everything was turned upside down.

# Chapter Thirty

*I am found out.*

So many people of all stations in Parisian life came to the Monkey House. Aristocrats came and fishwives, men who worked on roofs and men who worked in the sewers, men who composed operas and men who composed bricks in the brickyards. And so, in the end, it is not perhaps so extraordinary that a royal person should call.

The piece of royalty that came, for there was only one, was fourteen years old. A little girl. Paris and even Versailles were still caught up with Voltaire in those days, and this little majesty decided she wanted to learn a little more of this famous philosopher. This crumb of royalty evidently learned that the Boulevard du Temple was home to a hall filled with famous and infamous people, all made of wax, and accounted to be very lifelike – and among them was Monsieur Voltaire, in exact size and shape. Should her minor majesty be interested in getting an impression of the recently deceased, then this might be the place to visit. And so a little miracle occurred in my life, a wonderful bit of happy luck.

In she came, surrounded by her entourage. She did not arrange a visit, she merely came with her people in the morning, when we were closed. It was a very good thing that she did, for had she warned of her visit, I should not have been in the great hall dusting heads when the dead tailor's bell called out, I would not have drawn the bolts back, nor would I have been the one informed of who was here.

Madame Élisabeth Philippine Marie Hélène Bourbon, granddaughter of Louis XV, least significant child of the late Dauphin

Louis, sister to King Louis XVI, rose no more than four foot eleven inches from the ground. She was a little plump, with delicate grey eyes and a very fair skin, but these details can be skipped over. What was important was that her nose was quite large and bent in the Bourbon tradition. And her chin, her chin, was – how could I conceal my delight? – her chin was rather too long and prominent! Need I spill it out? She was not a pretty little girl. Need I spit it out?

I took my spectacles off.

The royal bit looked like me.

I looked like the royal bit.

Yes, I was seventeen. Yes, unshod I was four foot eight inches in length. I am ready to concede that my lantern chin, a good impression I believe of Father's, was wider and more jutting. I admit my eyes are brown, not so prettily pale grey, yes, yes. But regard the two noses, first the Waltner snout, and now the Bourbon conk!

They are very nearly the same.

As if the world had suddenly doubled itself up.

We recognised each other instantly. What could be done with this strange unsettling intimacy? I wanted to kiss her and shove her simultaneously. To shout and to whisper. To dance and to flee. What a person! Just like me – a clearer version, more expensive certainly, but my likeness without a doubt. Did she see it? Yes, I knew she had. I suspected she knew everything about me already. I wanted to cover myself up and to pull off all my clothing. It was as if I'd known her all my life.

How my heart joyfully, fearfully bounced inside.

Similarity sometimes breaks barriers, sometimes pulls them up.

Standing before her, I curtsied. But I could not keep quiet. I wanted to tell her all. 'My father died,' I began. 'He was behind a backfiring cannon. My mother died, very suddenly.'

'Her Highness, Madame Élisabeth of France,' announced one of the entourage as the widow came into the hall. The widow went white and bowed.

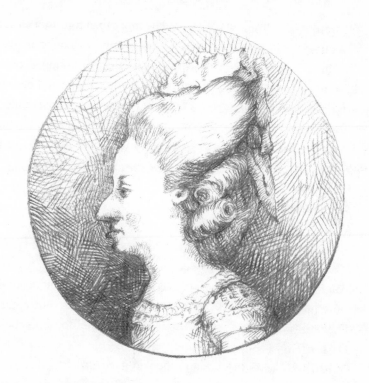

But the princess had heard me. 'My father died,' she replied in her quiet voice. 'And my mother. It was tuberculosis that took them away. Would you show me the people in wax?'

'Little,' said the widow, 'kitchen.'

But I did not listen. Instead I showed her. First Voltaire, then Doctor Franklin and Doctor Mesmer. It was in front of Mesmer that Madame Élisabeth turned and surprised me: she would like to sculpt, she said. Would I perhaps teach her wax modelling?

'Me?' I asked.

'She only does the hairs, Your Majesty,' said the widow.

'Yes,' I said, 'but I know much more.'

'Little,' said the widow, 'that's enough, go to the kitchen. Your Majesty, she is just a serving girl.'

'Would you like to see my work?' I asked.

'There is no work, Little,' said the widow.

'If you please, Your Majesty, this way, may I show you?'

'Jacques,' said the widow, 'take her outside.'

'Jacques,' I said, so bold with my new likeness beside me, so bold in my new spectacles, 'do not do it.'

And the princess said, 'I should very much like to see your work.'

I took her to the kitchen; with the thunder of my heart in my ears, I closed the door on everyone but the princess. I heaved my trunk out. I opened the lid. There were all my Edmond heads.

'I made these,' I said, 'every one.'

'Who are they?'

'A boy. From memory.'

'Who is he?'

'It doesn't matter now. He's gone away.'

'You did all this?' the princess asked.

'Only me.'

'They are wonderful!'

'Say it again,' I said.

'Perhaps you would show me how.'

I put the pieces back. When I opened the door everyone was there waiting. I showed her our wonderful murderers then, and here Jacques stepped forward and would not be silenced.

'Victor Joly cut up his brides!'

'Oh dear!' whispered Madame Élisabeth.

'Audrée Veron,' said Jacques, filled with his special enthusiasm, 'sifter in the dustyards, killed her sister Jacqueline, over something in the mud, over a broken watch. Slit her sister's throat with a rusted shard of iron.'

'Poor girl,' whispered the princess to me, 'to live with such things!'

'This here,' continued Jacques, who, having begun, could not now be stopped, despite the widow's troubled looks, 'Antoine-François Desrues. In a trunk he—'

'Stop! Stop, please stop!' called a member of the entourage.

'To live every day with such monsters,' the princess said, not

200

looking at our dear murderers but regarding my master, the widow, and Jacques.

She told me how she felt for me, how terrible it must have been for such a girl as me to grow up in such a place, with such murderers for company. She left soon afterwards. What a visit it was, what a holiday.

I smiled a huge smile, smiled until the door was closed and the bolts pulled across. But then the smile left because here came the retribution. The door of the kitchen was opened again and so was my trunk.

'What's this?' asked the widow.

'Heads, Madame.'

'They're wrapped in my muslin!'

'I admit I took some muslin, I freely admit it, and more besides. Why may I not? After all, I have never yet been paid for all my labour.'

At first, she couldn't see who it was in all those heads. How could she? She never saw Edmond as I had. In her eyes he was someone else entirely. My master, though, great knower of humans, he knew.

'Is it? Are they? Edmond? I think they are. Why so many Edmonds, Marie?'

'Who? Who!' came the widow.

She knocked my head very hard with a small wax bust of Edmond.

From wax I went to coal; I was put in the coal room.

I sat there for very long hours. Jacques came to visit.

'What are they doing?' I asked. 'What's happening?'

'The widow's breaking it all, smashing the heads.'

'That's her own son she's smashing. I'm to be beaten, I suppose, am I?'

'You're to have no food, widow's orders.'

'That's like her. For how long?'

'Doesn't say. The widow wants you gone.'

201

My master came to the door of the coal room.

'I am trying to keep you.'

'Thank you, sir.'

'Or find somewhere else for you to go.'

'No! I must stay with you.'

'I fear what the widow would do if you did stay. She is so energetic. I honestly fear she may hurt you. She particularly does never
like you thinking of her son. I fear the punishment.'

'Please, sir, I cannot stop.'

'Oh, Marie, I am trying to do everything right. I have had an
idea, I have written a letter.'

'I have to stay. This is my home.'

'Nothing is decided yet, Marie. It might go this way, it might
go that.'

But it was decided very soon. A man came, on official business.
The first I knew of it was Jacques saying I must brush myself
down and hurry to the workshop. Curtius and the widow were sat
next to each other at one end of the worktable, a stranger at the
other.

'You are,' the stranger said, 'Anne Marie Grosholtz, ward of
this house?'

'Ward, sir?'

'Yes, Marie,' said the widow, 'you are to say yes.'

'Marie?' I replied. I had never heard her call me that. To the
man I said, 'I am a servant here. I do the hairs.'

'I am to offer you a position, on a trial basis. Sculptor tutor to
Her Majesty Madame Élisabeth of France. Would it be acceptable
to you?'

I said nothing, no words, no words would come.

'It would not be acceptable to you?' the man asked.

I could not breathe. I could only, after a time, nod.

'I should think so indeed,' the man continued. 'Your guardians
shall be paid for your services by the month.'

'Yes, sir. But is it my money?'

'You must take it up with your guardians here.'

'I think it must be my money. You see, sir, I have never been paid.'

'That is not my business, Mademoiselle. Please may we conclude: I have set the date of your arrival at a week hence. I trust that that, too, is acceptable.'

'Yes, sir.'

'All accommodation and meals will of course be provided.'

'Excuse me, sir,' I said, beginning to understand. 'I would have to live there, would I?'

'You would indeed. That is necessary to the position. It is on a trial basis, you understand,' the man said to my master and the widow. 'Your ward may be gone only a week, perhaps merely a day. But, should she prove favourable, she may stay as Madame Élisabeth's household decides and in agreement with you as her guardians.'

'Yes, sir. Thank you, sir.'

'Your papers shall remain here,' he told me, 'at your guardians' request.'

'She belongs to us,' said the widow, all charm.

'Since Berne,' added my master.

'It is agreed,' concluded the man. 'Do you understand?'

'Yes, sir.'

The widow was rather quiet afterwards, a sourness upon her face. Once or twice I saw her watching me. Jacques kept his distance, but could be heard in the kitchen whining, scratching on the floor.

'I don't want to go,' I told my master.

'It is for the best. Until things are calm again.'

'Was it you who wrote to the palace?'

'The little Princesse was clearly so eager. The man came so quickly.' But he gave a slight nod; I might not have seen it without my glasses.

'Sir! How can I ever leave?'

'Marie, be good.'

203

In the evening, in the kitchen, the widow.

'There are royal people,' she said, 'at the palace. The queen, for example, she lives there, and is much adored by all.'

'I suppose so, Madame.'

'You may come upon them, such people, from time to time.'

'Yes, Madame.'

'You must behave well in all situations. You must not make us in any way ashamed of you. You must say only the best things about our work.'

'Yes, Madame.'

'And something more: you must gain an appointment for Doctor Curtius to cast the queen's face. We should like to have the queen from life. And all other essential people. But the queen most of all, she who is all fashion.'

'Yes, Madame, I shall try. Madame, may I ask a question?'

'You may.'

'How is Edmond?'

A reddening on the great mass of face, a rumbling of the mountain, the chin twitching, but the flame was quickly put out as she spoke.

'My son is with his wife.'

'Madame,' I said choking suddenly, 'I wanted to marry him. Could you not tell?'

'You! *You!*'

'How I wish that I had!'

'*Your* wishes – what are they? They are nothing. Edmond did not wish you. How could he? Who ever should? How could my son be with a foreign servant! Do you have no idea how the world works?'

'I am going to the palace,' I said. 'I have been invited.'

'You shall ever be our kitchen rat, Marie.'

I loathed her utterly, then and always, without end. Can I describe my hatred for her? It would poison these pages. I shall leave it out.

204

The night before I left, Jacques, like the old monkeys, began to hit the Monkey House. He smashed its walls with his fists, he smashed the fake wooden furnishings, smashing in one direction then another, kicking his legs and moaning in pain. He screamed as he did it; his riot dance could not be controlled. He moaned like a tortured animal. With my leaving, his fragile world was being upturned. Nothing would convince him that he wasn't being abandoned.

My master nervously let the storm exhaust itself; the widow went upstairs to calculate the damage costs. When his anger was spent at last, we put the house back in order. I swept up the broken pieces.

'Jacques,' I said, stroking his great head, 'it is just for a little while. But I do thank you, very much, for your tears.'

The next morning I set out with Mercier, a little more threadbare in those days, with Curtius, and with Jacques limping behind, carrying the trunk containing my clothes and Marta and Father's jawplate and my drawings, which, being kept in a kitchen drawer, had survived the widow's tempest. People stopped when my master walked past them on the boulevard, taking off their hats and bowing, as was usual then: 'Good morning, Doctor Curtius,' 'What wonderful weather, Doctor Curtius.' We made for the Place Louis-le-Grand, where Doctor Mesmer had once worked – what a vast space it was; it made me rather fearful; I wanted to cling to the sides of it – but Mercier gently tugged me on. I was bought a ticket for the *carabas*, the eight-horse Versailles omnibus, which people called the 'chamber pot'.

As he lifted me into the coach, Jacques whispered to me through clenched teeth: 'Don't let anyone hurt you. Tell Jacques if they do.'

'It's nothing but a colossal servants' hall,' Mercier said. 'Don't tarry long there; it never does anyone good to tarry there. But, Little, even I must admit: a great adventure.'

'Dear Little,' my master said, 'my own girl, you shall be so much missed. I shall call you Marie today. Marie, who shall do the hairs now? Who will sit beside me? Who shall I tell of my progress?'

'Goodbye, sir,' I said, 'thank you.'

And then the chamber pot was off.

Holding Marta in my lap, I watched Paris going nonchalantly about its business. The coach went far away from the Boulevard du Temple and the Monkey House, from Ticre's print-works, to the Porte de Versailles, out into the fields, and everything I saw was new to me and I was alone. I was to be teacher to Princesse Élisabeth. Versailles beckoned.

On Paris I turned my back.

## Book Four

### 1778–1789

# A Cupboard in Versailles

*It begins when I am seventeen,
it ends when I am twenty-eight.*

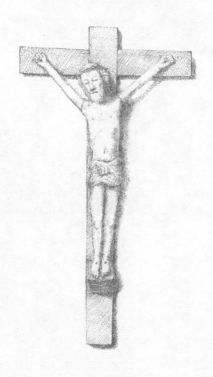

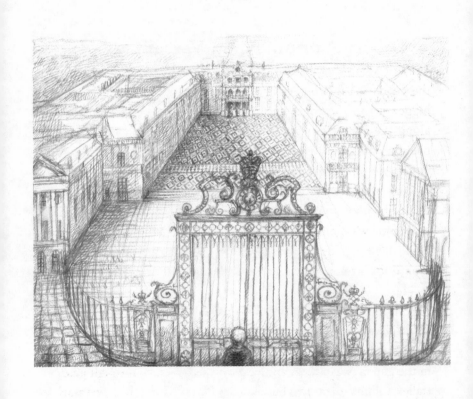

# Chapter Thirty-One

*In which I have a brief interview with my new employer,*
*and am shown to my lodgings.*

I saw it some time before I reached it, and as we advanced in the coach it grew bigger and bigger and then still bigger and bigger yet. So strange, when we finally did stop and bumped along the cobblestones as the palace took the sky away, to see ordinary humans there, of the size I was used to. It was a whole city made of a single building. How to navigate such a thing? It rearranges everything you'd previously understood about size. I felt like poor Jonah, one of Mother's people, only this whale before me was golden. Was ever such a place possible? And how could I be coming to live inside it? Mother, I wanted to call, look, look where I am! I am at the palace. I have been invited inside.

A footman in blue livery came for me. My trunk, he said, would be delivered separately. I was to follow him. He guided me over cobbles (the size of great tombstones, where people might lie down in the gap between them and never be seen again), through gates (taller I think than any building in Paris), through a servants' entrance (an opening as of some vast sphincter), along corridors (guts), past rooms and people (food being digested). The valet advanced at great speed. I trembled at the vastness of it all; everything loomed upon me, all the people and all the space. For a moment, distracted by a group of loud people, I lost the valet entirely, but he found me and told me, in a strict clipped voice, that I must cease to delay him further.

Look up: painted ceilings. Look down: wooden floors with patterns. Look ahead: the back of a valet dressed in blue, getting further away. Look about: people, people everywhere. Finally, in a quieter passageway, I saw that one of the windows was cracked. I was so glad to have seen that; I felt like I had a chance then. The valet opened a door. 'You're to wait here,' he told me. 'Do not touch anything.' Then he closed the door and left.

I looked about. I was somewhere on the ground floor, a room filled with expensive, distinguished, furious objects. I had never before considered that carriage clocks could be disapproving, nor had I supposed a candelabra might resent lighting me. I had never stepped upon a carpet that did not wish me there, nor felt the enmity of a marble mantelpiece. Nor had I come upon a gold-braided stool whose fat little feet seemed aimed at my ankles. Not before I entered this room.

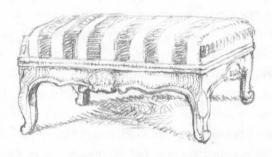

In the Monkey House, I had lived on a stage set. Now before me was a real carriage clock, not a piece of wood clock-shaped, but one that clicked away genuine seconds. Here was an actual marble fireplace, not wood got up in paint to give the impression of marble. Here real people lived, not imitations of people contrived from wax. But I felt then, and do still now, that I was much more at home among hastily contrived theatre props than with functioning objects built by masters. I stood in the centre of the room, stared at by these objects for a full half-hour, until at last another servant entered: a pale young woman who began to busy herself about the room. She did not look at me, as if I were not there at all.

'Am I to wait here?' I asked.

But the servant said nothing.

'Will she be coming soon?'

Still nothing.

'What's your name?'

Now she shook her head.

'Might I sit down?'

'Please,' she said, her look very troubled. 'I'm not to talk. It's not allowed.'

'Who can I talk to?'

'I'm only a bit-maid. You mustn't ask me anything.'

The door opened; the servant stood frozen. The voice of an old, imperious lady came from the doorway.

'Have you been talking, Pallier? Don't ever let me catch you.' And the servant was instantly gone.

Slowly the old woman walked around me and lowered herself onto one of the sofas. 'Why you are here,' she said – and it took me a moment to understand that she was not addressing the sofa – 'I cannot conceive. With luck it shall last only this day, and then we need never share the same room again. Madame has her little whims from time to time; the only consolation is that Madame is certain to find something else that interests her more than you, for you don't look very interesting at all. She will be here shortly. You are to bow, to call her "Your Majesty" or "Madame Élisabeth". You are to carry out her instructions precisely, whatever she asks. But do not *touch* her; you must never touch: that is not permitted.'

I heard the noise of running. A moment later, in came red-faced fourteen-year-old Élisabeth.

'Ah! There you are at last!' said Élisabeth. 'How lovely!'

'Your Majesty,' said the old woman, prompting.

'Your Majesty,' I said, bowing.

'I'm so glad you're here. I've thought of nothing else since I

211

saw you! Of all the things we shall do together. My own person, my very own body, that's what you are! My sister Clotilde – married now, to Charles Emmanuel of Sardinia; oh, and I'm to be married soon too – she never had her own person, not like you anyway. But here you are! I shall write to Clotilde and tell her. They tell me she's grown very fat. How I miss her! Well then, what shall we do? Shall we draw? Shall we hide and seek? Shall we go on a visit? I must tell you about my visits.'

'Your Majesty,' I whispered, 'I thought we were to . . .'

The evil carriage clock chimed and the little princess went very white. Her round face twitched; her grey eyes began to moisten.

'The time, Madame Élisabeth,' said the old woman with great severity.

'Oh no, no, no,' whispered Élisabeth.

'Your aunts, Madame Élisabeth,' came the old woman again.

'I have to go now. I've got to go, my *dear* person,' Élisabeth told me. 'My aunts must not be kept waiting at all, they hate that more than anything; Grandfather always kept them waiting and they abhorred it. I'm so glad you're here. You're very precious to me. I'll see you later. How wonderful that you're here! Show her to her room, will you, dear Mackau?'

With that, the little princess was gone and I was left with Madame de Mackau. 'No doubt she'll fail again,' she muttered as soon as the door was closed. 'I won't show you,' the old woman said without looking at me. 'Don't think for an instant that I will show you. Wait here.'

The old woman left and a few moments later a different servant appeared.

'Follow me, please.'

We went outside the room a little way and stopped before a very tall and wide double-doored cupboard fixed into the wall. My trunk had been placed beside it.

'You may open a door.'

I opened one.

'It is a cupboard,' I said.

'Yes,' she said, 'so please you, it is your cupboard.'

'I'm to leave my things here?'

'You're to live here.'

'In a cupboard?'

'You sleep here. You spend your time here. When she wants you you're nearby. You sleep on that shelf, and leave your things on the one above. You'll find it is plenty deep enough.'

'A cupboard?'

'Yes indeed. A cupboard.'

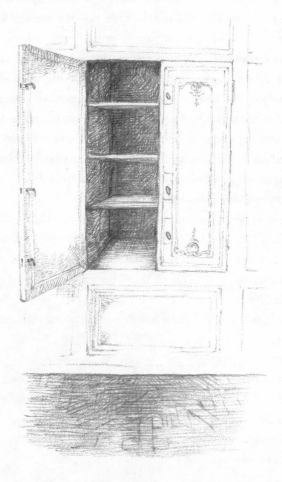

A cupboard is the resting place of objects; a bed is the thing upon which humans lay themselves down. I thought this was understood. But there were contrary ways in Versailles and I must learn them; my master had taught me this when we first came to Paris. It is necessary to learn the rules of new places. Perhaps this was not so very different from the windowless room I inhabited in the dead tailor's house. I wondered if people were kept in all the cupboards of the palace, if their drawers were pulled open only when they were required. What happens, I wondered, if your cupboard drawer was never opened and you just lay there starving, hoping you might soon be required again? Would you live on flies or spiders? Later I would come to learn that servants throughout the great houses of Europe were often billeted in cupboards, for the sake of convenience, to be close to their employers. George III of England stacked his servants in a chest of drawers outside his bedchamber; the Duke of Urbino kept a servant in a desk; the barons of Bavaria suspended their servants on custom-built coat-hooks; it is said that the Duchess of Blois had a beloved maidservant who lived for forty years in an empty water closet.

I felt such a sympathy for objects that day as I lay down upon a cupboard floor. How dark it was in there.

# Chapter Thirty-Two

*My little bit of palace.*

My cupboard doors could be opened from both the inside and out; there was a handle on both sides. Still, shut up there on my bed-shelf, I felt I might as well be in a coffin. Waking after a short slumber, I hammered on the doors in a terror that I'd been buried alive. I dreamed I was deep dead in the boulevard ditch. Even after I remembered where I was, I kept checking the handles to make sure I could get out. What a miserable night.

On my second morning at the palace, I was ushered into the same disapproving room. The old lady soon returned, and then at last Élisabeth, accompanied this time by a man in religious robes.

'Well, my person, we shall pray now.'

We prayed as instructed by her confessor, the Abbé Madier. I thought him rather a greasy piece of humanity; had God made him so? 'O divine heart of Jesus! I love you, I adore you, I invoke you, for all the days of my life, but especially for the hour of my death. *O vere adorator et unice amator Dei, misere nobis. Amen.*'

Afterwards she said to me, 'You pray wonderfully well.'

'Thank you, Your Majesty.'

'There's someone I want you to meet, someone very dear to me.'

The person she fetched now likewise lived in a cupboard, but this cupboard had velvet lining and was portable, and in fairness should probably be called a box. This person was made of painted plaster. Not very big – about a foot in fact – and not particularly accurate, this was an idealised human, simplified and sentimentalised. He was

215

made to represent the Saviour of mankind. I'd met him before of course, this fellow, or hundreds like him; he was very popular and very common, an old favourite of my mother's.

'You cannot hold him,' Élisabeth said, 'but you may look upon him.'

'I have a doll,' I said, 'she's called Marta. Would you—'

'I sometimes spend hours with him. I feel he's alive and is listening to me.'

'No,' I said. 'He's plaster. He's only painted plaster. He can't hear a thing.'

'I shall put him away now.' Jesus was returned to his box, but only after being kissed. I thought I should like her to kiss me like that.

'It is wonderful that you have called me here,' I said. 'I thank you very much.'

'That is not necessary.'

'I think we will do very well together. We are like twins, you and I.'

'I do not think that we look so very alike,' she said. 'There may be a passing resemblance, perhaps; I have heard some comment upon it. But you have, forgive me, rather a nose, haven't you? And a chin, upon my word! They rather peak out and are, all in all, a little alarming. But you must not worry; I don't mind how you look. No, though there may be a similarity, I don't think we can look so very alike, can we? I'm the king's sister. Oh, don't look so sad. What a silly creature you are. How can one feel sorry for something with such a face? I like you much better when you don't look so glum. Come now, I have something else to show you.'

She took me to a room decorated with many very amateur drawings, particularly of crucifixes and saints. 'Oh, but look at all these drawings!' she said with enthusiasm.

I looked at them and turned to Élisabeth.

'They're mine!' she said. '*I* drew them.'

I said nothing.

'What do you think of them?' she asked.

'I think, Your Majesty, please forgive me,' I said, 'I think we must begin our studies right away.'

'My person?'

I paused, but I felt I had no choice. 'You do not . . . *look*, really, do you? Not yet. I'm sure you shall. My master taught me to look, and it took a great deal of bread before I could see anything at all.' Her face was exceedingly red. 'I should not lie to you, Your Majesty,' I said. 'If we are to progress together, if I am to be useful, there ought not to be lies.'

'I am Princesse Élisabeth of France.'

'Yes, Your Majesty.'

'Well!' She stamped her foot.

I could not tell what she would do. There was a long silence. At last she said, 'I've had enough for today.' I was sent back to my cupboard.

When I was not needed, I had been instructed that I should spend as much time in my cupboard as possible. It was understood that on occasions I might need to venture out, but I should never go further than the bucket in the side room. It was a large cupboard and the shelf was not so very much smaller than my bed at the Monkey House. A person can get used to nearly anything.

It was comfortable enough in there, and I had so much time to think, more than I'd had before, and some of that thinking was inevitably about Edmond and how there would be no room for him to lie with me in that coffin-cupboard, and that that was perhaps how it should be, since he'd been stolen from me. I wished that I had one of the heads I had sculpted of him; I felt that might have helped me a great deal, but the widow had destroyed them all. I was not to think of Edmond any more. I was to put him away. He was not my business.

I did try very hard not to think of Edmond, but they left me alone such a lot that Edmond was the place I most liked to visit, though he was so married. I wonder if he ever thought of me.

How strange he would find it to learn that I was in Versailles, employed royally. I'd tell him that royal employment was not half so splendid as he might suppose.

If I stayed too long in there, however, I started wanting Edmond too much, until it felt like the ghost of him was growing around me, eating at my brain and slowing my heart. If I lay there alone too long, I might be haunted to death by that shop mannequin whose shape I so longed for. So I forced myself to look forward, to try to vanquish the ghost, to busy it away.

In Versailles, I could have candles whenever I asked; there was always an abundant supply. Lying there, I could listen to the noise of the palace, to the soldiers marching outside, and in the night, to the rats running along the corridors, and, outside, to the screeches of the feral cats who lived off the waste created by the great building.

And I could learn. I was given a card-covered booklet, the *Almanach de Versailles*, containing a vast list of the people who worked in the palace, from the House of the King to the Department of Palace Couriers. I read this dull little tome again and again in an attempt to stop the Edmond spirit from coming. I tried to picture against each name a person. I tried to understand the king's two dental surgeons, Bourdet and Dubois-Foucou, supposing that Bourdet might be a heavy gentleman, and Dubois-Foucou a trifle fond of himself. I passed through a list of fifty equerries to the king. I moved beyond to the section listed as BOUCHE DU ROI, 'the king's mouth', which pertained to the king's eating, and marvelled at the list of four men responsible solely for washing the king's plates. (I remember their names even now: Cheval, Colonne, Mulochor, and Rollepot. I thought I might have liked Monsieur Rollepot.) My finger traced long lines of worthies in the King's Household, pages and pages of people, until I reached the House of the Queen. (Among the thousands in that great army, I can still recall four: Collas, Mora, Carré, and Le Kin, the minor flank of sixteen of the Queen's *Fruiterie*.)

At last, I reached the MAISON DE MADAME ÉLISABETH DE FRANCE, two hundred and twenty-six pages into the tightly printed *Almanach*. I counted the people of Madame Élisabeth's household, the seventh house listed and by far the littlest. Seventy-three people for one fourteen-year-old girl. From her chaplain to her confessor to Madame de Mackau, named there as the Lady of Honour. Beyond that followed a gaggle of ladies-in-waiting (fifteen), a single Chevalier d'Honneur, four primary equerries. Under the heading *Chambre*, there were the principal women of the bedchamber (two), the secondary women of the bedchamber (sixteen), the valets of the bedchamber (four), the valet of the upholstery (one), the boys of the bedchamber (four), and the valets of the dressing room (four). Then out of the chamber there was listed Madame Élisabeth's doctor (le Monnier), her surgeon (Loustoneau), and her surgeon dentist (Bourdet, who also troubled himself over the king's teeth – a speck of insight into the great whole). Also listed were Madame Élisabeth's librarian, her reader, her secretary, her harpsichord teacher, her harp instructor, her painting teacher, and a host of other servants: her tapestry makers (two), wardrobe valets (two), porters (four), silver cleaner (one), and finally her bit-maid (one), the lowest of the household, used for sundry unmentionable tasks, name given as Pallier, Lucie. I closed the book, blew out the candle, sat dizzy in the dark. And I summoned the Edmond ghost again because I was so lonely.

# Chapter Thirty-Three

*Concerning my employment as Person*
*to Her Majesty, Princesse Élisabeth.*

On my third day, Élisabeth sent for me again – not for drawing, but for a game of hide-and-seek, the princess's particular passion. I was to close my eyes and count to one hundred and then try to find Élisabeth and her ladies-in-waiting. When I opened my eyes there was no one in sight, only the furniture, but it took only a moment to find them hiding in a nearby room, a throng of official ladies enjoying their wonderful joke. A few of the tallest demoiselles were gathered in the doorway; I pushed through them – indecorously, I was later scolded – to find Élisabeth eating from a plate of small cakes. They looked rather nice. I was not offered one.

'Cuckoo,' I said. 'There you are.' I touched her arm.

'No!' shrieked Mackau. 'No! Never! You do not touch.'

The old woman dragged me down the hall, to a plain parlour I'd never seen before.

'Put out your hands,' she instructed.

And I did.

I heard wind, and a cane bit into me. It was withdrawn, then came down again. The third time, I moved my hands.

'No! No!' the old woman snapped. 'It must be three!'

In tears, I put my hands out once more and the cane instantly delivered its message. I was not too old to be beaten. Perhaps it was my height that confused them.

'Next time it shall be ten. You do not touch. Repeat: you do not touch.'

'I do not touch.'

I turned around. Élisabeth was behind me. She had been there all along.

'It is I who say "cuckoo", not you at all,' she said. 'And the game of hide-and-seek should last at least a half-hour. You do not do it right at all.'

'Well,' said Mackau, 'we must grow up. We must all grow up.'

The following day, we set to work. I put paper in front of Élisabeth. She held a pencil; I could tell the two were not intimate. The first thing I discovered was that Madame Élisabeth was not clear on the subject of anatomy. The heart, for example, that most noisy of organs and thus the easiest to detect, was to her mind – doubtless inspired by many inaccurate religious paintings – found precisely in the centre of the chest. She wondered why two kidneys, why two lungs, and supposed that this doubling of organs might somehow be connected to the bearing of twins. She was amazed to discover that the insides of a person were generally placed in the same position from human being to human being. She absolutely insisted that the insides of a man were completely different from those of a woman, and would not be contradicted on this. I drew the outline of the human form and tried to show her the contents, but it was very hard to make her believe. She could comprehend the notion that some intestines are large and others small, but found it quite ridiculous that everyone, no matter their size, should have both. I decided the best course would be to find a human model to aid my instructions. I asked Élisabeth for assistance, and soon Pallier the bit-maid appeared.

'Hello, Pallier,' I said.

Pallier said nothing. The poor girl was not allowed to.

'Who's this?' asked Élisabeth.

'This is Pallier,' I said, 'one of your servants.'

'I've never seen her before.'

'Even so, here is Pallier.'

Pallier had been in Élisabeth's service for six years, but she did her work so quietly and anonymously that she had made no more impression than a ghost. The palace was filled with such people, I think, perhaps hundreds of them, who lived so quietly and usefully alongside the royal family that they had not yet been spotted.

'Pallier,' I asked, 'could you please stand in the middle of the room with your arms outstretched like so?' She obliged.

'This is Pallier,' I said to Élisabeth. 'We know what she looks like from the outside, but what is she like inside? What is kept inside the cupboard of Pallier? Let us pretend that her ribs are like cupboard doors, as if we might open them at the sternum, from the centre outwards. What do we see? What does she keep on her shelves?'

'Bed linen, I should say,' Élisabeth uttered.

I let this pass.

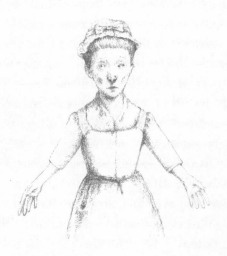

As I signalled hither and yon with my pointer, Pallier learned of many things she harboured within her, none of which she had known of before. Élisabeth learned too. Determined to stay away from my own cupboard as long as possible, I stretched our time together longer and longer, insisting that our lesson would not be complete until I had finished explaining the kidney, then the liver, then the heart.

'It's so hard,' said Élisabeth.

'But we make progress,' I said.

'Why must I worry over what a servant has inside her?'

'It is the same with all people, Madame. They have the same innards.'

'I hardly think so.'

'And yet it is true.'

'Are you sure?'

'Yes, Madame.'

'How horrid.'

She seemed to look at Pallier with a great resentment then. We walked around Pallier, who blushed and even jolted slightly as I touched. 'It's just your body,' I told her, 'just a human body like any other. There's nothing to be concerned over. Do keep still, we're trying to learn.'

And it did help, seeing a real body: it always does. As Élisabeth began to understand how a body worked, her drawing improved. I taught her how to leave off thinking about the rules and laws and passageways of the palace, and to concern herself with those inside the body. Now *there* was a palace to wander in. We burrowed, in our imagination, beneath the skin of Lucie Pallier, down among the organs and bones. Once we had finished the tour of Pallier, I had Élisabeth point to the appropriate places as I called out: 'Kidney! Bladder! Oesophagus! Small intestine! Lungs! Rectum! Heart! Spinal cord! Diaphragm! Pancreas! Spleen! Palmar fascia! *Anastomotica magna! Tuber omentale!*' And progress was made. Later, in the corridor, Pallier touched her abdomen and whispered to me with great wonder: 'Here, within, is my duodenum, which is short for *intestinum duodenum digitorum*.'

'Which means?'

'Intestine of twelve fingers' width!'

'Yes, Pallier, that is very well remembered!'

'Thank you, Madame.'

'Thank you, *Marie*,' I corrected.

'Thank you, Madame.'

At the end of our drawing lesson, Élisabeth would be greeted by her favourite ladies-in-waiting, girls she addressed as Bombe, Rage, and Démon, and I would be taken back to my cupboard. I lay there in the darkness thinking about Élisabeth, murmuring her name to the shelf above, until the ghost of Edmond came to lie beside me.

In those first weeks I had seen little more of the vast building than my cupboard, her salon, and our workroom, and I wanted to see more. I had seen so little in my life, but I'd heard many things and had glimpses of others, and the palace was really too much temptation altogether. I wondered what else there was beyond our small rooms. I was told I must never leave Élisabeth's apartment, but I wanted to – if only because I thought it might help me to keep the troubling ghost of Edmond away.

One afternoon a great opportunity arose in the form of a reprise of hide-and-seek. With Mackau occupied elsewhere in conference with the aunts, Élisabeth announced that she and her ladies-in-waiting should rush off and I should have the pleasure of finding them about her apartment. Off they giggled. I closed my eyes and I counted to one hundred, until I heard them bustle off into one particular room – and I took a deep breath and set off in the opposite direction. I went out into the palace; I found new geography; and my feet made noise upon it.

I ran this way and that through the royal maze, down unfamiliar corridors, into large and gilded rooms. Before almost every door in the palace were people waiting, people sitting down or standing up, all of them without exception holding papers in their hands. When I asked one man how long he had been waiting, he said, 'On and off, three years in November.' Another man was grey of complexion, as if by long exposure he'd absorbed the colour of the stone walls around him. I climbed stairways and opened doors, and many of these waiting people told me I shouldn't be where I was. When thunderous Versailles foot traffic came near, I grew uneasy. I began to wonder if the game of hide-and-seek was even still in process, or if it had taken a strange turn in which the hiders were forced to go in search of the lost seeker. I would have been happy to find Élisabeth, just then, for I was utterly lost.

When a group of men in blue livery rushed past, I hid myself behind a screen in an unlit fireplace to catch my breath and steady myself. As my heart becalmed itself, I became aware of a quiet knocking, and wondered if someone else like me was knocking his or her way about the doors of Versailles. Summoning some store of bravery inside myself, I decided that two lost people might be more comforting than one, and opened the door. The knocking ceased.

'Who's there?' said a man's voice on the other side.

'Please,' was all I could muster.

'You mustn't come in, you mustn't come in at all. It's not allowed.'

'Please, sir,' I managed.

'Private. Private. And not to be disturbed.'

'I'm not certain, exactly—'

'Who is out there? Who is it?'

I was stuttering now – not least because of the alarming, unnatural heat coming from the room. I began to wonder if I had disturbed some devil resident in the palace.

'Who are you there? Explain yourself.'

I tried to explain that I was the art tutor to Her Majesty Madame Élisabeth. I'm not sure how much of my mumbling was intelligible, but at last the voice in the heat replied.

'Oh, very well then, step in, step in.'

And in I went.

# Chapter Thirty-Four

*The locksmith of Versailles.*

Inside was rather a large man in his twenties, dressed in a leather apron, with his shirtsleeves rolled up, leaning over a forge, a small hammer in his hand.

'Well, close the door, or we'll have all and sundry within.'

I did as I was bidden. He went immediately back to his business, tapping on a small piece of metal. It was this, not a knocking on the door, that I'd heard through the walls. Engrossed in his work, he did not look up at me for several minutes. The Palace of Versailles was such an expansive place, I considered, that a great variety of craftsmen must be situated inside. I had stumbled across the locksmith; had I opened a different door I might have found the rat-catcher making traps, the clockman busy with his ticking, even the candle maker moulding wax.

I stood in the corner by the door and watched the craftsman before me, hoping that when he had finished his particular piece of business he might be willing to furnish me with directions back to Madame Élisabeth's apartment. The man had an almost comically high forehead, a sizeable Roman nose, full lips, and remarkable large blue eyes, which he often scrunched up and brought quite close to the red-hot objects he was working with – from which I gathered that he too might benefit from spectacles. He had a fleshy underchin and womanly breasts, all of which he stroked from time to time with his pudgy, knuckleless hands. He seemed not to breathe through his nose, but to use his mouth for the capturing of oxygen. With metal tongs, the man picked up the object he had been bothering

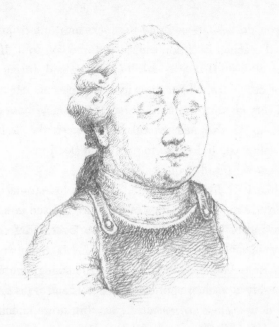

and dipped it into a deep basin of water, upon which the object hissed in complaint, a noise the locksmith greeted with a smile. He turned to me, squinted, nodded, delved into one of his apron pockets, pulled out a handkerchief, and carefully laid it upon a nearby table. Then he delved into another pocket, pulled out a crushed-looking piece of cold custard and pastry, placed this upon the handkerchief, and stood back to admire it. Finally, from a third pocket, he took out a handsome penknife, unhinged its blade, and bisected the custard pie, rather unequally. Taking up the major part in his tubby hands, he spoke at last:

'Don't tell a soul, and here's your reward.'

I stepped forward to take it.

'Do you really need all of that?' he asked, with crumbs on his lips, his portion already safe inside. 'There's a good deal there, and you are rather small. Come, what do you say I cut it in half again?'

Once more the piece of cake was fractioned, again not entirely evenly. I leaned forward to take the smaller portion.

'I say, you do hesitate so,' said the locksmith, interrupting me before I had reached it. 'I don't mean to force you to it. If you'd prefer, I could keep that for you till later,' he said, lifting up the last piece of cake, 'or shall I just pop it in here instead?' He brought my morsel very close to his mouth. 'Shall I?' Then, without waiting for my say-so, he dropped the cake in between the fleshy lips, chewed, swallowed, and kissed the air in satisfaction.

'Perhaps now,' I said, 'you shall be sick.'

'But I like it! I like it,' he said, stroking his stomach, very earnestly. 'And I'm forbidden it. "One piece a day," she says. "Only one and no more."' Then, in whispers, 'So I cheat. Of course I cheat. I've grown very cunning.' For a while he was quietly content, locking and unlocking his work, admiring it, making sure the lock was thoroughly dry, then applying a little oil and polish. At last he bowed down, close to me, and I saw those great blue eyes scanning me thoroughly.

'Well then, old thing, shall we install it together?'

'Yes, sir,' I said, 'I would like that.'

Taking my hand with one of his, and with the other picking up his new lock, he led me out of the little workshop into a long corridor. We progressed around the corner and stopped at a door missing its lock. Through the door I could see a fraction of what lay beyond: a great room, well lit, with an enormous painted ceiling and vast plates of mirror on one side, echoing the windows of the other, and peopled with various elaborate ladies and gentlemen, very engaged with each other. There never was a place so shiny as that one; it sparkled so much you were blinded by it.

'Is the queen there?' I asked the locksmith. 'Which one is she?'

I was to try to cast the queen – I hadn't forgotten my instructions, to bring a piece of this impossible shininess back to the dirt of the boulevard. The locksmith jumped a little at my question, looked into the hall, squinted, shook his head. 'No,' he said, 'no queen. Only decorations.'

The decorations – he meant the ladies – paid us no attention.

The locksmith laid his handkerchief on the floor, then got down onto his knees. I knelt beside him and took out various nails and bits of business from his apron pocket, which I held for him until they were required. He proceeded to place the lock into the door. It fitted snugly, and looked, I told him, very fine.

'Think so? I designed it myself. Yes, I like it rather.'

I heard people moving behind us, and turned to see several footmen and in between them the old lady Mackau. She motioned for me to come to her, and by the force of the gesture I understood her to be very, very unhappy. I bade goodbye to the locksmith, kneeling there on his handkerchief peering into his keyhole.

'You're off, then, are you?' he said. 'Please yourself.'

'I'll come again, I promise,' I whispered.

Seeing myself reflected over and over in those looking glasses, so out of place and far from home, I thought I might fall into that glass and drown. I walked slowly towards Madame de Mackau, who pushed me from the chamber and marched me down the hall. She insisted that she was quite speechless at my impudence – though she was far from speechless, lecturing me all the way back to Madame Élisabeth's rooms on how I must learn my place. Many guards had been sent out in search of me, she said, and had been told that a dwarfish stranger had been seen opening doors she had no right to open. 'This place was not built for your entertainment,' she hissed, her bony hand clamped upon the back of my neck. And then I saw the intimidating room – though it could no longer intimidate, now that I had seen that far grander chamber – and there was Élisabeth herself. 'Cuckoo,' she said, though without enthusiasm. Then, turning to the old lady: 'This is *my* person, Madame de Mackau, not yours.'

'She was found—'

'Let her go immediately,' ordered Élisabeth, with such confidence.

My neck was unclamped.

'Shall I have you beaten again?' Élisabeth mused.

I put my hands out.

'Send her away,' said Mackau. 'Beat her first.'

'You shall not go back to your home,' Élisabeth said, 'until you have taught me everything.'

'She has broken the rules!' cried Mackau.

'I should like very much—' said Élisabeth, with a wonderful new firmness, 'I should like us to resume the game of hide-and-seek.'

'We must grow up,' said the old woman.

'And this time, dear Mackau,' said Élisabeth, 'I have decided that *you* shall have the pleasure of hiding. We shall count to one hundred.'

'But I never do the hiding.'

'It has long been your turn, then. One . . . two . . . *three*. You must run, Mackau, and hide. You know the rules, do run along. We shall come and find you. Go and hide, and nowhere easy or close, or I shall be very cross.'

Mackau, uncertain, left the room.

'Sit down,' said Élisabeth. 'I have something to say to you.'

'That was very well done,' I said.

'Thank you, I quite surprised myself. It's you that inspired me to it. To run off like that! Only don't do it again, my person, my body.'

'No, I promise you.'

So we sat, two similar-looking undersized young women, upon a sofa designed for bigger people, and we talked.

# Chapter Thirty-Five

*The Poor Suffering Bodies of Madame Élisabeth, By Herself.*

'I am going to tell you about my people,' Élisabeth told me. 'The people I collect and put in here.' She held a beautiful leather-bound tome in her lap.

It was her brother, the king, who had inspired her to assemble people all in a book. He was always writing everything down, she said; he so loved lists; he knew the *Almanach* almost by heart. He had written down how many steps there were to the Queen's Staircase, how many windows there were in the entire palace, the number of times their grandfather sent for him. (Not very many, she recalled.) He knew the precise number of seconds, hours, days and years that their brother the Duc de Bourgogne had lived before he succumbed to tuberculosis of the bones, and the exact number of years, days, hours, and minutes after his birth that their mother had died. The king counted everything, it seemed, and wrote it all down. He had books and books of lists.

'I thought, in my small way, I might do like the king,' she told me. 'So I collect up my people. There are so many buildings beyond the palace, horrid, mean places, and there do I see such people. Oh, how awfully sad they make me feel. And I make a note of it, and I give a little money, and then I tell them that I, Élisabeth of France, shall pray for them. That's why I keep the notes you see here. Read.'

She handed me a long list, of people and their distress. Barse, Renaud: broken leg. Grulier, Madeleine: pains in the stomach. Gibier, Agnès: headaches. Billinger, Jean: his little finger, his daughter's nose. Enderlin, Odile: kidney. Roger, Roland: his mother shrieks. Pynson, Rose: discoloured skin on back. Parlant, Alphonse: hungry. Moulin, Dominique: pregnant again. Levesque, Pierre: son has died. Salvia, Huguette: corns, toothache, cannot see. Vincent, François & Olivia: cannot conceive. Cutard, Adeline: spots.

'I pray for them all,' she said.

Then I had the idea.

'You might do better yet,' I said.

'Have a care, my body, take warning.'

'You could *sculpt* the maladies.'

'Sculpt?'

'Yes! Think of it – the people's most grievous problems, captured in wax!'

'Miniature models? In wax?' She fidgeted a bit, as if imagining holding one in her hand. 'Oh – could we take them to the church? Good heavens! Might we? We could make them votive objects, couldn't we? Votive objects that are different? That are very accurate? Then God would be sure to listen. Then He would see how much good we're doing. Oh, my body, despite your unhappy face you are indeed a very clever one. Yes! Oh yes!'

Unsure what to say, I reached to take her hand.

'No! Stay back! No closer! But what a lovely idea!'

We never did search for Madame de Mackau that afternoon. She was found some hours later behind a tapestry by one of the queen's ladies-in-waiting. When she explained that she was hiding from little Élisabeth, the lady asked why – was she frightened of the princess? The story spread about, so widely that when the imperious lady appeared, people smiled at her in sorrow. Her authority slipped, and she slowly began protecting herself by summoning great blankets of imaginary maladies.

The next morning, I was awakened by a hammering on my cupboard doors before the sun was up. In the darkness I dressed and was escorted to that room where all Madame Élisabeth's drawings had been, though they were no longer there. A table had been

232

set in the middle of the room, covered with tools and wax and clay. I ran my fingers over the tools, touched the clay. And last of all lifted the wax to my nose.

'I shall call you,' Élisabeth told me as her hands moulded soft clay, 'I shall call you my heart.' And after a week she presented me with that object made in wax, crudely modelled but there it was. And I asked her if I might hold her, and she said I must certainly never consider it. But I was so happy I could not stop myself and asked again. And she said no again but quieter. So that I felt I might try once more. This time, I didn't ask permission. I put my hands around her and I felt her head resting upon my shoulder. And her smell, deep and warm, a tiny, perfectly grown cabbage. Only when Madame de Mackau's voice came from outside did Élisabeth quickly break away and return to her work. I slipped the heart into my pinafore pocket and have kept it among my possessions ever since.

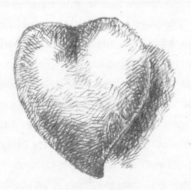

At my suggestion various animal organs were brought up from the kitchens, so that we may examine them, cut them open and draw them to help us get a better understanding of their place and function. A cow's heart, sheep's lungs, a pig's bladder. Initially reluctant, Élisabeth was soon happy to sink her fingers in. Great heavy books were brought also from the libraries, huge wonderful volumes with prints that folded out and showed just how the human is. Here was good instruction; we studied closely, and then we set to work.

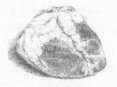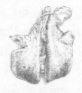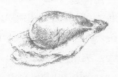

As we modelled, we opened up to each other. I showed her Marta and she told me her secrets. Élisabeth's greatest hope was to be married; her profoundest fear was to end up a spinster like her aunts. She told me that her hand had once been promised to the Infant of Portugal, but that somehow the proposed union had been broken off. The Infant of Portugal had been proclaimed 'not becoming'. The king said that someone else would certainly be found, that Élisabeth must just be patient, and so she went on being patient, and though she saw her brother often enough, her marriage had never been discussed again.

'Let me not be like my aunts Adélaïde and Victoire,' Élisabeth said. 'All they do is complain all day and eat and drink and talk of things that don't matter at all. They're just filling their days, it seems to me, one after the other, always the same, again and again, until one day they will just lie down and die. That's all they have to look forward to. Oh, my heart, I feel so much stronger since you've been here. I don't want my aunts' future. God in heaven, do anything to me, but save me from that!'

Madame Élisabeth had devised her own regimen of visits beyond the estate, in search of her needy, and each time she returned we made new anatomical votives. One day, I asked if I could join her. She frowned a moment but then happily agreed. Her poor and suffering lived very near the palace, she told me, but out of sight of it. Tucked away behind woods in miserable cottages in states of advanced dilapidation. We made the trip by carriage, accompanied by two guards. I asked why.

'For protection,' Élisabeth said. 'Sometimes the people are very unhappy and do not always hide it.'

At the sound of our carriage, people began to come out of their homes. The first thought I had was that their faces and bodies seemed of a piece with the distressed architecture. They approached the carriage. Élisabeth asked me to pull down the window.

'Hello, good morning to you,' she said.

They bowed, their hats removed from their heads.

'How are you? How do you do?'

And then, one by one, they came up to her and gave small details of their misfortunes, in some cases showing the maladies they carried with them. Only when they had spoken, revealed their agony, would Élisabeth pass them a coin.

'Do you find them fascinating, my heart?' she asked me.

'Are they starving?'

'I'm not certain. What do you think?'

'How did they come to be like this, so close to the palace?'

'Food is delivered to them.'

'But not enough.'

'And I make my visits.'

'What, I wonder, can it be like inside their houses?'

At this she stopped. 'Inside? I have never thought of it.'

'Aren't you curious?'

'Yes, I suppose I am.'

'Then let us.'

I opened the carriage door; how the people hurried back to let me by. Élisabeth followed. We walked up to one exhausted building, and I asked the derelict woman before it if we might go in. She said something I could not fully comprehend, but she shrugged, so I pushed at the door. So dark it was inside that it took a while to comprehend the place, despite its small size. Dirt floor. A bed propped up on bricks, stained blankets lying in a state of rigor mortis on top of it. Walls black with mould. A couple of dented pots. A stool much repaired. The whole place smelt like

235

the inside of some very rancid animal, long given over to despair. Nothing else save a tied-up dog, the woman's sole companion, who clearly followed her diet. Looking at the creature, you understood precisely how its skeleton was articulated. It raised its hackles, and with a look of profound outrage it showed its rotten teeth, and once it started barking at us it would not cease. Élisabeth clung to me. If the dog were loosed from its fetters, I was convinced that we might have become the first decent meal it had ever had.

'How horrid,' Élisabeth gasped.

The woman began to speak to us then, though the language was no tongue I had ever heard. Strange guttural noises, grunts and gnashes – but all the while, and this was the crucial thing, her mouth, that jagged slit, remained quite still. It wasn't exactly her who was calling out, in gulps and spurts: it was her body talking. Her neglected and failing corpus, making noise, involuntarily berating us. It was the muffled voice of some helpless spirit coming from within this poor creature's forsaken pelt. Then there came a tumbling from her, a sudden lurch forward, a bending in two, and we left in haste.

We had been inside perhaps half a minute before we were out again, inhaling the cleaner air. I would never forget that place, the miserable room and dog and lady.

Look away from the hovel; look anywhere else. Behind the village houses was a small chapel and a large graveyard with many fresh-dug graves.

We retreated to the carriage.

'How does a woman come to be like that?' Élisabeth panted.

'Not overnight, that's certain.'

'Can she be helped, do you think?'

'I wonder. In some cases, death itself is the only remaining help.'

'I must try to help. Heavens, my dear heart, what kind of soul was she?'

'Only a woman.'

236

'Oh! Horrid! What can I do? What can I do? The votives, more and more! Marie, I need your help.'

As we returned to the palace, it seemed colour had been restored to the world around us. I had never known the world to change so quickly.

With each excursion, the walls of the side chapel in the nearby church of Saint-Cyr were slowly being furnished with waxen human bits. At first no one worried about these additions, never imagining how their number would grow. We brought kidneys and bladders and lungs, arms and eyes and hearts, livers and stomachs. Passing this wax or clay flesh back and forth, we once or twice touched hands ourselves, and felt, I thought, such a comradeship there, a great closeness among the body parts.

Three months were gone already. I was to return to the Monkey House. But I was so nervous to leave; I should much rather stay with Élisabeth. When I told her that, she responded that it couldn't be simpler: someone would write to them and tell them that I could not be spared. My master – or probably the widow in his stead – wrote back to say that, in that case, they must be further compensated for my absence. They were. I never saw that letter. I was so relieved not to go. I never wanted to go back, not then. It was too sad. The longer I lived in that cupboard, the easier it was to forget I had ever been anywhere else.

# Chapter Thirty-Six

*Up on the roof.*

I spent ever longer days with Élisabeth modelling organs. I went into her bedroom as soon as she was awake; she told me all the business of her day, and asked me again and again if I was happy. Very happy, I said, very happy. And I was.

After a while, my presence was credited with somehow giving comfort to the royal child, and I began to be sent for at different odd times of the day. Soon enough I was given the strictest instruction never to venture far from my cupboard, for I could be needed at any moment. Should I require something, I must only call out and one of the other servants would come to me. Sometimes I would sit in the corner of that disapproving room of hers while she and her ladies-in-waiting ate their evening meal. Bombe, I discovered, was the Marquise de Bombelles, Rage the Marquise de Raigecourt, and Démon was the Marquise des Monstiers-Mérinville. They were three pleasant enough young ladies, I understood now, the princess's classmates; they smiled at me and slipped me a piece of chocolate or a biscuit or a lump of sugar and patted me on the head.

Before Élisabeth was to enter some official gathering, I would be positioned nearby, standing very still, very upright; the knowledge that I was near, ready to be looked at, had the effect of lightening her terror. I would sometimes be positioned by a footman in the strangest of places, behind screens in great halls, so that once or twice an evening Élisabeth might quickly glance at me there, pinch my nose or take hold of my chin, and so be put at ease.

238

One early evening I was rushed up to the roof of the palace by one of Élisabeth's blue-liveried servants and told to wait there, at a certain spot, until called down. From where I stood – pressed against the balustrade, midway between two large stone vases, just above Madame Élisabeth's rooms – I was in a perfect position to see the road to the church of Saint-Cyr, not to mention the Grand Canal of the palace gardens, stretching so far away, as if it were there to serve as a lesson in perspective. Although I lived in a cupboard, such vastness was no longer peculiar to me. I was instructed to keep to my position, so that Élisabeth, going by in her coach on some official venture, might pull down her window and see me up there, and be made happy because of it.

I stayed at my post, as I was bidden, and watched people drift away from the vast garden. It began to drizzle, but still I remained, for that was my instruction. After a while dusk descended, until I could no longer see the canal or gardens so well, and soon enough I could hear little save for a few laughs and cheers from somewhere within the palace and the shrieking of a few cats down below. I was beginning to feel certain that I had been forgotten when I heard someone else walking on the roof, and coming closer. Whoever it was stopped nearby and leaned against the balustrade, holding on to one of the stone vases for support, staring downwards. The figure began to busy himself with some sort of long rod. The next thing I heard nearly sent me over the balustrade and dashed upon the cobbles: my rooftop companion had lifted and fired a gun, directly at the cats below. I heard a great bang, saw a burst of light, and heard a shriek, which I took to be that of a cat. Then, shortly after, a second shot, no second shriek. Fearful of being shot myself if he should mistake me for a cat, I called out, 'Please, please, sir, I'm up here with you. Don't shoot me! Don't shoot.'

'Who are you? Who's there?'

The gunman hobbled over to me, his large white face becoming more intelligible as it approached. It was my old friend the locksmith, dressed in a large overcoat.

'It's you!' I said. 'I'm so glad. I'm sorry I haven't brought you any pastries yet – I'm kept so busy.'

'Oh!' he said when he was close enough to see who I was. 'Oh, that's all right.'

'What are you doing?'

'Don't be sentimental. There are so many of them,' he said. 'Cats everywhere. Hairs and smells in every corner of the palace. And so it falls to me, from time to time, to lessen the problem. Come and sit,' said the locksmith, patting the slope of the roof.

'It's beginning to rain,' I said. 'I wonder if I should go down.'

'Come, it's just a little wet. I'll wipe it myself. There. Come now, sit, sit. I insist!' And so I sat by him, and felt his warmth next to me. He shared his overcoat between us, and we sat, side by side, in the dark.

'Do you like it up here?' he asked, and continued, 'Well, I'll tell you, I love it. I come here often. It's really, I sometimes think, save for my forge, the only peaceful place in the whole pile. How I love moments like this. Ah!'

'Ah,' I said, imitating his sigh.

'Here we are. Up on the roof.'

'Up on the roof,' I said, 'and no one else anywhere near. We could pretend it was just us, that there's no one else downstairs. Only us and the night.'

'What an idea! I think I could do well indeed, if there weren't any other people. I'm a very practical sort of fellow. Not at all bad with my hands. I think, on the whole, if I found myself on a deserted island I'd manage excellently. I might even be happy with no other people. I'd know what to do then. But there are always people. Never an end to them. There's a wonderful book about life on a deserted island, I've read it countless times. Do you know it?'

'I don't think so.'

'*The Life and Strange Surprising Adventures of Robinson Crusoe, of York, Mariner: who lived eight and twenty years, all alone in an uninhabited island on the coast of America, near the mouth of the Great River of Oroonoque; having been cast on shore by shipwreck, wherein all the men perished but himself. With an account how he was at last as strangely delivered by pirates. Written by himself.'*

'That's a long title.'

'That's a wonderful book.'

'Let us pretend it is just us up here,' I ventured, 'and the rest of the world is flooded.'

'How marvellous.'

'Isn't it?'

'No laws, no battles, no meetings, no etiquette.'

'Noah could not have done better.'

'Of course, pastry might help, mightn't it?'

And so we sat, the pair of us, up there on the roof, quite alone, talking of empty islands, and of flour and butter and eggs combined and heated, and also of locks and springs, until a blue-liveried servant marred our peace a little by coming out with an umbrella. I thought at first that he had come to take me inside, but it was a different servant who did not talk to us at all or even make eye contact but only held the umbrella over us both. I thought this unusual but soon enough I forgot he was there, and the locksmith and I chatted on. We were on the roof together for perhaps two hours before Élisabeth's servant appeared. I had missed her coach returning. I said goodnight to the locksmith and left him there upon the bench upon the roof, with the liveried servant and the umbrella. And I thought, with the exception of missing the coach, what a very pleasant evening it had turned out to be.

# Chapter Thirty-Seven

*Concerning women, horizontal and perpendicular.*

More people noticed that Madame Élisabeth was showing improvement in society. At the same time, old lady Mackau was increasingly retreating to her bed, where she affected many noisy maladies while eating her favourite almond biscuits. One day, Élisabeth and I visited her in her musty third-floor apartment. She greeted Élisabeth as her 'wonderful loyal child', thanked her for coming to see her 'old friend', but to me she said not a word. When Élisabeth asked her where she hurt exactly, she was confused and could not exactly explain. 'All over,' was all she could manage, and that furiously. So Élisabeth entered those words into her book and we made an entire miniature wax woman and placed this beside the other objects in the chapel. We returned to her so that Élisabeth could inform her of this progress, but she only groaned and turned over in bed, showing us her back.

'Illness,' she said, 'knows no manners.'

That was the summer of Élisabeth's great freedom. Mackau's reign was coming to an end; she sniffed and sweated through the last weeks of her office, always promising to return, but soon her bed became too persuasive for her. The heavy mattress cupped itself around the old lady and became her bones and support, until she could not be solid without it. It sucked her in, sucked her dry – it sucked, I do believe it, all the fatness from the old form – and as the woman began to ail in earnest, so the mattress grew in health, becoming greater and puffier. What a beastly mattress that was, expanding and inflating, leaching the old lady of her life.

242

In Mackau's absence, as the old lady was slowly surrendering to her mattress, we had continued our visits beyond the palace, and afterwards made many more organs for the church. Once, when we asked if we might be allowed to enter a poor home, the wretched young man who lived there refused.

'He is ashamed,' Élisabeth said. 'That must be it.'

'Or perhaps,' I said, 'he simply does not want to let us inside.'

'Doesn't want? Why ever not? What's wrong with us?'

'It's his home. He's in charge of it.'

'It belongs to my brother.'

'Does it?'

'Certainly.'

'Then your brother should have it fixed.'

'My brother has the whole country to worry over. I go to the village. You know nothing about it. It is not your business.'

She was very put out. She was always struggling over what was the best way to react. There were so many contradictions between what she was told and what she saw that she could only hesitatingly move forward, lacking, as she did, power or knowledge. She was a girl trying to make her way. We both were.

In our great work of seeking out all the ill, we found, besides Madame de Mackau, another patient inside the palace. One afternoon, Élisabeth herself opened my cupboard door. 'Lamballe! Come quickly, my heart! Lamballe has fainted again!'

'Yes, I'm coming! But who is Lamballe?'

'Oh, you know nobody, do you! She is a lovely lady, but so delicate. Her husband died young and she's been a terrible fainter ever since. She once fainted because she happened to smell some violets. And once also for no greater reason than she saw a lobster in a painting. And when Antoinette complained she had a headache she fainted then too – in sympathy, it is supposed, for Antoinette. Simply everything makes her faint. Isn't it awful?'

'Will the queen be with her, do you think?'

'She's sure to be. Lamballe's her favourite. Poor thing.'

243

The collapsed fainter we discovered lay stretched out in some Versailles salon, still far gone. Her fellow women of court stood around her pale, limp form, whispering distractedly. I looked about.

'Where's the queen, Madame Élisabeth? Which one is the queen?'

'The queen, dear heart? Oh, I do not see the queen anywhere.'

A team of doctors milled around the slumped body, bleeding it. Élisabeth and I moved forward until one of the doctors stepped aside and we could get a better view. She was certainly still alive; her flat bosom was moving up and down. I leaned forward to have a good look. Here was the queen's person. I saw the blood of Marie Thérèse, Princesse de Lamballe, in a little porcelain bowl that a doctor was staring into.

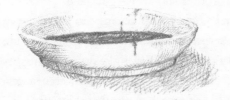

'Where does it hurt her?' Élisabeth asked.

'The nerves, Madame. Her nerves are too easily alerted.'

'Thank you,' Élisabeth said, trotting off. 'That's all we need for now.'

'Excuse me,' I said in whispers, 'shall the queen be coming soon?'

'The queen? What business is it of yours?'

'I am with Madame Élisabeth,' I said. 'It is Her young Majesty who wondered,' I lied.

'The queen had wanted to stay,' said the doctor, 'but I could not permit it. This unfortunate lady was seen to convulse, and convulsions bring about miscarriages, and so the queen, in her delicate state, was instantly removed.'

'How long ago?'

'Some five minutes.'

'But five minutes!'

'Come along, my heart!' called Élisabeth.

We made a wax brain for Lamballe, who recovered very shortly thereafter.

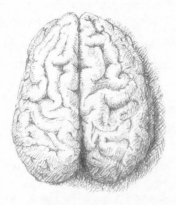

In our private times, Élisabeth asked me about men and their bodies. I told her everything I knew, and made models so that she might understand better, and there were books brought up for consultation. I thought of Edmond again, though his body seemed so far away and as lifeless as cloth. I must be sensible, I told myself; I was brought up to be sensible; I must try to let the pain go. We went once to see a dog and bitch put in a pen together, but Élisabeth did not like that at all and it just made me feel ill and irritable. Still, she said, she was to be prepared for marriage, which she always insisted would be very soon.

'Will you marry, my heart?' she asked.

'No, Madame, I doubt it very much.'

'No, I didn't think you would. I asked anyway, out of politeness. When I am married, I shall send for you. You'll always be near.'

She had me draw her a pair of male lips for her to practise kissing on.

'No,' I said, 'no, that is not right at all. You are pecking, Madame. Have you never kissed a person before?'

'Of course! Certainly! No, well, not in that way. Have you?'

'Yes, I may say that I have.'

'Oh, my heart, have you truly? Someone such as you?'

'Yes,' I said, 'I will teach you.'

I kissed her.

'You kissed me!'

'In instruction.'

'Very well.'

I kissed her again, more fully.

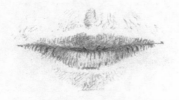

Likeness of the lips of Madame Élisabeth.

'Yes, that is how it is done,' I said.

'Are you certain?'

'Most certain.'

'Horrid.'

'Not really, no it isn't.'

'Well, then, let us try once more.'

And we did. And every now and then we tried again and kept our practice up behind closed doors. And sometimes, too, we should gently point and stroke the place about us where we kept our fellow organs.

'Show me, Madame, where I keep my heart. Touch there.'

'Show me, my heart, where are my lungs, my womb.'

What a royal body it was, and I, her twin almost, joyed in it. Our hearts, little women's hearts, playing the same music to each other all alone.

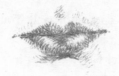

Lips for practising.

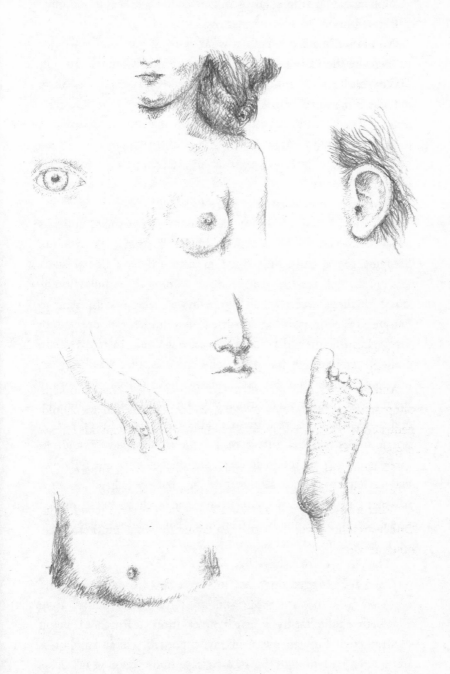

One morning, at long last, Madame de Mackau was found quite suffocated upon the bloated mattress.

Even after Mackau herself was taken away, a heartbeat seemed to linger in the mattress for a time, until it finally shrank from its obesity back into the modesty of its former days and was burnt outside in a courtyard. And so, from the summer of Mackau's illness, we entered the ghastly autumn of Madame de Guéménée.

Guéménée the Rod, Guéménée the stickler, Guéménée matron of misery, her chin barely there at all – a lack of chin that must have made her furious all the time, for her scowl was perpetual, her attention continuous, her stare indelible. Pleasures were left behind then; Élisabeth was to be made into a woman, and this process, it was instantly clear, would hurt. Playthings: thrown out. Skipping ropes, balls, little dogs, miniature horses: all banished. 'Sit up! Sit up!' was the call of those autumn days. Silly Bombe was forbidden access; when Élisabeth was caught whispering to her behind a door, what lecturing her misdemeanour caused. Simpering Rage could be seen but once a week. Insipid Démon could remain, if she was quiet, and she was; that was her role, always the silent one. My rival, plaster Jesus Christ, was out of his cupboard almost all the time. When Élisabeth lost her temper, and at first she did so a great deal, Guéménée allowed her to pound floors and kick furniture, but the chinless lady would not be beaten. A cane in female form, she opened wide the windows and invited my princess to bellow out, but no help ever came. Élisabeth, swollen-faced and miserable, had no choice but to quieten down. Once, when she bit Guéménée's hand, she was slapped.

'I am a princess!' she screamed.

'Then be seen to behave like one.'

Guéménée tugged out what joy there was inside the girl and replaced it with sitting upright, with quietness; before long Élisabeth could hardly join a conversation, terrified of being contradicted. Stowed away in my cupboard, called upon less frequently, I adapted to this new strict autumn, keeping my dress clean and curtsying at Guéménée whenever I could – and so I was allowed to remain, though the princess and I both feared that I would be sent away. In those autumn days of her last rebellions, and into the winter of her acquiescence, Élisabeth was never left alone. Someone was always sitting beside her, finding fault with the way she held a cup, or how much she ate, or how she carried herself. But at times, if I was careful, I still held her hand, or sneaked a hurried kiss in the modelling room. I told her often that I was her person, her body, that I should not be going away. As if in proof of this, I found my name printed in the new *Almanach*, the lowest member of her teaching faculty.

M. le Roux, *Bibliothécaire de Mad. Élisabeth*
Mlle Payan, *Lectrice*
M. Simon, *Maître de Clavecin*
M. Boilly, *Maître de Harpe*
Mlle Grosholtz, *Maîtresse de Cire*

I studied this page a great deal. In solitary moments, I read it out loud to myself. And soon, not long after it appeared, I found myself at last in the presence of the queen.

# Chapter Thirty-Eight

*Small incidents connected to a National Event.*

It began in the early hours of the morning with the ringing of bells of the Chapel Royal, of Saint-Cyr, of all the churches of Versailles, followed by the arrival of the Princesse de Lamballe in our corridor. I opened my cupboard a little and peeked out from my mound of blankets. It was December, we were under the weather of Guéménée, and I was very cold. With my bedding wrapped about me, I saw the astonished princess arrive with a great deal of fuss, trailed by servants and women, all looking alarmed.

'Madame Élisabeth!' she cried, knocking on her bedchamber door. 'The queen! The queen is in labour!'

In our own small way, Élisabeth and I had already been preparing for the coming expansion of the royal family. We had made some twelve small wax babies, laying them out in a perfect line – a dormitory of them – in Saint-Cyr. We set all other requests aside for a while; the birth of the royal child was all we could possibly consider. 'Everyone in the palace,' Élisabeth said, 'is quite desperate with expectation.' And now at last the moment had arrived, and the bells were sounding, and so was the Princesse de Lamballe.

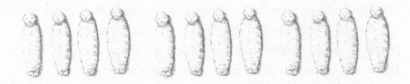

As Lamballe scurried off in a high state of agitation (something like a bony chicken shrieking through a farmyard), our corridor bustled with activity. Sitting in my open cupboard, still in my nightdress and sleeping bonnet, I dangled my legs off my shelf, pulled my blankets about me, and peered off to my left and then my right. The cracked windows along the corridor had been sealed off from the winter cold, but this was only partially successful; when I breathed, I could see the results.

At length Élisabeth appeared, fully dressed and trailed by three of her ladies. As she made her way towards the place for royal births, the servants on either side of the corridor bowed as she passed. I bowed, too, but Élisabeth stopped.

'Oh, my body, my heart, what are you doing? I shall need you today more than any other. You must dress yourself and quickly too. Should the queen need our prayers, you must hurry to our workroom and quickly assemble in wax a little baby to be rushed to Saint-Cyr. Do stir yourself, my heart, my person!'

And so, on the day of the birth of the first child of Marie Antoinette of Austria and Louis XVI of France, I dressed myself in public, in that chilly corridor, with many looking upon me and urging me to hurry. When I was ready – and not a moment too soon, they made quite clear – little Élisabeth marched on, intent on being an aunt. I brought up the rear of her procession, just behind the Marquise de Monstiers-Mérinville. The further we travelled, the harder we must push, for the whole palace was desperate to be as close as possible to the birth of the new Bourbon. Élisabeth, being the king's sister, caused a parting in the sea of people, and Moses-like we pressed on, the waves of people crashing back behind us as soon as we passed. I felt the palace, not without pleasure at first, growing warmer and warmer as we journeyed towards its centre. The population had been moving in since the bells sounded, people growing thicker and thicker and louder and louder and hotter and hotter the closer to the birth room we progressed.

The hottest location of all – a baker's oven of a place – was the queen's bedchamber that very early morning, and the hottest part of that boiling address, the very red burning coal of the Palace of Versailles, was the swollen belly of Queen Marie Antoinette. French law mandated that various selected people must sit in on the queen's birth to ensure that the child born was genuinely from the queen's womb.

We were in time. The child had not yet arrived. Élisabeth took a seat near the front, with other important personages upon chairs with armrests; only benches had been provided for lesser attendees. I was left to fend for myself. I could not yet see Élisabeth's eldest brother, the prospective father, the king himself, but he must be somewhere in the room. I squeezed around, pushing a little against some very noble sightseers, until I had a tolerable view. There – at last – I saw before me Maria Antonia Josepha Joanna, or Marie Antoinette, or the Queen of France.

The royal head was sweating under the strains of the moment. It was a long head with pale-blue eyes, rather far apart; I lost sight of it, then by manoeuvring a little found it again. A sizeable prominence of aquiline nose, a lower lip that stuck out rather more than the upper, a nicely rounded chin; I lost sight, then found it again. Above all else, a great expanse of forehead, covered at this moment with many beads of sweat. In that hot bedchamber, I had quite forgotten my chill of the morning, or that this was December.

The queen sat up, causing a good stirring from all around, as we all strained to see her better. What a creature! What a long white neck. What sloping shoulders. But then she took a gulp of air and lay back down – to another stirring from the populace – and I lost her entirely from sight.

I looked around for a place where I might be guaranteed a good view. There were no windowsills, and the few benches in front of the windows had already been taken. In that busy room and its objects – mostly people by now – there seemed to me only one place where I could be guaranteed a truly unrestricted view. In one corner sat a mahogany chest rising five feet from the ground, an object with a top, which I might term a roof, and I thought I might happily sit myself there and observe all without fear of visual interruption. I tried to climb up its marquetry walls, but they were highly varnished and I didn't get far up before slipping down. I tried to open the drawers, thinking I might climb them like steps, but they were locked, the object holding its five jaws firmly shut. And yet I was certain this was the place for me. I waited anxiously, and all the while still more people came in, and I could see less and less of the queen, gathering only that I had not yet missed anything very much; she had not yet said more than a few muffled sentences, and the royal people nearest her had made only a few muffled replies, but there was no yelling nor any screaming of baby, so I was certain I still had time.

At last my opportunity arose. There was a great commotion – not the birth moment, but a sudden scramble to secure the tapestry in the room, lest the crowd somehow dislodge it and send it toppling atop the queen. There was a deal of fussing, and most everyone stood, and I seized the moment to borrow a chair and drag it over to the chest, where I added to my height by standing upon it. At last I managed to heave myself onto the roof of the chest. And there it was.

A perfect uninhibited view.

There were by now more than fifty inside the room, I now could see. The queen lay in her bed, surrounded by doctors and her family, talking a little and trying to pretend, I think, that there was no great crowd of people waiting for her to entertain them. And so we all waited, and we watched the region of that hot belly, which was covered at the moment by loose sheets, but still nothing happened. After a time my gaze wandered about the golden room, and I began to study the crowd of nobles beneath me. Cravats had been loosened; every forehead was clammy; ladies jerked fans about them; make-up began to run. The Princesse de Lamballe, in the second row, looked particularly agitated by the warmth. Then, quite close to the front, I saw someone I recognised: it was my friend, the palace locksmith! How wonderful, I thought, that this man so beloved by the people of Versailles should be permitted entrance to such an event.

253

Then Queen Antoinette made a loud groan, and the real performance began.

There was much activity and much noise from Antoinette, and much advice given by the doctors, and the Princesse de Lamballe began to look extremely white. People whispered to themselves, shifting about to attend better every cry and moan, every push and wince, every strain and gasp of the queen. The poor woman puffed and panted and went very red in the face and heaved and yelled, and yet no child was forthcoming. The baby would not come out; indeed it stayed inside a good while longer, and during the intervening moments of quietness, as the poor queen lay panting, the audience sat down again and talked among themselves, only to be roused to their feet again by groans from the queen. So it went on, the audience rising and falling with the tides of the queen's labour, until at last, sometime after eleven o'clock, a baby began to appear.

Soon there was a whole red head, and then a pink and red body, and two arms and two legs. And with it, to much joy, came the baby's first noise. Up there on the roof of a chest, I thought to myself, I know that: there's the umbilical cord, just as Doctor Curtius said it would be, and there's the mucous membrane he spoke of – and there, after a while, as my master had described, there was the placenta! How marvellous it was! What new lessons I was learning! What miracles may a woman perform: look, look at the new life come out of her!

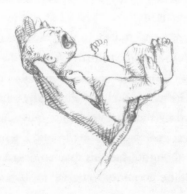

The room had grown fearfully hot and filled with an awful reek of vinegar and essences, on account of the doctors. I had undone my bonnet and loosened my dress, and many other people had made similar adjustments. During those last moments, as the baby came out into the world, the audience pressed further and further forward. But as soon as the child was free it was hurried out in cloths by the medical scrum; the king must have been among them, I suppose, though by the time I thought to look he was nowhere to be seen. Then, after the room had cleared a bit, I was able to see the queen once more. Suddenly she had become only the second most important person in the drama. She had grown appallingly white, I saw, and I wondered if she had perhaps died – there was certainly blood on the sheets – until she sat up and called out through the heat.

And no one noticed.

The audience was clapping and clapping, for nature is such an astonishing thing, especially when it applies itself to a queen. But then the audience began to worry, very much out loud, what sex the child was, whether a boy or a girl, a dauphin or dauphine. And the word began to go around in a whisper, a disappointed whisper: 'a daughter, a daughter, a daughter, a daughter'.

But no one noticed the queen.

From my perch atop the chest, I waved to get people's attention. 'The queen!' I called out. 'The queen!' For I could see, from my vantage point, that Her Majesty was having convulsions.

And still no one noticed.

In a moment, someone else had. The Princesse de Lamballe, always very pale, always on the brink of fainting, her hands flailing wildly about, had seen the queen, but traumatised as she was, she was unable to get the words out. Standing up, I suppose, to try to collar someone and alert them to the danger, Lamballe began to totter, and those great eyes began to go blank, and then she collapsed in a great swoon, falling backwards and knocking into whatever was in her path, which was quite a lot, and which caused several loud crashes, and this had the result of centring everyone's attention on the collapsed princess, distracting even further from the troubled queen.

And so it was only after the Princesse de Lamballe was carried out, and I became quite desperate with my hand waving, that at last someone noticed me. It was the locksmith. Standing right there, in the thick of the crowd, he couldn't hear me through the deafening noise, but I caught his eye and pointed urgently to the queen. Seeing Her Majesty suffocating upon the maternity bed, he launched himself bravely through the crowd, but not in the direction of the queen; rather, he set out in the opposite way – perhaps this was all to do with their no touching rule, and he could think of no other way to be useful – pushing people aside until he reached the windows, sealed like those in my corridor against the winter cold. With his brute strength, he started to strip the seals away, and at last the locksmith had them open and fresh air was coming in. Then many other people, of a lesser bravery and lesser strength, tugged other windows open, and December came hurrying. But those other people had no idea quite why the locksmith was ripping the windows open; they seemed to think it was to call out to the crowds in the courtyards below; and so now the heroic locksmith had to force himself back through the room to reach the queen where she lay still upon her bed, very white, sheets soaked with blood for all to see. And all did see then.

Great commotion followed; hot water was called for but never arrived; the doctors prodded her white majesty, at first to no effect. They began to bleed her from her foot. They drew five saucers full, considered the correct amount, and at last the queen showed some life. And all this time the locksmith, hero of the moment, never left her side. There were tears, unmistakable tears, in his eyes. Was she dead? But at last the queen gasped, and all was well again. And the locksmith looked enormously relieved. He put his handkerchief to his face to hide his tears. It had all been very exciting indeed.

When the locksmith stood up from the bed, people bowed to him, out of thanks, I supposed. Then I saw him turn around and look at me, and, very briefly, nod. The bowing continued, and it was only then that I began to understand something new, something incredible.

The queen had married a locksmith.

The locksmith she had married was called Louis XVI.

I wanted to cheer. I wanted to tell someone. But who could I tell? I couldn't tell Edmond. Who then? I made up my mind to write to my master to inform him, to tell Jacques about this very opposite of a hanging, but then came the worry: if I did write, Doctor Curtius would be reminded of me, and the widow would wonder why I had not yet secured permission to model the queen. Still, how marvellous it was: I knew the king! I did! Little! And so I did a little clap, just as Curtius would.

This king I knew, this king I had almost shared pastry with, now called for the room to be cleared at once. The queen was to be left alone. Everyone was ushered out. This king, my roof companion, my umbrella sharer, had his servants rush everyone from the place and then rushed off himself, with his unsteady gait, to be with his little daughter. By the time I looked for her, taken as I was with my extraordinary discovery, I saw that Élisabeth and her ladies had already gone. They had left me there.

When the nursemaids came in, the queen called out for her baby. They calmed her. The baby, they said, was perfectly healthy. She wished to see him, to see the new Bourbon, the heir to France she had produced. No, they told her, not an heir, not at all, a girl, a daughter, not an heir I'm afraid, yes we are sure, Madame, a girl, a very pink, healthy girl, but a girl all the same, yes, yes we are quite certain. And then the queen, exhausted from the day and the crowds and the result, began to weep.

I had a suspicion then that I no longer belonged in this room. It was becoming a private place. And yet I remained, the last member of a very noisy public. I thought to leave, and yet before

257

me at last was the queen, and she was less busied now, things were getting quieter all the while, so I wondered if now, after all, might in fact be the time to approach her for a casting. Not to be done instantly, of course, but perhaps I could make an appointment for Doctor Curtius. These opportunities, after all, do not happen every day. The room was growing quieter and quieter, the queen's sobbing grew more controlled, and I counted this a sign that the moment was propitious. I quietly clambered down, dropping the last few feet to the floor, with a little bump. This little bump caused the eyes of the queen to open and look at me. I smiled and took a few steps towards my goal, grinning now I suppose, almost laughing, but before I could make my gentle proposal, the queen opened her mouth and uttered these very inappropriate words:

'A devil! A very devil!'

And all hope was gone from me in an instant. I was frightened, and she increased this fright by screaming, and in a torment of upset, of cruel disappointment and horror, I rushed from the screaming locksmith's wife through the doors, through the remaining people, all the way to my cupboard. I hurled myself inside, slammed the doors behind me, and hid under the blankets.

# Chapter Thirty-Nine

*A servant and a king.*

Far from the cramped darkness of my own cupboard, closer to the core of the palace even than the queen's bedchamber, I found myself two days later. Never show your back; bow down; speak when spoken to; do not approach closer than three and a half feet; certainly do never touch. I had met the king before and had even felt quite relaxed on those occasions; I had conversed with him freely and had even once shared a portion of his overcoat; but then the king had simply been the palace locksmith, one of many in France, thousands I should imagine, since so many people insist on locking things away from other people. But there is only ever one king to a country. That is a rule. Otherwise bloodshed.

I had seen portraits of the king; his profile was stamped upon every French coin. But the king's head on coins and the king's head eating pastry seemed to have very little resemblance, and so I had not known him.

Nevertheless, at this moment, His Majesty the King of France Louis XVI by the Grace of God was sitting in a chair before me.

'Well, Marie Grosholtz,' he said.

'Your Majesty,' I said, bowing very low.

'Well, I must say the queen is much better now. Next time it shan't be like that. Next time we'll have nobody present who isn't strictly necessary. Nobody at all, for example, on top of the furniture. Next time: private.'

'Yes, Your Majesty,' I said, thinking all the while: those are the king's lips, beyond them the king's teeth and tongue all together in one royal cavern, and the king's epiglottis, and the king's salivary glands too, and a royal passageway called the king's pharynx, deep down into the depths of the corpus majestic.

'Tell me,' he demanded, 'did you have no idea who I was?'

'No, Your Majesty. I thought you were a locksmith.'

'I am proud of it. But on the roof, the footman wore my livery.'

'But your sister's footmen wear blue also.'

'Élisabeth's very fond of you, isn't she? She's coming out of herself at last. We should never have allowed Madame de Mackau to look after her. Our parents' death was a terrible thing for her, our brother's too. We were quite thrown together for a while. She can be, you see, a little nervous. Tears and things. But she's better, I like to think, of late – better certainly. Which is another way of saying, well done. And thank you. For Élisabeth, and for your recent attentions on behalf of the queen. Is there anything in turn I might do for you?'

Here was my opening, opened by the king himself.

'Before I came here, Your Majesty,' I said, 'I was employed with a wax modeller, a very gifted one, in Paris. I know that it would be the prize of his collection if Your Majesty should grant him permission to cast your face from life.'

'Oh, I don't like the sound of that at all.'

'You would be most impressed with his art.'

'Would I? I wonder. And you were his pupil?'

'Yes, in Switzerland, in Berne, where I come from, he taught me.'

'We have our guards from Switzerland, positioned around the palace inside and out, for personal protection. We should not do without them. I am not ignorant of Swiss, no indeed. Your master, was he a good teacher?'

'Oh yes, quite wonderful.'

'And were you a good student?'

'I studied very hard and learned much.'

'Well, then, you can model me yourself.'

260

'I, Your Majesty?'

'Yes, you.'

'You cannot mean it.'

'I absolutely do.'

'No, no, I could not.'

'You could not?'

'Well, that is, I could, but I must not.'

'Why must not?'

'No, it wouldn't be right at all.'

'If I say it is right?'

'But please, sire, it is for my master . . .'

'I say it is for you.'

'It would hurt him so.'

'Then let him hurt.'

'He would never forgive me.'

'He will. You shall say it is the king's word.'

'It is so far above myself!'

'Then grow, girl, do grow to it!'

'It would be a crime, sire.'

'It is now, Grosholtz, or it is never.'

And so, so help me, I did it, myself.

We were in one of the king's private chambers, his little forge close by. At first we ate raspberry tartlets. The king took off his brocaded jacket and pulled on a simple frock coat. The room was bedecked with globes, and a great quantity of maps; there were scale models of strange-looking buildings, and a great many different ingenious devices: telescopes and microscopes and sextants and theodolites and orreries and all sorts of instruments I had never heard of. And around the room, between globes of the earth and of the planets, were hundreds of books, all in the correct order. Among these was the entirety of Diderot's *Encyclopédie* and also — how I longed to tell him! — *Paris in the Year 2440* by L.-S. Mercier.

I cleaned the king's face. I oiled his eyebrows, I patted them down. I put straws up that large and royal snout, I did it. I laid plaster on the face, I covered the face of the king as if blanking it out, I did it. How quiet everything was, just myself and the king. Alone in the world after all. I took off the plaster, cleaned his face. I took certain necessary measurements of him. Thickness of head from ear to ear: eighteen inches. Girth of neck: twenty-two and one-third. Marie measured.

I had the king's head, then, but not the queen's. I feared to ask for more and yet I must.

'Your Majesty, may I ask something else?'

The king nodded.

'I would be most obliged to you, Your Majesty, if you might help me get an appointment so that my master might make a cast of the queen's head.'

Of an instant, the king was overcome by a fury of protection. 'The queen is not to be disturbed! The queen is not an object to be pushed and pinched, to be prised open at public will, to be gaped at. She's not to be exposed. There's no decency any more. No, no, the queen is not to be disturbed.'

'Yes, Your Majesty.'

'I won't have it.'

'No, Your Majesty.'

'It upsets me.'

'Yes, Your Majesty. I thank Your Majesty.'

He looked around the room, agitated, as though losing his bearings amidst so many globes. 'We shall not have our talks again,' he declared, shaking his head. 'That would hardly be right. Not at all correct. I was confused. When we first met, in my forge, you see, I thought you were my sister. I should have known it then by the spectacles, but I see now you are not. Not at all, you are a caricature of her. Perhaps you are not to blame. Well, it shall not happen again. I am the king, and you are merely Grosholtz. Good morning. Good morning.'

I would not see the king up close again for several years.

Later, in the workroom, I told Élisabeth all.

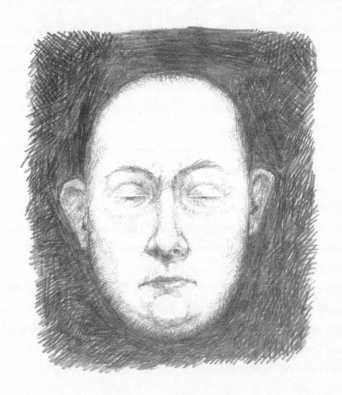

'I, Anne Marie Grosholtz, have smelt the sweat of the king.'

'You are very crude, heart. I should not have to remind you that you are my body, my body alone, not anyone else's.'

'I have cast the king, and must send the mould to my master in Paris.'

'You are my body, aren't you?'

How easily she was made jealous.

'Yes, dear Madame Élisabeth,' I was quick to reassure her. 'Of course I am.'

'You're not going to leave me?'

'I am not, not until you wish it.'

'I shall never wish it.'

'Please say that again.'

'I shall never wish it, heart.'

'Then may I kiss you?'

'I think you may.'

I had the cast packed into a crate with straw. Inside I put a letter, one it had taken me many tries to write to my satisfaction. In the end I wrote:

*Dear Sir,*

*I do hope all is very well with you in Paris. I think of you often, and of all the wax people. I trust the business is well. I am very busy here and work every day for Princesse Élisabeth. I do not think I exaggerate when I say that I have become her favourite and, sir, I think she would very much like to keep me here with her always. I would be very happy for that. I am most grateful and sensible of the care you have put into my education and I most humbly thank you for it. I shall always think of you with great gratitude. May I also say, in a whisper, that I have served you, without pay, for a long time and that I do hope my work has given you some satisfaction. In short, sir, will you please release me and have my papers sent here?*

*I enclose in this box a cast, from life, of His Majesty* LOUIS XVI. *His Majesty insisted that I cast him and that there would not be another chance. I asked for him to send for you but he would not allow it. And so I had to go about the business myself. Please forgive me in this, but I do hope you will see that I have done the casting most correctly. And that it now requires your great brilliance to complete. Please may you accept this as payment of me, and may you write to the palace and give my service officially over to Princesse Élisabeth and so send my papers.*

*Thank you,*

*Yours most sincerely,*

*Little, formerly Marie Grosholtz, your old servant from Berne*

It took two weeks for a reply to come, and when it came it was not from my master.

*Little creature,*
*You have upset your master more than you shall ever know. The trouble I have had with him these last days. I thought he should die.*
*Understand your name is filth here, and your papers shall not be given over.*
*I acknowledge receipt of the cast. Years it has taken you to give us this little. It makes me sick to think of it.*
*What use is a king without a queen? Get the queen, and quickly too, or you shall be dragged back here and how we shall work you then.*
*Get to it!*
*In sincerity,*
*C. Picot (widow)*

I carefully folded the letter, which seemed to contain a very powerful unhappiness, and, with the help of a ladder borrowed from Pallier, put it on the top shelf of my cupboard where I never visited. Still, even so high up, it came to me in my sleep three shelves down.

# Chapter Forty

*Regarding toys and their owners.*

Very soon there were new circumstances, that, in our daily intimacy, I had forgotten to worry over.

'Oh, my dearest heart,' Élisabeth said, opening my cupboard door, 'something incredible has happened! I was sent for. I'm going away. It's going to happen. I shall be married! I shall miss you, dearest heart, but I am to be *married*! I shall go away from here. I shall leave all this behind. All will be well. O Lord, I thank you, I thank you from the bottom of my heart.'

'No,' I said, for this was my region, 'hardly from there.'

'It has been announced! My husband is to be the Duke of Aosta. The Duke of Aosta!'

To my mind *Aosta* sounded very like *aorta*. The aorta is situated above the heart. She showed me a portrait of her duke; he did not look much of anything to me. When Élisabeth was too busy to join me in the workroom, she said I must spend my time copying the portrait, that she should like to have another copy, one that she could fold up and keep with her always.

The drawing grew smudged and creased after constant attention.

Another day, Élisabeth knocked on my cupboard door. 'I'm not supposed to spend so much time with you any more.'

'Has Madame de Guéménée proclaimed it?'

'Madame de Guéménée has been appointed governess to the dauphine. It is Madame Diane de Polignac who looks after my house now. Rage has been sent away, and even Démon is to be rationed to twice-monthly visits. I have new ladies-in-waiting. I am growing up, I feel it.'

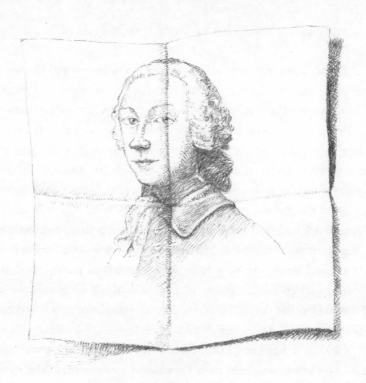

The Duke of Aosta.

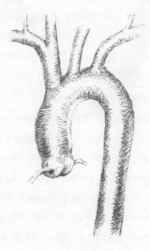

A human aorta.

'And me?' I asked. 'What has Madame de Polignac said regarding me?'

'Oh my heart, my own heart, it is such a new beginning! My heart, we're so cramped in here. Would you like me to find you a proper room? It would be a little further away but perhaps it would be better.'

Pity the poor toys, for they are generally loved for such a short time; they get broken, or other things come along to replace them, and they are taken to distant rooms set aside for unloved objects. Generations of dolls are left to decay in outbuildings. Seeing new parts of the palace, now, it seemed to me no longer the golden leviathan I had first encountered, but rather a vast skeleton, the remains of some beast that had been killed, and that we lived within its expired body. My new location was a whole room, cold and empty; you could not warm it. I tried to think up the ghost of Edmond in that sorrowful place, but he would not come. He had disappeared on me, never to visit again.

And yet it has been known that discarded toys are sometimes taken up again, and held with a rekindled passion; that familiarity is very helpful in despair.

Then, as suddenly as talk of the Duke of Aosta had begun, just a week after I was shown my room forty minutes' walk away, it all ended, with two small words: he, too, was 'not becoming'. Élisabeth must make do with that. And instantly I was remembered. The cupboard was open for business once more.

It was a quieter Élisabeth who emerged from the tears and the shivers on the evening I was returned to the cupboard. That evening Élisabeth gave up on herself; she declared that she was rededicating herself to the poor suffering people, that from now on she would expect nothing for herself. She instructed me to fetch the plaster Jesus from his cupboard, then held that object in her lap like the babies she would never be having. Thenceforth our days were to be religious days; from now on there would just be us: Élisabeth, myself, the plaster fellow. And if ever I tried to kiss her, I was gently pushed away.

# Chapter Forty-One

*Pain is to be found at the church of Saint-Cyr.*

Afterwards, time came to be measured in trips to the church of Saint-Cyr. In that church, in various side chapels, could be found a growing populace of body parts, nailed one on top of another, and ever less wall. Élisabeth's *Poor Suffering Bodies* advanced into its third volume and months went by and the year changed at last; and the next year began, which would be very much like its predecessor; and so would the ones that followed it, and all time was very much alike and bodies were grievously poor and endlessly suffered and showed us with their tears or clenched teeth where it was that they hurt. They really did hurt in those days and years, very greatly, and there seemed ever more of them. They were not always glad to see us, and sometimes took Élisabeth's money with cold looks. One reason for this, we supposed, may have been the poor weather and the bad crops; another may have been one of the men, a former stable boy now lamed by a horse. One day, this poor man had come limping into the palace grounds to beg for alms. He was beaten and sent away by the guards, and he died from his wounds. Money was given, but no matter: when the man expired, their spirit declined. But Élisabeth never stopped her visits, and we took note of the people and rendered their difficulties in wax. And we grew older. And though we could still be considered young, and Madame Élisabeth was always the youngest, layer by layer the dust settled upon us and Élisabeth turned by degrees into a spinster and put away all thoughts of any other kind of future. Inside, her body was drying out.

We were moved also.

Princesse Élisabeth's new household was to be found at the very end of a corridor in the south-west wing of the palace; this was so that she would not be so disturbed, but in fact it was so that she might be forgotten. From the windows of her new rooms we could see the Grand Canal, but more importantly the road to Saint-Cyr, the direction we always looked. We were situated on the first floor; beneath us were the great apartments of the queen, above us the rooms of the master of the horse, whom we could always hear pacing back and forth in his great boots. All around us we heard the life of the palace, but it was never with us. The new household consisted of eight rooms: the antechamber, the second antechamber, the bedroom, the grand cabinet, the billiard room, the library and the boudoir. Outside the bedroom was my new wall cupboard; it had one shelf fewer than my old space, and was not clean when I arrived. Its previous tenant had not cared for it, had left boot marks and scratches on the interior walls. I cleaned it out and climbed inside. Ants lived there with me, and a mouse to begin with, on and off, on the bottom shelf.

These were the long seasons of Madame de Polignac. Diane de Polignac, sister of the queen's newest favourite, was an ugly woman, hunchbacked and slovenly, with sallow skin and wet lips; she swallowed when she saw men. She did not care for Élisabeth, a fact she made perfectly plain once she had secured her position. She peopled Élisabeth's corridor with her own harem; they laughed at Élisabeth loud enough to be sure she would hear. Her only companions were myself and the cupboard Jesus.

Whatever difficulties had marked the successive reigns of Mackau and Guéménée, they had undertaken their work with good intentions; their methods, however wayward and defeating, were truly designed to benefit Élisabeth. By contrast, Polignac was concerned only with herself. It was Polignac who demanded the billiard room; Antoinette had taken to this entertainment, and everyone had to follow. Élisabeth retreated and retreated. Elsewhere, the palace bustled with society; there were great parties and fêtes and gambling,

270

but I never saw any of it myself. Below we heard laughing and happiness; above we heard marching and slamming doors. Though she was only seventeen years of age, Élisabeth seemed thirty.

'Don't ever leave me, my body. Don't ever go.'

We lived our quiet lives and made friends of the side chapels of the church of Saint-Cyr. Each of these chapels was named after a saint. I came to learn my saints very well in those days. Mother would have been most pleased.

Saint Vincent de Paul was an ancient man who devoted his life to the poor and had houses built for them. We filled his chapel with our wax pieces, until there was no room left for another hurting kidney or broken finger, not even space for a cloudy eye. Saint Martin de Tours was an ancient man who cut his cloak in two to give half to a beggar; in his chapel soon were smashed legs, swollen arms, bruised trunks, dented heads, torn noses, blistered mouths – all in wax, until there was no longer space for even one more crumb of grief. Saint Denis was the first bishop of Paris, and in his chapel appeared, in wax, rent ribs, burst lungs, exhausted hearts, spent livers, stinging bladders, useless ovaries, twisted testes, yellow skins, tender stumps. All that pain, all that suffering, so much poverty.

The bishop was worried: his church was being taken over, his holy place remade as a wax butcher's shop. But Madame Élisabeth and I could not be stopped. Just as Saint Cyr himself, who had never grown into adulthood, had had his head smashed against a wall for insisting he was a Christian, so Élisabeth was martyring herself upon the hurt of others. Élisabeth hungered after pain, other people's pain to dull her own; the pain of those poor everyday people fed her life. She had become addicted to misery. We piled up organs. My cupboard door was knocked upon at different hours of the day, sometimes at night, before the sun was up, to summon me to work. Élisabeth believed in those little wax objects – they were evidence of her intention – even if to the poor and suffering they meant nothing at all.

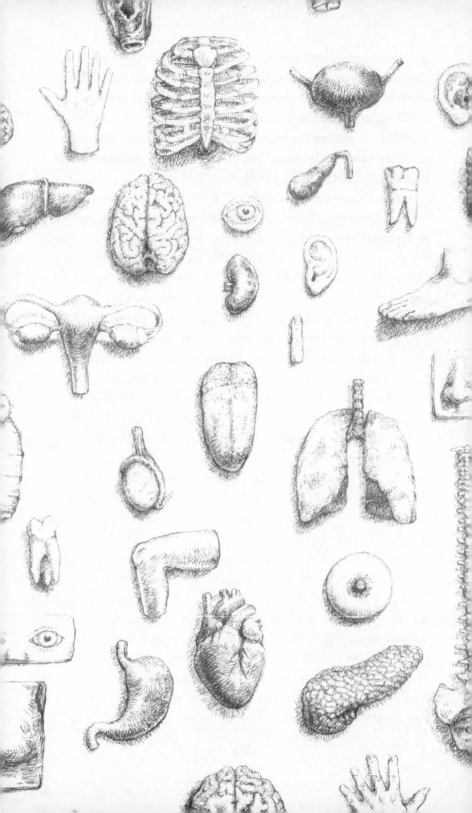

'Come, come, my heart, we must be busy.'

I grew older in Versailles. I shifted shape, I grew thinner, I grew sharper angles, I was quieter. I drew in my cupboard home by candlelight, and when I made mistakes – and I did still make mistakes – I rubbed the marks out with a ball of vegetable gum, the latest tool for the artist; Élisabeth always had the newest and best of objects. Goodbye, bread.

Élisabeth and I dwelt together in rooms of body parts, within a vast many-organed home of wax flesh, our days filled with prayers made tangible.

# Chapter Forty-Two

*Marie Fecit or fourth heads.*

Sundays had by habit always been my most free day at the palace. On Sundays, Élisabeth was almost entirely with members of her family within the walls of one or another of God's sacred barns and I was not required then.

Most Sundays I spent an hour or so washing my cupboard and airing it out or having a little ale with Pallier. We spent time together discussing bodies, Pallier and I. One Sunday, when she was away because one of her relations was poorly (we prayed for him and made a wax oesophagus), I was feeling a little lonely. Though I had not ventured out for so long, at last I went beyond Élisabeth's rooms. Polignac's servants, smirking, let me pass, and I was out and free. I found myself walking the same path towards that place of royal births, following a crowd of visiting Parisians hurrying in that direction. Having no other engagement, I decided to join them. We herded into a great queue by the King's Guardroom and stopped in a throng just outside the Queen's Antechamber, a room also known as the Antechamber of the *Grand Couvert*. Here there were guards who would let us into the next room only after inspecting our dress. Having passed their scrutiny, in we went.

At first the whole fuss seemed to be about nothing more than a circle of Swiss Guards, each with three white feathers in his hat. But then, when I peered between them, I spied a horseshoe-shaped table, surrounded by high-backed chairs, and upon those chairs was the entire royal family.

They were eating.

I wondered at first if these were not some expertly crafted clockwork versions of the royal people, so mechanical did they seem as they brought their soup spoons to their mouths, or cut their meat into pieces. Then I saw the queen blink. Then I saw the king swallow. Then I saw the Comte de Provence, the king's younger brother, smile broadly, and the king's youngest brother, the Comte d'Artois, smile back, and then these two, unlike anyone else, began to talk. There, too, I spied Élisabeth, who ate her food in fits and starts. Two older women sat beside her, one thin and one fat; I took them to be the aunts. Most of the royal family were playing with their food rather than actually eating it, and behind them were other people to help the royal eaters with their royal eating. It was most clear that the royal family was not enjoying itself, that it did not appreciate being so stared at, but most of all, something else: that these royals were mere humans, and that watching them was fascinating.

Soon enough we were pushed out of the room again.

'That is the *Grand Couvert*,' Pallier told me. 'Every Sunday it happens, did you not know?'

'Every Sunday?'

'Unless they're away.'

'And can just anyone go?'

'You must be properly dressed. Men in sword and stockings and wig. But if you don't have such things they can be hired at the gate when you come in.'

'Everyone can see them?'

'If properly dressed.'

'But *why*?'

'Louis XIV's rule. He declared that the royal family should be seen once a week by an appropriately dressed public, as a family.'

I went back the next Sunday. And every Sunday thereafter. At first I told myself it was in order to be closer to Élisabeth, but

275

later I admitted that what I truly wanted was to see the whole royalty of France at feeding time. I would slip beyond Diane de Polignac's ladies-in-waiting and rush along. We must all file past in a queue, our observations interrupted at regular intervals by the Swiss Guards, who served as the barrier between us, the common people, and them, the royal ones. I never tired of the ceremony, waited eagerly for Sunday to come, and soon I started taking paper and pencil with me, making quick sketches and pages of notes.

Now, when I closed my eyes, I saw royal mastication. I saw food munched to a pulp, I saw swallowing, I saw crumbs on royal lips. The entire royal family did not take part; the queen's gloves remained on her hands, and the plates put in front of her so carefully were never so much as looked at. How interested my master would be in all this, I thought.

In my boredom, in my cupboard, I began to turn my notes into sketches for the heads of the royal family. I should not have done so, for soon, like my master before me, I began to yearn to make those heads. When I held a wax lung in my hands, I yearned to give it a nose; when I held a liver, I longed to give it a mouth.

Once I had my idea, I could not stop myself: a group of people in a scene together. Whole figures. Close to each other. Reacting to each other. That had never been done at the Monkey House before; that was something new. And the scene? Why, The Royal Family at Dinner. Royal mouths open, royal cheeks bulging, royal jaws up and down, all those royal Adam's apples bobbing.

I sketched them every week. I never told anyone about it. Month after month after month. Until a pile grew up. Over time I began to worry that my master might not understand my markings, and that perhaps it would be wiser if I made the heads myself, just to be certain. They could, I reasoned, adjust or discard them later on, as they wished. In this way, I set out to make the royal family. In this way, I lied to myself.

276

Once I had begun I could not stop; the heads took over my life. I did not tell Élisabeth about them, hiding my work in my cupboard. We grew very crowded in there. I helped myself to everything in our workshop. We went through so much clay already that no one noticed me taking more. In time the same could be said for plaster and even for wax. I ordered more and it was always delivered promptly, without question. In truth, the people in the palace had no real sympathy for objects; they never properly considered them, leaving them here and there as if they should never run out. Of wax and its subtle talents, they were entirely ignorant. They never properly comprehended the dignity and sadness of a stick of candle. They never sat long hours with objects, quietly encouraging them. They didn't know and couldn't care.

Head. By head. By head. Mouth by mouth. Swallow by swallow. I caught them. I moved the clay, went back each Sunday and checked and changed and started again, stopped and gave up and started again. And slowly the eaters came to me. Back again the king's chin; back again the queen's earlobes; back again the comte's forehead. Back again, back again. Look, look harder, that's not right, not yet, scrape it back, pull it all down again, look harder, concentrate. I'd never do it. I'd do it. I'd never do it.

It took me months. No, it took me years. I worked when Élisabeth was away with her aunts and often while the palace slept. Only four at first: king, queen, king's brothers. Four heads with armatures nailed into planks, damp cloths over them, hidden in my cupboard after my night's work; after they grew too numerous, secreted in cupboards in our workroom. Just the heads. The bodies could be supplied later.

The shape of each head came quickly enough, but then followed months of adjustments. Towards the end I might stare at the clay head for hours and make only a single small change, add only a single moist crumb of clay the size of a rice grain over two hours, then repair to bed to dream of clay heads. But their skin was clay skin, and clay skin smoothed down and finished is poreless, and

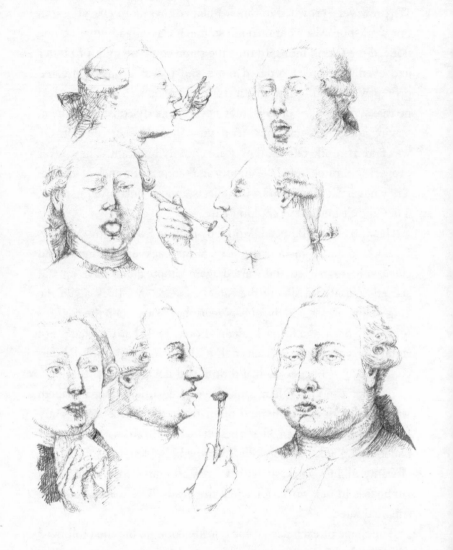

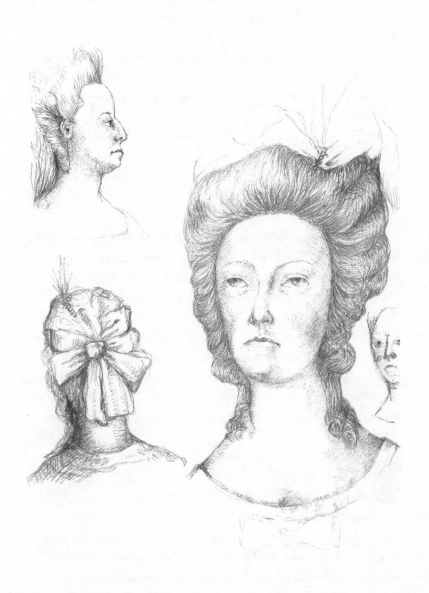

human skin is pitted and pored: my spectacles insisted upon it. In order to make my royal family more real, then, I asked Élisabeth if I might eat some oranges in my cupboard and she had them sent up for me. Orange skin, like ours, has pores. By making a cast of an orange's skin, I discovered, you may imprint the negative of that cast upon the clay flesh of royal heads, giving their skin all the detail, all the small dents, of a truthful real head. I stood back. I clapped.

In this way, I cast them. I covered those clay faces with the deadening plaster, as if I were murdering my own work, and ruined the clay heads taking the plaster away. I mixed the wax, poured it in the mould, and opened the mould – and there, there! What had been clay was now wax flesh. Is that the queen? High forehead, pronounced lower lip? Close my eyes, open them again. Is that the queen, not cast from life but sculpted from observation? Close your eyes. Open them again. Yes, I thought it was. The very queen.

These were my marks. On my own. These hands, these thoughts. There's the queen, but not only she: there's Marie Grosholtz too, both alive in that head. The moment I understood this, I couldn't stop. It was all I wanted to do.

I danced around the queen's head. I made you. I did. Welcome.

'What's the noise? You'll wake everyone!' There was Pallier. 'What's going on? What are you do— Why, that is the queen, isn't it!'

'Say it again.'

'That is the queen!'

'Once more, beautiful Pallier!'

'That's the queen!'

It was, and then followed the king (once more), the Comte d'Artois, the Comte de Provence. My royal family. At night, or when Élisabeth was away, I sat with the royal heads and talked to them, as if I were a part of that family. I would rather spend time with my heads than with real people. For a while I kept them; they were so dear, my first heads. They would be greeted as a triumph at the Cabinet, my royal family, so I told myself in my cupboard. Once they had the heads, I thought, I would be allowed to stay here. I would ask my master again if I could be released. That's what I told myself. I lied, of course. I wanted to be appreciated. Who does not? We all do.

And so I betrayed myself.

I sent the heads away.

I wrote a letter explaining who each head was and enclosing my many sketches. Each wax head was placed inside its own mould, the halves of the mould were tied together with rope for protection, and they were crated up and sent to the boulevard. I closed my eyes, trying to imagine them opening up those heads. I was almost sad that I could not be there to witness it, but here was my home, here was where I belonged, in a cupboard, in the workshop with Élisabeth. I must forget about those royal heads now, I told myself, and concentrate upon the other human pieces I had so loved before. But how I missed them, how dull life was without them.

A week later came a letter from my master:

*Dear Little Marie Grosholtz,*

*The Widow Picot and I shall be at Versailles Sunday next to observe the* Grand Couvert *ourselves and to judge the likenesses. We expect you to meet us at the gate and to show us the subject of your long exile.*

*I remind you that I am your master,*

*Curtius*

# Chapter Forty-Three

*My family at Versailles.*

The coach discharged its passengers. There was no mistaking them. Versailles people obeyed rules and were very strict and though they wore many colours they were not necessarily colourful. Monkey House people were loud and triumphant and were noticed a good deal off. They didn't suit Versailles; they weren't made for palaces; it wasn't the sort of architecture that should contain them. Before me were two worlds colliding.

There was Doctor Curtius looking very stretched and strained, an old heron in a gleaming new suit, quite out of place for the palace, and with a large black spot on his left cheek.

'Sir!' I cried. 'Here I am!'

'Is that you?' he said, a dear grin cracking his face apart. 'It is! It is indeed! How old you are!'

'Sir! Doctor Curtius!'

'Marie, Little Marie.'

'Little! Just Little it is,' came the booming voice.

The widow, red-faced and agitated, striking out with a stick, awkward in a large hooped dress. She was smoking a cigar.

'Madame!' I said.

'What trouble you have put us to.'

'Little!' came a bark.

There was Jacques, hobbling, struggling in a waistcoat. 'Yellow nankeen,' he said. 'From Japan!'

'Oh, Jacques,' I said. 'Dear Jacques. What murders have there been since I last saw you? What hangings?'

'Such! Many!'

The whole family had come, except Edmond of course; he was neither present nor talked of. And there were other new people, boys all dressed identically in suits, all with a red rosette upon their jackets with a 'C' embroidered in its centre. Jacques had one who served under him, a rough-looking lout with a shaved head.

'Who are these?' I asked.

'Who indeed!' said the widow. 'We have grown much since you left us and there are many more in our employ. We couldn't wait for you to come back to us.'

'Of course not, Madame.'

'We have another four and twenty, and not just the Monkey House either. We've grown buildings!'

'Buildings! Good heavens!' I cried. And it seemed to me that the widow had kept up with this extraordinary growth of architecture herself, that her body had likewise developed real estate. 'I never thought of it.'

'You think of very little, as I recall. Isn't that why you're called Little?'

Two of the boys were carrying heavy card boxes.

'What are those?' I asked.

'Never you mind,' huffed the widow. 'Come along, show us in, let us see it all. We have not come all this way to look at you. I should think not indeed!'

I showed her which windows I had looked through, pointed up to the roof. Before long, the bells of the royal chapel sounded, and it was time to go inside. The widow's eyes darted all around. My master was wearing a hired sword, and with it he looked like a greyhound with an excited tail.

'Did you like my heads?' I asked.

'It's actually quite dirty,' she said.

'It is so big, you see,' I said, 'so very big that it's hard to keep it all clean. There are wild cats. In my cupboard there was a mouse. My heads?'

'Do they let just anyone in?' asked the widow, observing the crowd forming for the *Grand Couvert*. 'Of course, we're different,' she said in a loud voice, 'our girl is sculptor tutor to the Princesse Élisabeth. What's through this door?'

'It is time,' I said, 'for the *Grand Couvert*. We must hurry now.'

'No one hurries me. Do they, Curtius?'

'Oh no, Little, she will not be hurried.'

In the guardroom where everyone else was waiting, the boys with boxes began to hurriedly unpack them. They contained, I saw, my wax heads of the king and the queen.

'No, please!' I cried. 'You should not take them in with you. You must not!'

'We must,' the widow said, 'to judge their accuracy.'

I could not stop them. I never could. In they went. First the widow, then Curtius, then the boys with the wax heads, then Jacques and his boy. I did not press towards the Swiss Guards as usual, but kept close to the windows and so avoided most of the commotion that followed.

Unlike my previous visits to the *Grand Couvert*, there was no timely passing of people from one room into the other; instead, a major block had formed before the horseshoe-shaped table. Now the talking was only on the public side of the Swiss Guards. On the other side, the royal side, there was only staring, not at the food but out at the common people.

I saw the heads then, my heads, but I was not holding them. There they were, king and queen, and before them King and Queen. Likenesses doubled! Where first I had admitted happiness and ownership, however, now a sudden doubt crept in, spreading and infecting. The heads held up had no bodies to them; worse than that was their baldness, for they wore no wigs and so appeared scalped. They were terribly naked and unadorned. And where their eyes should have been, there was nothing, just empty sockets. It was as if these heads had come straight from the dissection room, as if the king and queen were seeing their very own deaths. I hadn't meant that. That wasn't right. A terrible mistake. They should never have come together, my king and queen and the originals.

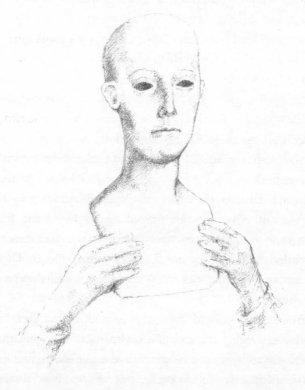

Only then I heard a very definite clapping. It was from Curtius for certain. And I thought, How wonderful! How wonderful it was after all! But then there came a wail, a woman's wailing, and then a bark, like a dog, and then cries and shrieks and screams.

I ran away.

I fled.

I hid.

# Chapter Forty-Four

*Closing the cupboard doors.*

Polignac's bit-maids found me out at last, hiding in a courtyard where they kept the dogs. I was hurried back inside to Élisabeth's rooms, pushed into my cupboard, the doors locked behind me. Perhaps an hour later, the doors were opened and Polignac herself pulled me out. Two servants tugged up my dress and Polignac lofted a cane and gave me twenty hard strikes. To be treated so like a child, though I was not so many years from thirty! When she was done I was put back in the cupboard, panting and stinging and pulsing.

There in my cupboard, locked away with no candles, I lay in the darkness peering through the keyhole. No one ever stopped. Élisabeth came by once, running to the cupboard, but one of Polignac's people was following her, and she was moved on before she could speak to me.

Through the keyhole I saw the workroom of Madame Élisabeth being emptied out. All the wax and paint, the jars of turpentine and oil, all the tools, they were taken away. I called out and banged my feet against the cupboard door, but no one came.

When the doors were unlocked at last, Pallier was there, telling me kindly not to speak. How strange that was coming from her. Then I noticed something hanging from my cupboard door: a wax object, suspended from a string. Élisabeth had come not to talk to me, as I had thought, but to pin something to my door. It was a single, well-modelled object.

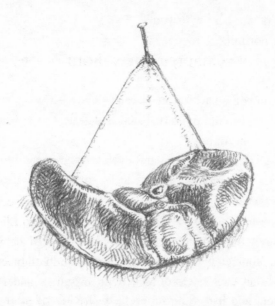

'I am a fine teacher,' I said. 'There is no doubting it.'

The sign beneath the wax organ said:

INSIDE THIS CUPBOARD

IS THE SPLEEN

OF PRINCESSE ÉLISABETH

DO NOT DISTURB

Pallier whispered that Élisabeth would see me now.

In I went. The room, disapproving at best, seemed especially vehement now.

'You're going home,' Élisabeth said.

'This is my home,' I said.

'I was only lent you, for a time, and now that time is over.'

'I don't understand.'

'Your master has need of you.'

'But I don't want to go.'

'That doesn't matter.'

287

'I should stay here with you.'

'You're not mine.'

'I have much more to teach. There's so much more.'

'All done.'

'But I can come back once a week? I can visit you?'

'Grosholtz, listen; my body, listen. I will never see you again.'

'That can't be right.'

'Those terrible heads, bald and eyeless. The queen was deeply upset. Faces with mouth agape, cheeks stuffed. Like people in a common tavern.'

'It was not my intention . . .'

'It was not *yours* indeed, it was never yours. You never asked. You took. Your employer has been fined. It was only because I intervened that they were not locked up. One of your people was quite violent and had to be suppressed. We looked after you, we fed you, we were ever loving and attentive. And in return you showed us as pigs in a sty.'

'No, just as you were. Just exactly as you were.'

'It is not for you to judge us.'

'I did not.'

'You must not look at us. A servant may not look upon a king and a queen. What a thing to have done, Marie. How could you have made those heads?'

'Please, Élisabeth, please believe me. I could not stop myself. I am sorry for it now, very sorry, but when I was working, I had such a need for it that I could not stop myself. I shall not do it again.'

'No, you shall not.'

'I do promise.'

'It is too late.'

'My place is with you.'

'No, no longer.'

'Madame Élisabeth, you are not throwing me out?'

'Marie Grosholtz, it is not just your master who insists you leave.

288

I have to be grown up now. I have to put you away. I'm not going to see you any more. I've done with playing. They are saying I have been left too long to myself.'

'To yourself? *I* was with you!'

'It does no good to be alone so long. I am to spend more time with my aunts now. Goodbye, Marie Grosholtz. Think of me. No, no, you must not touch. You must not.'

'It's me, your heart speaking. Listen to me, I beg you. I want to be with you.'

'No, I won't cry today, I've lost the trick of it.'

'*I'm* crying.'

'Servants should not have feelings. It is a cold you have. I'll pray it improves. Whatever you feel, master it, keep it inside. It mustn't be seen. How odd-looking you are. Were you always this un-comely? Perhaps you were. I must have become used to it.'

'How shall you manage? What will become of you?'

'To think you once thought we looked alike. No one should say that now.'

'You'll be an old aunt by the end of the week.'

'Goodbye, Marie.'

'You'll call for me. You always said you'd call for me. I shall be waiting.'

'Goodbye. Goodbye.'

'Can't I say sorry? Can't you see I'm so, so sorry?'

Her final gift to me was the wax spleen.

'Élisabeth!'

So I learned not only that your loved one may be forbidden you, given away to someone else, but also that though you love someone they may run from you, and you may open your arms but they shall not come in. The Élisabeth I loved was no longer. What was left was a shell, a plaster personage. Hollow. Inside was nothing but stale air unable to get out. How I wished to crack her open.

I was allowed to empty my shelves.

I am tucked in the world, into the smaller parts of it. I do not impose myself in any grandiose way. I find the gaps and inhabit them. Now another gap had closed.

I put my things neatly in my trunk. The trunk was taken down. I opened the door to her bedroom and saw the home of the cupboard Jesus.

'You're coming with me,' I said. 'Be careful not to fall from a high window.' But when I opened his velvet-lined cupboard, he was not inside: he was out with her. He had beaten me. An hour later, when I went to say goodbye to Élisabeth, there were footmen guarding the room where all her furious objects were kept, and I was not permitted entrance. I needed one last head; I could not leave without it.

'Madame Élisabeth! Madame Élisabeth!' I called out. 'Please, Madame Élisabeth, I never took your likeness. I must have your likeness – not for anyone else, only for myself. Oh, please. Madame Élisabeth, it's your heart calling for you! Your spleen if you must. Do but answer me!'

A lady-in-waiting came.

'Démon! Démon! Thank heavens it's you. Let me in, will you?'

'My name, please to note, is the Marquise de Monstiers-Mérinville,' she said. 'We do not know you. Was there ever such a person in Versailles?'

'Please, Démon . . .'

'Do not address me.'

'Please, I must say goodbye to Madame Élisabeth.'

'You are no longer required.'

'Can I see her face? Just for a moment.'

'You must go now. This was not the place for you.'

She turned away, Démon did. So solid, as I had not seen her before, quite an adult. The final favourites, Démon and the painted plaster man. Servants took me downstairs, one at each arm, escorting me out in a rush.

As I was hastened along the corridors, I saw that I was not the

290

only person packing up and leaving. The corridors were littered with trunks and servants running here and there with objects wrapped in linen. 'Where are they all going?' I asked. 'Why are they all leaving?' But I was not answered.

Jacques was waiting for me at the gates. I was glad to see him, but he had two black eyes and a cut on his forehead, and he was stiff and awkward with me. His fierce-looking boy was beside him, similarly bruised.

'Did they hurt you, Jacques? Oh Jacques, I'm very sorry if they hurt you.'

'Can't hurt Jacques,' he said. 'Can't be done.'

As the coach began to move, I thought only of love. I had loved Edmond Picot before he was taken away from me. Now, I had a heart in one pocket and in the other a spleen. And that was all the proof I needed. I had imposed myself upon the world. I had left little marks in wax. She will send for me, I thought, she is certain to send for me.

'My cupboard!' I called. 'I want my cupboard!'

But my cupboard was locked from me, and I could never get it back.

## Book Five
### 1789–1793

## The Palace of People

*When I was twenty-eight, until I was thirty-two.*

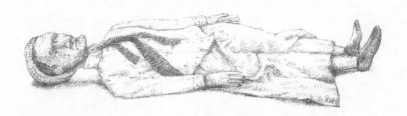

# Chapter Forty-Five

*In and out.*

Jacques stared at me as we journeyed back into Paris, likewise his crop-haired boy. If there was to be any conversation, I saw, I must be the one to make it.

'Who's your friend, Jacques?'

'This is my boy. This is Émile.'

'Hello, Émile, I'm very happy to meet you. I'm Marie.'

Émile curled his lip.

'He's just like you!' I exclaimed. 'You used to do that!'

'He does copy me a bit. I don't mind. He's my boy, he's paid to help me out.'

'He's paid, is he?'

'We all are.'

'What changes there must be, and so many new people.'

'Oh yes, it's much bigger than before, and I have my Émile, and we do get along wonderful well.'

Émile growled at me.

'She's all right, Émile, she's a friend. Been gone so long.'

'I'm here now.'

'Yes. There you are.'

I thought at first that Jacques Beauvisage had put on weight, but it was not fat he had accumulated, I think it was fondness. He had grown an attachment; parenthood had put a tiny touch of softness to his face. In my absence he had found somewhere else to put his love; it was only fitting, I suppose, but still it smarted.

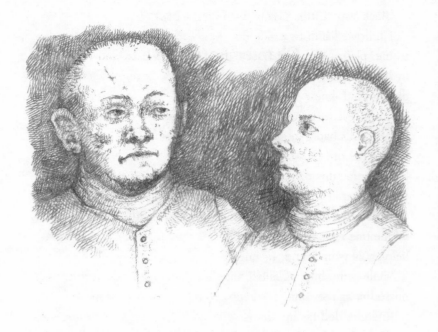

Back into Paris we went, along the crooked, crowded streets, more dismal than I remembered, all the way unto the boulevard. And there it was.

The Monkey House, grown so large in my absence.

I was shy of it. It was like seeing an old friend after a decade, once slender but now gone over to corpulence. Once young, now middle-aged and thick with it.

There was not one but two great doors at the front, one labelled IN, the other OUT. Our old neighbour on the boulevard, the Little World Theatre, had been pulled down and onto its land the Monkey House had spread. To the right, on the fallow ground where the chess café had once stood, more additions had been built. All this progress was protected by tall metal fencing and a large spiked gate, which Jacques ushered me through. High atop the gate was hung the old bell of Henri Picot. I walked towards the door marked IN, but before I climbed the steps Jacques took my arm.

'Back way, Little. Come through the back.'

I followed him to a side door and entered territory unfamiliar to me: plain walls, dirt floors, boys running back and forth deep in business. Near this back entrance were several stacked shop dummies. I knew these! They were the last remnants of dear Edmond Picot, gone over to the Ticre print-works. One of the mannequins had a moustache. I was shocked to see them. Jacques tugged me on.

'To come this way,' he said. 'Now to come. Must not keep them waiting.'

There was Florence Biblot in the kitchen, still shiny and now with more folds and creases, and with a small, thin girl in an apron helping her.

'Hello, Florence!' I called. 'Do you remember me? How I have missed your cooking!'

'Ddddd, dddd,' she said, giving her little laugh, just as before.

'Now, Little, come fast. Must not upset them.'

I was taken into a study. The floor was dotted with metal pails, many of them filled with cigar ash and stubs; the walls and the large desk in the centre were covered with prints, portraits of different people. Jacques told me to wait there and was gone.

I've done this before, I thought; it's like my first day at Versailles. Only what a different place this was, what a different room. A moment later, the heads on the papers seemed to shiver in terror as the door opened and the Widow Picot entered. She was massive and mole-ridden, proudly hairy, profligate of eyebrow and of lip, a great handsome toad in a pretty dress, indomitable, brutish, and bad-tempered. Her hair remained tied up, out of sight beneath her great lace bonnet, but her clothes, I noticed now, looked a little dirty and careworn.

'What a nerve to show your face,' she said. 'Why should we have what the palace spurns?'

'I want to go back,' I said. 'I'd rather not stay.'

'But you never can go back, little creature, so buck up.'

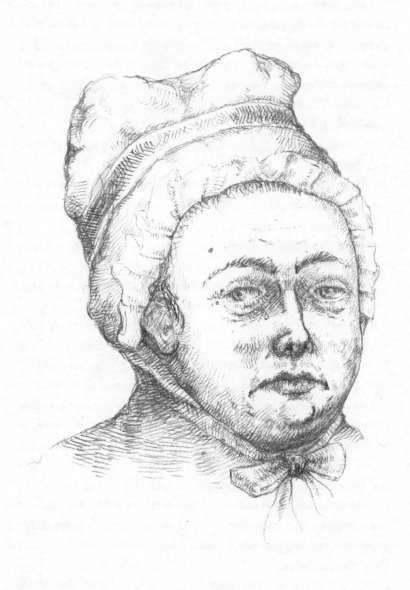

The door opened once more, the heads on the pages shivered again, and here, done up in silk and powder, came the cadaverous form of my own dear master, quite wasted away, his clothes and jewellery new and shining but cloaking something old and hurting. The beauty spot, now migrated to his chin, did little to improve the spectacle.

'Dear Widow Picot,' he said.

'Doctor Curtius,' she nodded.

'Quite well?'

'Fit! Fit!'

'I prosper myself.'

'I am glad of it.'

From which I understood that the widow and my master did not see each other every day.

'She is come back.'

'I wish to return to Versailles,' I said.

'But they won't have you, Marie,' my master said. 'They sent you home.'

'I've told her already. She wouldn't believe me.'

'Élisabeth *will* call for me,' I said.

'What trouble you have caused,' chimed in the widow. 'It was Swiss Guards that hit Jacques. His head was bleeding. People from your country!'

'I am sorry for it.'

'I should think so!' she said.

'Am I to do the hairs, as before?' I asked.

'You shall do what you are told,' said the widow. 'You may have come from a palace, but here's another, one called the Great Monkey House. I don't want to hear anything about any other.'

'No, Madame.'

'I'm afraid you cannot have a key to the wax cupboard, Marie,' Curtius added.

'Certainly not,' confirmed the widow.

'There is still more for you to learn, Marie, but there are so many heads and hands to be made that you must be thrust into service.'

'I must?' I asked. 'Thank you, sir. I do thank you for that.'

'Don't get above yourself,' added the widow, 'and don't go where you're not needed. The attic is dangerous, the rooms are not safe. Step up there and you'll fall to your death. The architects of the Great Monkey House have advised us never to let anyone step up there.'

'No, Madame. Please, sir, Madame, may I ask something? Will you be showing the royal family at dinner?'

A silence before the widow muttered, 'There must be some compensation for Jacques.'

'You will, then?' I whispered. 'You will!'

'I don't like her noise; I never did.'

'And I shall be paid like anyone else. Now I shall be paid?'

'I am done with this interview,' said the widow. 'I was not looking forward to it, and it has put me in a foul temper. I'm stepping out. I'll return this evening. It may not be until late. Send a boy if you need me. I'll be with the better people.'

She left, taking words away with her. My master and I stood looking at each other, neither knowing what to say. At last my master, stroking his beauty spot, muttered, 'She's gone to the Palais-Royal. She has rooms there. She is blessed by the Duc d'Orléans himself, who gave his permission.' I said nothing. He continued. 'She's mostly there these days, smoking her cigars. We keep all the best waxes there, all the good humans in polite society. It's very grand, actually. Such an address and such rent! While here we have all the criminal and dreadful countenances. You see? Only the bad here, all the good there. She looks over the good people and I master the other tribe. It's an accommodation, you see. It's how we live these days: divided.'

'It has all grown very much since I left, sir.'

'Yes,' he said dolefully, 'we do prosper.'

'Excuse me, sir, I can't help noticing. There's something on your chin.'

300

'Is there?' he murmured, touching the dark circle. 'Oh yes, I quite forget it's there sometimes. It's supposed to make me look more attractive.'

'And does it, sir?'

'I wear it for her. Do you know, Little, it cost me thirty-five livres? It's the very best quality, you see, black taffeta. I'm never quite sure where to put it. Sometimes I have it on a cheek, at others upon my upper lip. Recently it has come to rest upon my chin, where I think it is happiest. But it's scarcely worth the bother, Marie, for she never notices.'

He went silent again, then let out a long melancholy sigh, shaking himself a little. 'Come with me, then.'

As we walked, not into the old Monkey House but through a part of that swollen building I had not known before, I asked him, 'Did you like the heads? My heads? A little?'

'I am a collection of pains and twitches.'

'We've come a long way from Berne, sir.'

'Berne? I do remember it, Little. Yes, a long way – and yes! I have come so far.' He was walking faster now, as though we were being chased. 'May I tell you something, Marie? I have been dis- covered. I am the great leveller. I equalise the people, you see. People have written about me – and I have read it! – and that is what they call me, Little, the great leveller.' Then his eyes fell back on me, and it was as though he were waking from a dream. 'Oh! Dear Marie,' he said, looking me in the eyes and smiling at me for the first time, 'I should not say it in front of her, she is so mighty, but I am happy you're home.'

'I am glad to see you too, sir. But, also, I will say that I am sorry to leave the palace. I grew so fond of Élisabeth and she of me. I think I must go back again, very soon probably. You will spare me, won't you?'

'Versailles is being emptied, Marie. The aristocrats are packing up.'

'Are they? Are you sure? Why would they? I don't understand.'

301

'I don't know if anyone does, except the widow perhaps: she studies that world so. No one understands it better than she. Everything's in chaos, Marie, haven't you heard? People are being very argumentative. I wish they wouldn't be, but they are. It upsets her so. Monsieur Mercier runs around as if he has the worms. Nothing is certain.'

'Was it for my own good, then, that I was sent away?'

Curtius didn't seem to hear me. Instead he asked: 'Did she love you, your Élisabeth? How nice to be loved. Come along.'

Versailles, packed up? Could such a thing be possible?

I wondered if anything would ever be certain again.

# Chapter Forty-Six

*A new beginning.*

'There are heads, new heads to be thought about every day,' said my master. 'The Monkey House has grown so big, we can't stop it now, even should we want to. Through there, Marie, is your workshop.'

'My own workshop?'

'And with you, every day, will work Georges Offroy.'

A boy stepped forward.

'Hello, miss,' he said, bowing.

He was addressing me.

'Hello, Georges. I am very pleased to meet you.'

What a cheerful, healthy face, what crooked teeth. I liked him instantly. An ordinary thirteen-year-old boy. Since when did I know such creatures?

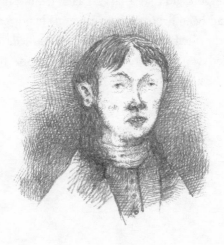

'I'm to do what you say,' he said. 'I am at your service.'

'I'm very glad of it,' I said. 'I didn't know I was to have an assistant. I've never had one before.'

'I mean to do well by you, miss.'

'And I'm sure you shall.'

'I saw your royal heads before they went off to the Palais!' he exclaimed. 'They're famous, they are! What heads!'

'Thank you, Georges!' I cried. 'And that's where they are? At the Palais-Royal! My heads! May I see them?'

'You must get on, Little,' my master said. 'You must be busy. So much to do!'

My workshop was a small room connected to my master's on the ground floor of the new extension. A store cupboard that had been cleared and fitted out with a table and two chairs. It had no access of its own; it was only reachable through my master's workroom. There was one window, high enough that I should have to get a chair to look through it. But it was my room, my workshop.

That first afternoon, my fingers touched all those tools and jars, even wax. Georges and I were to make some wax hands for a figure my master was finishing, while the heavy body was being assembled in a different workshop. Great spades of hands were our first charge, huge sausage fingers, and so a large baker from Charenton who fitted the bill had been brought in to have his hands cast for a fee. The head for the fat hands was very pockmarked, with a huge unkempt, clotted wig. He looked like a lion gone to seed. The Comte de Mirabeau was his name.

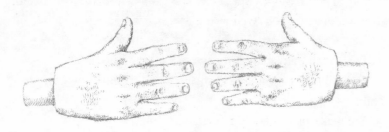

That first day, those fat hands so occupied me that after a while I almost forgot to think about Élisabeth in her corridor with her plaster man. My mind was on other things. As we worked, I turned to my assistant. 'Excuse me, Georges. I don't mean to pry, but are you paid for your work?'

'Certainly, miss, regular like clockwork. I shouldn't stick around otherwise. I go to the counting room and am given my due. It's good employment.'

'Do you think I shall be paid, Georges?'

''Course you shall.'

'Do you think so! I wonder, Georges, if you would show me the counting room. It's new since my day and I don't know how to find it.'

'I'd be happy to. Right now? Certainly. Nothing simpler.'

We went along the corridor and turned a corner and suddenly we were in the old house I had known so well. As we climbed the stairs, we were greeted by the dummy of Henri Picot, now wearing a fine white shirt and a silk waistcoat of bold stripes.

In the place that was called the accounting room stood a tall metal strongbox. The body of this cold personality was filled with the Cabinet's great fortune. There were three keys, I would learn; one for the widow, one for Curtius, and one for the bookkeeper. This very bookkeeper was perched upon his high stool when we arrived, a man in his middle twenties, prematurely balding, with brown hair, brown eyes, and a pasty face lacking warmth.

'This,' said Georges, 'is Marie Grosholtz. And this, miss, is Martin Millot. He keeps the figures.'

Martin pointed at my spectacles and said, 'Twenty livres.' Then, after a moment: 'You lived at the palace.'

'Yes, I did.'

'For which there came fifty livres a month,' he said.

'Fifty livres!' I wondered at such a sum. It seemed to me a great deal.

'We make that in a few hours sometimes.'

305

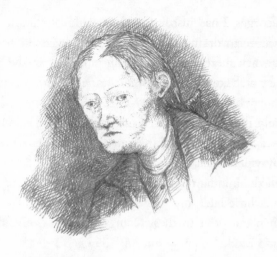

'Is the money mine? That came from Versailles? May I have it?'

'Have it?'

'Since it was in payment for my services.'

'I have no authority to release such funds.'

'But it was for me, was it not? For my wages.'

'That may be, but I have no authority.'

'Excuse me – will I be paid now?' I said. 'Now that I am back. Am I to have a wage?'

'I have had no word of it, either one way or the other.'

'The royal family at dinner – I made the heads. They were my work.'

'Were they? And what then?'

'Shall I not be paid?'

'What do you want me to say, miss? I've had no word of it, neither for nor against. Without word, the money does not migrate. How miserable you look. Don't trouble yourself so much; I say, it's not my doing. I add, I subtract. I cannot say what sort of figure you are. I ask you, please, to calm.'

'Shall we return to our work, miss?' asked Georges.

'I suppose we must, Georges,' I said.

'Do not be so down, miss.'

'No, Georges. I had just hoped.'

We had been working for several hours, and the evening had come on, when there came a growing humming in the building, followed by a shaking of the objects in the room.

'It's the public,' explained Georges. 'The doors have been opened, and they've come in. We generally get shaken around a little, tossed and turned, until they go. It's a good noise really: the widow says so. She calls it prosperity.'

The whole building rattled with the life of people from beyond the gates. A little later, my master put on his coat and went out.

'He often goes out in the evenings,' Georges told me, 'with Jacques and Émile.'

'Where do they go?'

'I couldn't say exactly. Dark places, cockpits and such, dangerous drinking holes where there are fights, murderous places. But now that he's gone, would you like to see them all? There's a spyhole.'

Georges took me by the hand down the backstairs and along a dark corridor. Another new man passed us by.

'What are you doing, Georges?' he asked.

'Just showing Miss Grosholtz around.'

Did I need showing around my own old home? I did.

'*Should* you be doing it?' The other boy's face came into view, half sunk in his abundant collar. He had a severe squint, and his eyes were placed so far apart on his head that they seemed entirely unacquainted with each other. 'I'm not sure you should.'

'I am Marie Grosholtz,' I said.

'Are you?' he replied. 'And so what?'

'I made the royal family.'

'And there was I thinking it was God what done that.' He looked, one eye on each of us, before sneering away.

'That's André Valentin. He's a ticket-taker. We have nothing to do with him generally.'

'So much the better.'

'Here it is then.'

307

He showed me a hole that had been drilled in a wall. Through it could be seen the colossal business – people of wax! – and the people of flesh here to see them. What a populace!

'I think,' I said, 'that the rest of Paris must be empty now.'

'I think it must be.'

The old theatre props were gone. Everything was very dark and poorly lit. The walls seemed to drip; great black shadows crept across the hall; all the murderers and their murdered were grimly about their business. This was the Salon of Great Thieves. Here were all the most horrible accommodated. Figures everywhere, standing proud in their mischief. And living people moved about these stillborn souls and screamed and laughed at them. Benches were distributed here and there, where a person might sit down and rest from all the infamy.

'Do you see,' said Georges, 'a person sleeping at a bench?'

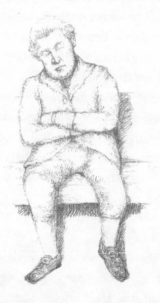

There in the hall was a middle-aged man, his head slumped on his shoulder. Two or three people approached him, pointing and smiling; finally, one stepped forward and tapped the man upon his knee. When he failed to move, he was jogged a little more. Then the little gathering gave a shriek, and I heard the announcement: 'He's wax!'

'A wax man pretending to be the public!' I exclaimed.

'That sleeping fellow,' said Georges, laughing, 'is a wax replica of Cyprien Bouchard, painter of porcelain. He won the lottery.'

The lottery, Georges told me, was drawn every six months. A very public occasion: names in a sack, and the name pulled out became a waxwork. There had been three lottery winners so far: a scullery maid, a coiffeur, and a painter of porcelain. They were placed among the exhibits, to mingle with the celebrated and infamous. Scullery maid with assassin, coiffeur near a thief, porcelain painter by drowned bride.

'What an idea!' I said.

All the sounds and humming of the expanded Monkey House, all its chattering and hammering, its odd knocks and reverberations, were so new to me. I lay alone on my pallet in my own workshop that night, after the public departed, and listened to the building breathing, making so many odd sounds – how the house talked, it always had, but in different sounds now, a new complaining, so that just when I thought I might drift into sleep at last, some new noise would waken me. And sitting up, I was certain I heard footsteps nearby.

# Chapter Forty-Seven

*A visit.*

The sounds came back night after night as I lay upon my pallet, thumping, scratching. Sometimes, half awake, I thought someone had come into my room; I would sit up in fright and look at the door, and sometimes it would be open, though I always closed it before going to sleep. My master, I said to myself, must have been up in the night.

One early morning when I awoke, daylight just coming in, I was suddenly aware that I was not alone. Someone was sitting at the bench before me.

'Hello,' I said.

There was no answer.

'Who are you there?'

The person kept very still.

'Is it you, Georges? Don't fool about now; what are you doing?'

But the person only looked on. As more light came I saw the slightest outline of a bonnet. It was a small woman sitting there.

'Is it?' I said in a rush. 'Élisabeth! You have come for me!'

But she said nothing.

'Cuckoo?' I ventured.

And there was no response. The daylight rose and slowly I saw the person with more clarity. She was wearing a black dress and a white bonnet; upon her chest was a red rosette with the letter 'C' in the middle, such as all the workers wore now. Slowly, slowly I saw a little more. The woman was staring at me with shining dark eyes.

'Who are you? Why have you come?'

But she sat still and stared hard.

'Please talk. Speak to me. Why are you here?'

But she just stared.

So I leaned forward and pushed her, and she tumbled forward and fell to the ground and lay there, very still.

I leaned over and touched her hair. The hair came off.

I screamed.

By then I could see: the strange bald woman was not of the living; no, she was indeed very dead, and had never been alive, for she was a doll. A doll of an undersized human, made of not wax but wood, wearing a cloth dress, with glass eyes set in her head. I sat her upright; how heavy she was, and awkward, her limbs falling this way and that. Someone had put her in my room to frighten me.

What a horrible, mean-looking face. How it stared at me with its lifeless eyes. I put back her hair, though I hated to touch it. As I righted the wretched doll, the door moved and someone, some shadowy form that had been there all along, darted out through my master's workroom and along the corridor. I rushed after it, following the creaking of the floor, as if the house itself wanted me to find the culprit. I stopped at the foot of the attic stairs in the old house, at the very edge of the forbidden territory. I didn't care if the attic did kill me then; nothing would stop me.

I creaked up, very careful, very slow. As I stood upon the top step, looking in the darkness, I saw no one. But then, after a long time, after my breath grew quieter, I saw a small patch grow a little lighter in the gloom, and that patch came drifting towards me. And its name, oh its name, yes its name was Edmond Henri Picot.

# Chapter Forty-Eight

STICK NO BILLS.

Edmond Henri Picot. With a moustache and grey in his hair and haunted eyes. My hands over my mouth to stop the screaming. The figure came right up to me, so soft in motion that it might have been the wind stirred by a spider, and whispered:

'Catarrh? This powerful treatment makes cure certain. Nazalia. Cleanses and purifies all the breathing organs; penetrating to the innermost crevices of the mucous membrane of the throat and nose, dissolves and removes all crusts and phlegm, disperses the catarrh, stops buzzing in the ears and cures partial deafness.'

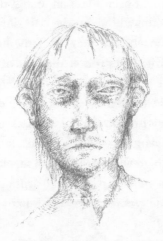

'Oh, Edmond!' I cried. 'What has happened to you, my very dear Edmond?'

'Do you suffer from skin sickness,' he continued, 'in the form of skin shine, pimples, spots, and redness, that may lead to eczema with its terrible burning and itching? For an absolute cure for eczema, is two livres too much?'

'Edmond, what has happened? Do you live up here all alone?'

'A laxative and refreshing fruit lozenge. Most agreeable to take. Tamar Indien Grillon for constipation, haemorrhoids, bile, headache, loss of appetite, gastric and intestinal troubles. Tamar Indien Grillon.'

'Oh, Edmond, what have they done to you?'

'Mouse traps!' he said. 'Rat traps! No more vermin!'

Think, Marie Grosholtz.

'We won't talk about it. We'll just sit here a while. Let me catch my breath.'

'An oriental dessert in Paris – pistachio nuts.'

'Yes, Edmond, yes, of course.'

I could see about the attic rooms now. They were . . . populated. Edmond had placed a shop doll in each lonely space. There were plates and cups, a small table, even a tablecloth. So then I supposed something else.

'They know you're here? Everyone below, I mean. You're not really in hiding, are you, Edmond?'

I held his hand. Every one of his fingers was stained black with ink.

'Stick no bills,' he whispered.

'They do know, don't they?'

'Bill-posters will be prosecuted.'

'Yes. They know.' Someone had been bringing him food. 'It won't do, Edmond.'

I touched his face. His ears were pale and cold. I touched his timid moustache.

'Wait there, Edmond. I will be back in just a moment.'

I took a sharp knife from my workshop, and some soft soap, and with a bowl and water I removed Edmond's moustache. 'There,' I said, 'that's better. You look more yourself already.' But

313

in truth he looked like very little without the moustache there. 'You do know me, Edmond. I know you know me. You left something in my workshop this morning. I do not know what has happened to you, but you shall be well again.'

'Stick no bills,' he said.

'Quite right,' I said.

A bell sounded downstairs.

'I must go now, Edmond, but I shall be back later. I have people to talk to down below. Yes, I do. But I'll return!'

Downstairs in my workroom, Georges had arrived.

'Edmond Picot,' I declared, 'is in the attic.'

He said nothing, but looked uncomfortable.

'Where is the widow?' I called.

'Please, miss, she went out early today.'

'Then where is Curtius?'

'He is likewise gone out, very recently. You've just missed him.'

'I believe you. He heard me up there no doubt and left to avoid any mischief.'

'It is possible.'

'Then Jacques?'

'Has not come in yet.'

'Tell me, Georges, does the widow know about the person in the attic?'

'Yes indeed, miss. It was she what put him there.'

'Oh, the wretched woman!'

'He would not stop crying.'

'The poor dear man! Georges, tell me what has happened.'

'He went down with a brain fever, miss, total nervous exhaustion, and when the fever was done with, his brain had left him.'

'No one told me!'

'Forgive me, miss, but was there a reason they should?'

'He is kept on his own in the attic?'

'He is less panicky there, on his own. Have you seen this wooden doll, miss?'

314

'Yes, I have. It gave me quite a shock.'

'He made it. Do you know whom it is of?'

'Edmond made it? Did he? No, I do not know.'

'Truly, you cannot tell whom?'

'It is a horrible-faced woman and it makes me shudder.'

'Honestly, you don't know?'

'No, Georges, I don't. I'm certain I've never seen anyone who looks like that.'

'Why, it's you, miss.'

'Me?'

'You.'

'I look like that?'

'Something like that.'

'Oh.'

It seemed to me the very worst news.

'You're very quiet, miss.'

I was.

'I thought it would be flattering,' he said, 'you know, to have a portrait done of yourself.'

'That is how he sees me.'

'Done from memory.'

'I'm not a vain person. I never was.'

'How he toiled over it.'

'It has my old clothes, I see that now, and my measurements, I suppose.'

'Indeed it is unmistakable.'

'Is it?'

'He took a deal of trouble over it.'

'Did he? *Did* he?'

'Shall I tell you a story?'

'Yes, Georges, do.'

'There then. I shall tell you about this doll. Perhaps it will help. Now, here I go. Whenever Monsieur Edmond came to visit here, he would sit with his mother a while, or with his father's dummy-shape, but later he started climbing up to the attic. There, after a time, visit by visit, he carved. He made you, by himself, up in the topmost rooms, when he was away from his wife. He carved your head out of one of the joists in the attic, though the attic complained of it so. He tugged the joist away, and since then I believe it's slumped a bit, the attic. Afterwards, whenever he came to visit, he would sit upstairs beside you.

'When the widow at last found the doll, there was great noise. The doll was smashed about a good deal. He came less often afterwards – his wife would not allow it – and there was some shouting, I recall, between Madame Cornélie and the widow. But the widow found her own uses for the doll. She put it in the windows – I'm sorry, miss – to scare the boulevard children when they came spying. And sometimes it was used as a weight, to press things down. It has propped doors open also. Jacques sometimes lugged it out onto the steps to sit beside him. The doll was let stay. And that's the story, miss, of the doll, if you don't mind.'

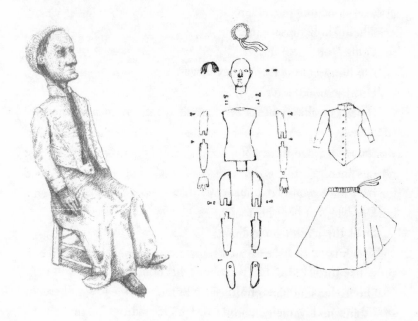

Tears, tears for Edmond then and for me, snot and sobs.

'Is he very broken?' I asked. 'Do tell me, Georges.'

'I believe so.'

'And Cornélie threw him out?'

'We don't see her any more. The Ticres brought him back. Madame Cornélie would not own him in such a state. She broke the marriage. In court, she did it proper. She protested how unhusbandly Monsieur Edmond was. And when the judge asked Monsieur Edmond to speak he just muttered his nonsense, and so the judge broke the marriage and he came back here.'

'With a moustache and with his fingers dyed with ink.'

'The widow cannot have him around the public. He is an unhappy sight. He disturbs people.'

'She hides him.'

'The wax people terrify him. He is happier in the top rooms. Food is taken up to him, and when he tries to come downstairs one of us boys will guide him back up. Those rooms are his; they are always spoken of as dangerous, but only so that he will be left alone. He is quite happy by himself. Much happier than he was. It was thought that you might distress him, so you were told never to go upstairs.'

'But he found me out.'

'Yes, he found you out, miss.'

'He talks such nonsense.'

'They're advertisements, miss. Bills they did at the Ticre printworks. He learned them all. It's all he ever says these days. He just repeats them, so many different ones, over and over. He is good for only light duties, and not really those. Sometimes he is given a little needlework, but he does prick himself.'

'Does the widow go to him?'

'Sometimes. But she is such a proud lady, she does not like to show her softer side.'

'She leaves him alone up there?'

'I think he is quite content.'

317

'We shall see,' I said.

I went up and down to him all that day and brought him his food. He kept very still there, muttering words from the printers.

When at last she came home, I was waiting. I went upstairs, took Edmond's hand, and led him back down. Into her office, without a knock.

'It's Edmond,' I said to her. 'This is Edmond!'

With trembling, furious face, with clenched jaw she hissed: 'Get him away! Back up to the top! Visitors are expected any minute!'

'Stay, Edmond!'

'GET HIM OUT!'

A boy came.

'This is your own son,' I said. 'Will you not own him?'

'NOW! OUT!'

'Polite notice,' Edmond said louder than usual, 'no trespassing.'

He went of his own accord, silently from the room. The boy followed. I was left alone with her.

'Do not presume to know me,' she said. 'Get in my way again and I shall smother you. With my own hands I will do it. I'll throttle the life out of you; I'll extinguish you and be the happier for it. I could do it now. Who are you, a speck, and who am I? Get out!'

I got out, but that was only the beginning of it.

I washed Edmond's fingers every day. I fed him. I went up and down the stairs for him. I lured him back to the workshop. I would find him again, I resolved; if Edmond was in there I'd find him.

'Edmond, you know me,' I said. 'You do. I'm back now. I'm here again.'

'Ship's chandler.'

'I won't leave you in the attic.'

'We buy teeth.'

'I'll have you downstairs with me.'

'Very convenient premises, apply within.'

'I'll have you about me, you'll be my society again.'

318

'Containing an area of about six thousand feet.'
'And somewhere in all those words . . .'
'Frontage about one hundred and thirty-one.'
'. . . some genuine Edmond will fall out.'
'To be let on lease.'

# Chapter Forty-Nine

*Everyone is inside.*

Louis-Sébastien Mercier came to visit. He sought me out in my workshop where I made hands with Georges. Edmond sat mute in the corner.

'There you are again, Little! Back on the real stage!'

'Not too loud, sir, if you please. It isn't good for Edmond. See him there. See what has become of him.'

'Ah yes, I had heard. But, Marie,' he said, brightening, 'I've seen your royal ones!'

'Have you? How is Élisabeth?'

'I mean of course the waxes. So bold. To show them so!'

'Thank you. And how are you, dear Monsieur Mercier? How are your shoes?'

'We are kept at it. How we are kept at it!'

As Georges and I worked on, Mercier told us how the times kept him running from place to place, these days, as if all of Paris were in continual earthquake. Sometimes, he said, he saw the widow rushing about too, breathless, gathering information. He took off his shoes and passed them round. They were indeed worn very thin. He showed us a little booklet he had recently finished, its subject the CELEBRATED SALONS OF WAX, and read to us a passage from it:

> *'In these new and fast-paced days, the Cabinet of Doctor*
> *Curtius is the essential sight at the Palais-Royal and on the*
> *whole of the boulevard. Some go so far as to say that nothing*

*can beat it in the entire capital. Curtius's is an excellent enter-*
*tainment for men of any profession, for children, for women, for*
*the aged, for the curious, for the uninformed, for the brave, for*
*the uninspired, for the tired of life, for the understimulated, for*
*the overdressed, for the ragged, for weaklings, for the powerful,*
*for masters and for their servants, for the daring and for the*
*proper, for the natives to understand quite how their capital*
*works in these shifting times and for the foreigners to under-*
*stand an unfamiliar city.*

*'There is scarcely a person in Paris for whom Curtius's is*
*not relevant these extraordinary days. No matter how well you*
*think you know the city, Curtius always holds surprises for you*
*— as if it is Doctor Curtius himself who decides who is in and*
*who is out. All that is well known, all that is the greatest, all*
*that is extraordinary and inspiring, all that is abominable, all*
*of that is kept concentrated in the Cabinet. Where famous*
*living personages may disappoint in real life, appearing briefly*
*and at too great a distance, at Curtius's they never disappoint.*
*In his establishment, the most exclusive of ladies and*
*gentlemen have time for simply everyone.*

*'For this is true: Curtius, in his great hall, has abolished*
*privilege! Curtius has dismissed all laws of etiquette. Curtius*
*has done away with class. Where else in the world might a*
*pauper approach a king? Might the mediocre touch genius?*
*Might ugliness draw close — without shame — to beauty? The*
*Cabinet is the only place.*

*'It is true that his certain magic works only within the*
*confines of his places of exhibition; once outside, the gravity of*
*everyday pressures and worries and hopes instantly reasserts*
*itself. But who can complain when they have seen the wonder*
*of a schoolboy coming face to face with his latest hero? Who*
*can complain when they see a scholar from the Sorbonne*
*approaching in reverence the figure of the great deceased author*
*whose words so move his life? Who can complain when an*

321

*ordinary law-abiding matron can behold in terror and prox-*
*imity the greatest murderer of the age? Who indeed can*
*complain when any subject of the country of France may visit*
*the Palais-Royal and see, at his own convenience, on any day*
*of the week, the royal family seated for dinner, and step closer*
*and closer still, and feel a connection to the king or the queen*
*that has never been felt before, and may even, for the cost of*
*three livres, if he should be so brave — and few are — even dare*
*to . . . TOUCH?*

*'So be it!*

*'Even the mystery of royalty is solved at the Cabinet of*
*Doctor Curtius!'*


'Thank you, Monsieur Mercier,' I said, taking the slim volume.
'I shall treasure it.'

'Do you think, Little, do you think now they might consider a
new bust of me? For the Palais-Royal, of course, not for here. Do
you think they would?'

'Who can say?' I said. 'It is not up to me.'

'You don't think so, do you?'

'I do not know,' I said.

'No, no,' he muttered. 'I try each time for the wax lottery, put
my name with the others.'

'Pure milk, new-laid eggs,' said Edmond.

# Chapter Fifty

*In which heads are stolen.*

The widow changed the uniforms of the Monkey House staff. Silk suits were removed and in their stead were black cotton coats and black hose, simple black three-cornered hats, but all adorned still with 'C' rosettes. This sombre outfit was a replica of the dress worn by the representatives of the common people at the newly formed parliament.

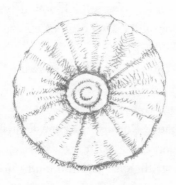

One Sunday, not long after my return, bells sounded all about the city, clanging far longer than was usual. We laboured in our workshops through the morning, thinking little of it, though the bells continued to sound and Edmond paced back and forth in his attic. I went up to calm him, but the noise had disturbed him and he was very wretched. I held his ears; that always helped. I told him that the bells were bound to stop soon, but they did not.

And in the late afternoon the widow, screaming, returned to the Monkey House, bursting into my master's workshop.

'Stolen! Stolen! Property taken! Heads! Our heads, Curtius!'

What a red-faced, sweating widow it was.

'Madame!' cried Curtius. 'What troubles you?'

'Heads! Heads!' she panted.

'Yes,' said Curtius. 'Any in particular?'

'Yes,' she gasped, struggling for breath, 'ripped from us at the Palais-Royal!'

'A robbery?'

'In broadest daylight. Hundreds of them!'

'Hundreds of heads?'

'No, people! Hundreds of thieves, all demanding the same thing.'

'Was it heads?'

'Yes, Curtius! Our property taken from us!'

'But whose heads?'

'Ours!'

'But which?'

'Minister Necker and the Duc d'Orléans.'

'Whatever for?'

'To hold them high and parade them through the streets for a funeral march.'

'But they are ours! Why did they?'

'You must keep up, Curtius! You must open your ears. The minister has been dismissed, and the duc banished, and the people are marching around the city, holding high our heads. Since the actual men are absent, the heads in proxy must take their place.'

'They should get their own heads of Necker and Orléans. Those ones are ours!'

'They chanted, banged on the windows, pushed themselves into the salon with no ticket between them, demanding heads.'

'And what did you do?'

'I gave them over. They would only have taken them anyway, and done who knows what damage. They wanted the king, too, but I begged them not, saying the king was a whole figure and very heavy while the other two were only busts.'

That king was my work. 'I'm glad the king is safe,' I said. 'Thank you for saving him.'

The widow shifted so her back was towards me.

'We'll have them arrested,' groaned Curtius. '*I* made them! Private property!'

'I took two names. François Pépin, a pedlar, and André Ladry, a *limonadier*.'

'They will be charged!'

'They promised to return the heads.'

'You should never have let them go.'

'You weren't there,' she whispered – quietly, but I heard her. 'I was the only one there, and I was frightened.'

Such a silence then, a silence like a hole, like a ripped opening, as if the widow had come unstitched and with it our world.

'You, frightened?' Curtius whispered. '*You?* I'll never believe it.'

'I thought they would kill me, these people. It would be easily done. They'd step forward and nothing would stop them if they wanted to. Take a sharp knife, thrust it quick in and out, and I'd be spilling. I might have died, I might have. It's luck, I suppose in the end, Philippe,' she said, and tears came out of her.

'You never called me Philippe before.'

That was the second shock.

I think we were all frightened then.

# Chapter Fifty-One

*Concerning Captain Curtius.*

Wax is used upon muskets, upon rifles and shotguns. It greases the triggers to make them sharper; it smooths down the barrels to help the shot and powder pass through efficiently.

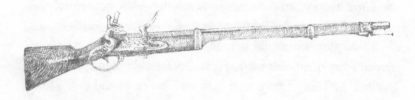

There were noises throughout the night. Shouting on the boulevard; glass smashed. A distant report of shooting. These sounds were picked up in the Great Monkey House, and the Great Monkey House made something of its own of them: it twisted them and elongated them, bounced them and seemed loath to let them fade. They played a misery upon Edmond and stole his sleep from him. I do not know how many doors and windows were smashed that night, only that the Monkey House gates stood firm.

In the morning all the bells of the city sang together, calling to one another across Paris. In the Great Monkey House, nothing. The gates were kept shut up. The staff who lived about the city did not arrive for work. Only the bookkeeper, Martin Millot, appeared, anxious to see that all was safe. Slowly, distractedly, we who remained worked in the back rooms. Millot counted money, Jacques cut cloth, the widow stitched busts, my master made heads and I hands. Edmond kept away because his mother was present. As the day went on, lost in wax or hairs or wood or canvas, we forgot everything but what was before us.

It wasn't until nearly afternoon that our own bell rang. Jacques went to the gate. He returned with two boulevard businessmen: the beanpole Monsieur Nicolet, master of funambulists – his brick building was the Grands Danseurs de Corde – and flame-headed Doctor Graham, he of the Celestial Bed. I hadn't known it until he spoke, but Graham was a Scot – a foreigner like my master and me.

These two men had come, they said, because no place in the boulevard was as famous as the Great Monkey House. They knew that the events of the night must have terrified us, who had so much to lose. Wasn't it a terrible thing, they asked, that no one now held the reins to the city? Unless something was done, and soon, the city would be driven into the abyss. Anarchy would spread from quarter to quarter; the city would burn and all inside it would be lost.

'We know about loss,' said the widow. 'Yesterday, two of our heads were taken from us.'

'Necker,' said Curtius. 'The Duc d'Orléans.'

'The men who stole from you, who marched illegally, were fired upon and dispersed.'

'And our heads?'

'There's blood now on the streets of Paris. Order must be returned.'

'Will we get our heads back?'

They had just come from the Hôtel de Ville. There had been a meeting; that was why the tocsin had sounded. These were desperate times, the two men agreed; it was easy to stay at home and pull the bedcovers over your heads, but if nothing was done, someone would rip the bedcovers from your face and tug you naked into the street. This last opinion was delivered specifically to Curtius.

327

In the meeting at the Hôtel de Ville it was proposed that a citizens' militia be formed, a militia large enough to protect the city from both those uniformed terrors outside its walls and the un-uniformed ones inside. The men paused, then spoke slowly and clearly: it would be a great relief to the people of the boulevard and the surrounding district, they said, if Curtius, as its most prominent personality, would volunteer himself to be the local captain of the people's militia. Will you do it, Captain Curtius? they said.

There stood Curtius and the widow. Through my glasses, they both appeared shrunken. There was a dripping noise that seemed to come from inside my master.

'You are mistaken,' he responded at last. 'Philip Wilhelm Mathias Curtius. Or Doctor Curtius. Only yesterday Philippe. Never darling, it is true, not dear one. Plain Curtius is acceptable. Nothing else.'

'*Captain* Curtius,' they insisted. 'No one would be more fitting.'

'His place is here,' the widow said, 'among wax people.'

'Yes, yes indeed,' they said, 'and to protect such a distinguished populace, this district must first be protected.'

'No,' said the widow. 'No, this is not right.'

'Captain Curtius,' they said, 'it is a great honour to be elected captain.'

'He does not need this honour,' the widow said to the two men, 'nor your cowardice.'

'His name is already written down at the Hôtel de Ville.'

'Forgive me, Curtius, for what I am about to say,' she said very quietly before turning back to the men. 'Does he look capable? He couldn't do it. He has no understanding of such things.'

'Advance to your duty, Captain Curtius.'

'Captain Curtius?' said my master.

'Captain Curtius, they are waiting for you at the Hôtel.'

'No,' the widow said. 'He shall not go.'

'There is a possibility then,' said Doctor Graham, 'that he shall be arrested.'

328

'There is a possibility then,' said beanpole Nicolet, 'that your property will be raided. We couldn't stop it.'

My master stood up, silent.

'Someone must go in his stead,' the widow announced. 'I shall go!'

'No,' they said. 'No, not at all. Dress. Skirt. No, no.'

Then my master spoke.

'Captain Curtius,' he declared. Statement. No longer question.

'Philippe, stop!'

'Thank you *very* much,' the men said. 'We salute you.'

My master actually saluted them. No army should employ such a salute: it was the vaguest approximation, the briefest wave across the face, as if to shoo a fly.

Even in defeat, the widow always knew what to do. 'Jacques, you shall go with him. Don't let him out of your sight.'

'Yes, I will!' yelled Jacques.

'Let no one touch him.'

'No, I won't!'

'Widow Picot,' my master said, 'I'm a captain. What would you say to a captain? Shall I get a uniform? I should like one. I shall go away to the people. They all know me. They shall say there goes Doctor Captain Curtius.' He took the beauty spot from his chin and placed it on the front of his tricorn hat, as if it were a military decoration.

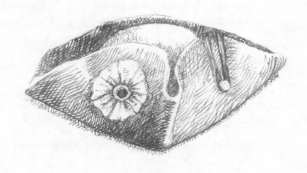

'Today,' said my master to the widow, 'I shall call you Charlotte.'

'Please, Philippe, you must not go!'

'Charlotte, O Charlotte, I'm going out.' He threw up his hands, the wingspan of a heron. 'Keep the doors bolted, let nobody in – that sort of thing. Bye-bye, Charlotte.'

'Sir!' I called.

'Philippe!' The widow was in tears!

I wondered if I should ever see him again.

They set out, Curtius with his old guard dog before him, limping, leading the way. Towards the Hôtel de Ville, along the boulevard towards the old Saint-Antoine gate – long pulled down – where he and I had first entered Paris. At the end of the boulevard they would turn right at the Rue Saint-Antoine, at the fortress there. On that fourteenth of July.

# Chapter Fifty-Two

*Unholy child.*

The noises reached their height a little after five. There had been cannon fire before, but now there was an almost constant roar of voices. When I could no longer concentrate on my work, I went to the backstage rooms, then up the old Monkey House stairs, past the tailor's dummy of old Henri Picot. I had not heard Edmond for some time and wanted to check on him. He wasn't in the attic; he wasn't anywhere. I looked out the window, hoping to see the source of the noise, but all I could see was a shaft of empty boulevard. Then I heard a clamouring roar of people, growing louder. The crowd must be coming closer; if I stayed there in my attic post I should witness it first-hand.

Only then did I notice Edmond. He was down below in the courtyard, within the Monkey House gates, walking back and forth and waving his hands. His mouth was wide open – was Edmond screaming? It was too loud by then to hear anything. As loudly as I could, I called out:

'Edmond! Edmond, come back in!'

But I do not think he could hear me. He went up to the fence and put his head to it. He banged his head against the railings. And then he banged so hard that his head went right through – and stayed there. Edmond's body was one side of the railings, the Great Monkey House side. His head was on the other. And a great crowd was coming on.

'Bring your head in, Edmond! Bring it in!' I called.

But he just crouched there, with his shoulders against the railings

331

and his head stuck out onto the boulevard. I rushed down the stairs, out the back door, and into the courtyard. It was very different outside. The people were gathered like a darkening storm, and growing thicker; the buildings rattled with echoed noises. And there was Edmond, his head through the railings, and the crowd coming on.

'Are you stuck, Edmond? Are you stuck?'

'Lemon vinegar lozenges!' he said.

'Edmond, I shall try to pull you out!'

It was no use.

'Edmond, you won't come free!'

'Potato cakes from Savoy!'

The crowd was in sight by then, such a great mass, a vast organ of people. A great, loud, many-mouthed beast it was, a king rat, stumbling forward on several hundred limbs. Some of the crowd were dancing, some held old pieces of cages above their heads; they were agitated and excited and I wished they'd be gone. When I got to the gates, they were packed close against them, so close that they took my breath. What new creature was this?

'Here's another head,' someone yelled, and then there was laughter.

'No, no, everything is all right,' I said. 'Please, do pass along now.'

'Has he got his head stuck?'

'Help! Help!' I cried back towards the Monkey House. 'Help me!'

'It's true! Another head!' someone yelled.

'Look at that head, would it like to meet our others?'

Then, with some cheering, they hoisted their trophy objects above the fray. Heads. Two heads, on sticks. Very well made, I thought for the smallest instant; perhaps Curtius had made them? Were these the heads the widow was missing? Only then the truth became suddenly clear: these were not wax heads, not at all. These were flesh heads, made by their parents. Real heads. One was shoved now level with Edmond's, as if for comparison, as if they might converse. Edmond screamed, his body bucked and rode, but his head would not come free.

One of the boys from the Monkey House came out.

'Wax,' I shouted at him. 'Bring wax, as fast as you can!'

Wax, I thought: wax would do it. Only wax, rubbed along the bars, would release Edmond in full. Wax is a lubricant; it stops doors and windows from sticking; it works on metal as well as wood. It can be used on humans as well as metal. It stops a hinge from screaming. It might stop Edmond too.

Now the widow was outside. 'Edmond!' she cried. 'Edmond, come in at once.' She pushed me away and tried to pull him back, but even her command wouldn't move him.

'Come away,' the widow ordered me, white and shaking. 'Let them pass along.'

'Bring wax!' I cried. 'Wax to loosen his head.'

'Wax! Wax!' bellowed the widow. Monkey House boys rushing.

'It's the house of wax – I been there,' said some voice in the crowd.

'Seen all the famous bodies!'

'What about ours, then? What about these famous heads? Not bodies, certain, but heads. Heads everyone should know.'

'Launay, governor of the Bastille.'

'Ex-governor.'

'He shot at us!'

'Won't any more.'

Boys came running, carrying wax. I cut some off and started rubbing it along the bars, around Edmond's ears. The widow pushed me out of the way.

'I'm here, Edmond! I'm here,' she cried.

'And this here's Flesselles – he made the people starve.'

The crowd dangled the other head before Edmond. How he recoiled.

'There'll be no more starving!'

'Fat merchant!'

333

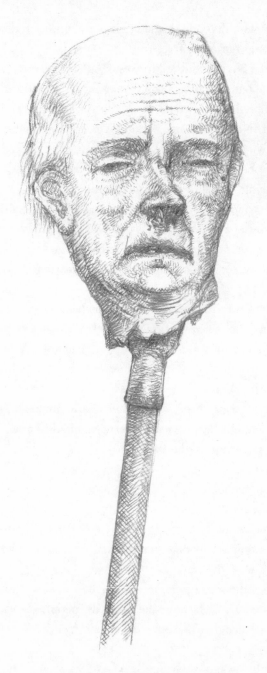

The elongated neck of the Marquis de Launay.

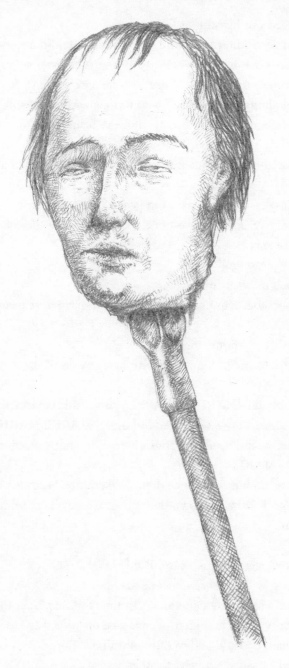

His travelling companion, Flesselles.

'We tugged out his stuffing.'

I'd never seen a murder before, never in my life. I'd never even seen the heads before they were cast. But now here we were, of a sudden, so close to them. So close to some new truth. I couldn't bear to look, but then I couldn't bear to look away. And still poor howling Edmond, in such dismal company, would not come free.

Wax will do it, I prayed. Wax will. Wax must.

'You should have *our* heads in wax,' some voice shouted at the widow.

'Go, please go along, leave us in peace,' she groaned.

'Not yet. Not until you've done the heads. Take these heads. Do them. In wax.'

'No! No, please go!'

'Don't tell us what to do.'

'We'll not stop. Not unless you want us to have *three* heads on pikes.'

'Cut it! Cut it! Slit his throat.'

Edmond screamed again, now with new reason. What a sound he made.

'Marie!' he said. 'MARIE! MARIE!' Real words! His own words, again and again – *my name*, over and over! 'MARIE! MARIE!'

'I'm here,' said the widow. 'Right here, Edmond, your mother.'

'MARIE! MARIE!'

There was nothing else to be done. 'I'll cast the heads for you,' I said at last. 'Follow me down the railing. Come along; bring the heads to me.'

'MARIE!'

'Run, boys; get Curtius's case. Run!'

'How long will it take?' someone asked.

'Minutes,' I said, 'a few minutes, just time for the plaster to dry. I shall be very quick and then you may be on your way.'

'Better had, or we'll add to our collection.'

'No need,' I said. 'No need for that.'

My master's bag, always packed by the side door, was hurried out.

336

'I am ready,' I said.

A man clambered onto the shoulders of a companion and passed a head, still on its pike, over the gate to my side. I was so surprised by the weight that I nearly dropped it. I must cover this item with plaster. Just the face.

'It will not take as long to cast these two heads as usual,' I said. 'They need no straws in their nostrils to breathe through the plaster, and if handled roughly they can be guaranteed not to complain.'

Right there in the Monkey House courtyard, I set about my work. Martin Millot helped me, his hands shaking.

'Some soft soap,' I said.

The head in my lap was the merchant Flesselles. He seemed to look at me with foggy eyes. I knew I should not be holding this head, that I should probably hurl it from me. Was it rubbish, was it filth? How could it be filth when only a moment ago it was the thinking, seeing, hearing, tasting, chewing ball on top of a human body? Are we instantly filth, then, as soon as we die? The unhappy object so missed what so recently was beneath it. How striking we are when fractioned, how odd-looking. And – oh! – the horrible sad heft of a human head. A weight that should never be learned. Poor sphere. I was not cruel to it. For Edmond's sake; for its own.

The second head was that of the Marquis de Launay, governor of the Bastille. This was not in such good condition as the last, though it was the more recently acquired. My lap was soon very damp. Order, I told myself, order. Say it like your master would. Don't miss a thing. Like when you were in Berne. Show your training, boast of it.

'The Marquis de Launay's neck,' I said out loud, as the widow applied more wax around her son's neck and head, 'is cut in jagged lines. There is a rent across his right temporal fascia; the muscles around the inferior maxillary region are badly slashed. The cartilaginous framework of his nose is very collapsed; the whole of that organ is bloody and pushed over to one side; a shard of shattered cartilage is peeking out from the left nostril. The point of

337

the pike has been driven right through the hole, the foramen magnum, at the base of the skull and has progressed considerably into the skull case until it could go no further. The very tip of the pike now rests on the very interior apex of the parietal bones, that is to say at the superior sagittal suture – this fact confirmed by a little cracking I feel just now, on the exterior of the skull, through the marquis's scalp.'

Thus I sat upon a stool just outside the Great Monkey House, casting two bodiless heavy heads for a wild audience just beyond the gates, while above me the sky grew greyer and greyer. And as I completed my work Edmond came free at last, and all of him, one hundred per cent, was back within the gates of the Great Monkey House, exhausted in the panting widow's great lap. The widow was sobbing. I'd seen a grouping like that before: it's called a pietà.

Saved, saved by wax.

When the plaster was dry, Martin passed the two heads back over the gate and the crowd marched away at last, their excitement on the wane. My dress was covered in blood and gore and plaster; I turned aside and was suddenly sick upon the paving stones. I wish it hadn't happened. I should have done better. They're only bodies, after all; it's perfectly natural. But my thoughts were slowing.

'Edmond, Edmond!' I said. 'You called me!' But he was already inside.

It was beginning to rain. I was glad of it. I stayed there, being rained upon. What a thing to have done, I thought. Before long everyone else drifted inside, but I was happy to be alone a while.

When at last I returned to the Monkey House, all three doors were locked.

'You're not to come in,' the widow called. 'I shan't have you inside. Stay out! Unholy child!'

338

# Chapter Fifty-Three

*Flea bite.*

For three hours I stayed in the courtyard in the rain. I shivered upon the doorstep until at last Doctor Curtius and Jacques returned. My master had spent the day at the Café Robert upon the Quai Saint-Paul – Jacques had put him there to keep him safe – and so he had missed everything. Curtius rang the bell and Millot came out, the widow standing behind him at the door.

'She's not to come in!' she bellowed. 'I won't have such a person in here. Disgusting! Unholy!'

My master heard what had happened.

'You cast these severed heads?'

'She did! She did!' called the widow from the door.

'To get the crowd away from Edmond. I thought it was right,' I said.

'How could it be right?' she called.

'It's not right, Marie,' he said.

'I had to give the crowd what it wanted,' I said. 'What else could I do?'

'That was a matter for *me*,' he said.

It took a moment for me to understand him.

'You were not here,' I said.

'I should have been sent for.'

'No one knew where you were.'

'I could have been found.'

'You were with the National Guard. You were needed there!'

'Well . . . I am most upset,' my master said.

'I am more upset,' the widow insisted. 'She kept the murderers here at our gate, while Edmond's own head was caught between the railings.'

'I would never do anything to hurt Edmond,' I said. 'I was trying—'

'Filth! Vermin! Who do you think you are?' she cried.

'A sculptor's assistant.'

'Vile, disgusting, dirty!' she spat.

And I shouted back, 'You do not frighten me, old woman.'

'Both of you, please. Calm,' said my master.

'How can I be calm,' cried the widow, 'with that abomination before me?'

'Come inside,' said Curtius quietly. 'Come inside and get dry.'

'She must not!' screamed the widow. Then she came at me, slapping me about the face, with the front of her hand, with the back.

I wouldn't have that. Not after everything else. I swung my little fist around and struck back at the flesh of her face. That stopped the slapping. And then, in my sudden anger, I struck again. A jab of fist thrust in her face. I did it. I.

I thought I must have pulverised my hand.

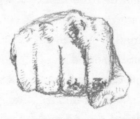

What work! Blood on her lips. The shock of that. I did it. How good it was, the cut upon her lip, the cut on my knuckles from contact with her teeth.

'Murder!' she screamed.

'I *could* murder you,' I shouted, for there was no calming me then. 'I've thought of it often enough. How I've imagined it!'

'Marie! Little!' said my master. 'Have a care! Poor Charlotte!'

340

'I've taken as much from her as ever I'm going to. Maybe I will have *her* head on a stick. How many years have I listened to her small words? I shan't any more. I'll be paid – oh, heavens, I'll be paid now. This very day!'

'Little, you must apologise. You know you must.'

The widow had turned scarlet. 'It's just as Nicolet said: anarchy!' she yelled. 'This is how it spreads, law turned upside down, rebellion in the home.'

'You have a fat lip, Madame!'

'You must beg the widow's forgiveness.'

And then all my hurt over all the years boiled over and came vomiting forth. Those heads had done it: cannonballs of anger, of pain.

'And you!' I said to Curtius, and I turned and kicked him in the shins. 'And you too. How much have I done for you? And what then have you done for me? If it wasn't for me, you would never have had any murderers. I gave you that idea. I got you the royal heads. I am dirty? How could you ever scrub the dirt of guilt from your skins? How many years have I mopped your floors? How many years have I yes-sirred and no-madamed? And what have you done for me? Not even thanked. You could not even speak up for me. So difficult a thing that was for you. What little for Little? Once, woman, you saw a little happiness, a little love growing in your doll's house, and you snuffed it out without a thought. You'd smother anything beautiful with your mean thinking. And now this is the welcome I receive for saving Edmond. I can take so much, but no more.

'You should thank me! I've earned my place! Look at you, red to bursting! Burst, then! You ruin everyone who comes your way. How you bullied Edmond into nothing more than a dishrag – all for that dummy on the landing. Burn that thing and save us the agony! You've reduced my master to a carcass, eaten up with love for you. While you sit around, so heavy with dead love, making such a meal of mourning. Stand back, Widow Picot! Stand back or I swear I'll relieve you of your head!'

'The bitch! The little bitch!' screamed the widow, trying to catch her breath. 'Do something, Curtius! How dare she? Without me you'd all be on the streets. Without me there would be none of this. I do everything in this house. I keep it going. And do you know what a burden that is? Do you know how it is killing me?'

'Die then!' I shouted from the corridor, then marched to my workshop and slammed the door so hard I hoped the whole house would tumble in. I sat for a while, weeping in my bloody clothes. Then, once I had calmed, I started packing my things, certain now that I should be dismissed.

At last Jacques came, carrying a bottle of wine. My master followed soon after.

'Important documents, those heads,' said my master.

'Is that all you can say?'

'Well, Marie, you were very cruel.'

'Anything else?'

'Thank you, I think. Thank you?'

'Anything else?'

'The widow is with her son.'

'Anything else?'

'My shin hurts.'

'Well, it would.'

'I don't know what came over you, but it shall not be ignored. You must apologise, but not yet. For now, leave her be.' He sighed. 'That was not like you at all, Marie.'

'Well, I'm waking up at last, I suppose.'

'I've never seen such a thing. What is happening to us all?'

'I was pushed to it.'

'Marie,' he said, 'will you help me now with the heads?'

'Yes?' I said at last. 'Yes, I will do that.'

And we did. And there they were, all over again.

'Sir,' I asked my master as we worked, 'how was it there? At the Bastille?'

'It was, I think, very terrible.'

'You must have been very brave, sir.'

'Yes. I must.'

'Were you not frightened?'

'Let us concentrate on our work.'

'Missed it,' said Jacques. 'Sorry to say. Should like to have seen it.'

'You missed it, sir?'

'Well, Marie, we were not far away.'

'We was at the Café Robert,' said Jacques, 'on the Quai Saint-Paul.'

'Sir, is that true?'

'Put him there,' said Jacques, 'to keep him safe.'

'Truly, sir?'

'It's heads I'm best at, Marie. The captaining business – I'm not made for it, I'm afraid. Heads, though, I'm quite at home with. It is where I belong, you do see?'

'It was well done, Jacques.'

'Though am sorry to have missed it.'

'Heads, you see, like these.'

Those two heads had provoked a newness in the house. They found my temper, and they split the widow's lip and my knuckles, and they did another incredible thing: they brought Edmond down from the attic. The widow had him moved back to her own bedroom. She wouldn't let me by him that night, but the next day I brought up a bundle containing some material, a little white linen, some thread, a needle, and a pair of scissors.

'What are you doing here?' the widow demanded, blocking the door. Was there just a little bit of fear upon her?

'These are for Edmond,' I said.

'You do not belong on this corridor.'

'I think he might like these.'

'You cannot come in.'

And then from inside the room: 'Marie. Marie.'

'He's calling me. I hear him. Hello, Edmond.'

'Marie. Marie.'

'It's all he ever says,' she admitted in her fluster. 'He's not right.'

'He calls my name. He wants to see me.'

'No, no, it's just a noise. It has no meaning.'

'It's my noise. The noise that means me.'

'Marie. Marie.'

'He does call me. Hello, Edmond! I have brought something for you.'

'Nonsense. He must not have them. He'll hurt himself.'

'I do not think he will.'

'Who cares for your thoughts? When have you grown so bold and important?'

'Since you shut me out.'

'You're an ugly little woman.'

'Yes, Madame? Is that your worst?'

'You have nothing to do with my family.'

'That is hardly true.'

'Get downstairs.'

'Yes, Madame. But only because I decide to. Goodbye, Edmond, just for now. I am glad your mother has noticed you again.'

And though she did not give him the bundle, she let him have some pieces of linen, and out of them Edmond formed a human figure, a new doll Edmond. That was something. He braved himself to the banister and dropped the doll into the hall so I should find it later. What in-house rebellions there were!

# Chapter Fifty-Four

*I am busy.*

Beyond our walls, unrest ruled the streets. Jacques Beauvisage took my master's place patrolling the boulevard with Émile Melin and other muscles. Coming home, small blood on his shirt, he hugged us all and shouted, 'All are citizens!' Soon he had proved himself so thorough in his business that he was appointed head of the National Guard for the boulevard section. My master retreated to the Monkey House until his brief tenure as captain was overturned, whereupon he returned to work in the Cabinet.

Word had got around about our heads of Flesselles and Launay. Now, when a person was cut in unequal portions, we were known as the ones to call on to get a good copy, so that afterwards, when passions had calmed and the sun had come up, the results might be judged with a more rational eye. In this atmosphere, I took command. Every person at Curtius's was primed. Every one of us, no matter how great, nor how small, played his or her role, handing buckets, scrubbing floors, mixing plaster, stirring wax, stitching in hairs, adjusting glass eyeballs, moving plinths, taking money.

Though the widow still would not let me near Edmond, I was emboldened by his voice calling my name. I could do heads; I had proved it. So I did heads, and my master let me. He stood back while I lugged those heavy balls onto my lap – the ones that had come away from the body, and been left, late at night, in our care. No one else wanted the labour, and I didn't mind. No, that's not it: I was glad of it. I felt I was living, such great living. I'd never been in such demand before. These were the most popular of my days. I quite impressed myself. I quite came into my own.

'Truly, sir, may I do it?' I would ask Doctor Curtius.

'Yes, yes, Marie, you may.'

'You do not want it for yourself?'

'I confess I am a little tired.'

'It is a fine head. Do look at the lips, the teeth within.'

'I find I have not the appetite.'

'You say that!' I couldn't help but grin. 'They're just bodies, sir.'

'Of course I know that.'

'Entirely natural.'

'But their ending was not, perhaps.'

'Of course it was! Isn't it a natural thing for a human to kill a human?' I stopped then, listening to myself. 'But . . . yes, sir, yes. Poor man. Poor fellow. It is terrible, isn't it, sir?'

'Very terrible. Murder is, you see.'

'Yes, sir. But I ought to do the head, oughtn't I?'

'Yes, I think you must.'

'I do not mind the work.'

The staff, all those new people, how they looked up to me! They nodded when I came near and kept their distance, such was their respect. I asked them to do things and they did. I'd never before had that experience. Georges was very busy working alongside me; he was not so talkative as before, but that was because there was so much to be done. And we were doing such important work, getting the heads down, putting them in the hall so people could come and see.

Even if the widow did not let me see Edmond, she began to show me new respect. She stopped ordering me around, and soon withdrew from the Monkey House altogether during the day, spending her time with Edmond at the Palais-Royal. She left me alone.

With all the incomings, there was also one outgoing. There was the young fellow of sixteen called André Valentin, the one with the wide-set eyes. It was not his eyes that got him thrown out but his character, for Martin discovered that Valentin was stealing from the cash box. The poor boy was terrified. The widow summoned us all into the great hall and asked Valentin if it was true. He tearfully nodded and begged to be given another chance. The widow stood before him for a moment, then she leaned forward and ripped the 'C' rosette from his breast.

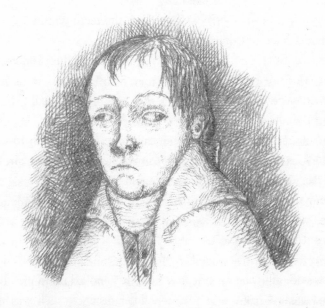

'No! No!' the boy cried. 'Sir, please!'

Curtius only shook his head sadly.

'Put him out,' the widow said.

'Please! Another chance!' he cried, looking both this way and that.

Jacques's boy, Émile, marched him to the gates, shoved him to the other side.

'This is not the end of André Valentin!' he screamed. 'One day I shall return, and then I shall pull this house down!'

I felt for him, poor boy, headed now towards the ditch. But I had no time to wonder over his poor fate. We had wax people to show. We had never been so popular. Men and women every day, hundreds of them, paying three sous each – reduced price for *Vainqueurs de la Bastille*.

# Chapter Fifty-Five

*Some love stories.*

This is the story of a shop. The story of a business, of its highs and its lows, of its staff coming and going, of profit and loss, and sometimes of the outside world and the people that came knocking on our doors. So then. Let me explain.

The royal family, including Princesse Élisabeth – most especially my Élisabeth – were moved from Versailles to Paris. A vast mob of women from the markets had come to the palace demanding bread, and the king, surrounded, fearing for his life, was bullied by a great gathering of common folk. The palace was shut up. I would have been frightened for Élisabeth, but I knew nothing of the bloody upheaval until it was over. A head was brought to me – that was how I knew.

A cloud of fishwives from Les Halles arrived on our doorstep with a parcel wrapped in an apron. They spilled it onto the table. One head, inexpertly severed.

'Here,' a woman said, 'I brought this specially.'

'Well,' I said, 'who is it then?'

'A guard from Versailles.'

'A Swiss Guard?'

'Yes, one of them.'

'I don't recognise this face. I doubt that his own mother would.'

'Make it over in wax.'

'It has been kicked, I think.'

'Ddddd, ddddd.'

That was Florence, the cook. Florence, among them!

348

'Florence, have you been there? Did you go?'

'Ddddd. Did. I did.'

'Oh.'

'Do it,' Florence said. 'Make the head.'

'I wish you had brought it to me before it was so tossed about.'

'Do it.' No smile about her now, none at all.

It was Florence who told me that Élisabeth had been moved. They were so proud of their work, those women.

'Your old home has been shut up,' she said.

What emptiness then. Has there ever been such emptiness as Versailles abandoned? And then: where to put all the people who had lived there?

'I am sorry to hear it.'

'Sorry, are you?' asked Florence.

'Well, for Élisabeth's sake.'

'Sorry? She says she is sorry?'

'No,' I said. 'I can't be, can I? I'm just a servant. I only do what I'm told.'

'Then do that head there.'

'Yes, Florence.'

'And later I'll bake you something nice.'

The next morning I went to the Tuileries Palace, where the royals had been taken. How my heart thumped as I walked through the gardens. There were Swiss Guards and soldiers in formation before the palace and a great thronging of Parisians hoping for an eyeful. I pushed my way to the front – children are allowed to do this, and I was still small as a child – and confronted the guards. I am a former servant of Madame Élisabeth, I said, a special servant. A friend, even. Would they let me in? 'Tell her that Marie Grosholtz,' I said, 'her heart and her spleen, is waiting just outside.'

'Go away, miss.'

'Just tell her. My name. She'll want to see me.'

'No visitors. Get away!'

Someone in the crowd spat at me, then, and another shoved me,

349

and then Georges was beside me, picking me up, come to fetch me because a new head had arrived. And so I hurried home, telling myself I'd be back later. Such unlikely things happened in those days, after all: the people had challenged the royal family. I had challenged the Widow Picot. And this: Edmond was out of the attic. Élisabeth was closer. We lived in Paris, all three of us: he and she and I.

'I shall go soon,' I told my master. 'Make use of me now, while you still can. Once I'm gone, you shall have to take the heads and make them. I'll have no more of it.'

But Élisabeth was not quite ready for me yet. I returned to the Tuileries, but the guards would not even speak to me.

Parisians spent money at the Cabinet of Doctor Curtius. They came to see the latest heads; they talked of citizens and liberty; they looked at each other and at the heads. So many people viewed the new displays of Parisian life; some wept at a distance, others couldn't get close enough. Their money was taken upstairs to Martin Millot, entered in the book and then into the strongbox. I saw it all, for I could walk into the great hall whenever I wished. When the widow went out, she came back a little redder of face, once or twice shaking her head, once even in tears, shouting at everyone.

Beyond the Great Monkey House, there was to be a huge festival.

'What men are these new Parisians, Little!' Mercier said. 'A tableau of concord, of work, of peace. This is the greatest spectacle ever seen. All divisions of citizens are there, preparing for the *Fête de la Fédération*. The multitude of the city has come out to work selflessly in common cause, readying the Champ de Mars for the celebration. All are brothers and sisters, fishwives and aristocrats. Little, we have lived to see it: the perfectibility of man! All will come! All will cheer!'

'Will Princesse Élisabeth be there?'

'Everyone! Everyone!'

'How I should like to see her.'

The rain fell in torrents on the *Fête de la Fédération*, but it did not matter. Thousands of people swarmed into the city, and many of these visited Curtius's wax populace, marvelling at the times they lived in. In that brief moment at the festival, people loved each other and shook hands and kissed their neighbours. A great lightness marked the city; these were miracle days when everyone was beautiful and young, when this city of Paris was briefly utopia. Even Jacques Beauvisage and his Émile thrived within it, roaming the streets, finding and feeding stray dogs, Great Danes and poodles, spaniels limping along the thoroughfares, elegant dogs hastily abandoned by aristocratic owners. Curtius sat with the widow in her office, making her small wax ornaments of fruit or flowers. She did not display them, she kept them in a drawer, but she did not throw them out.

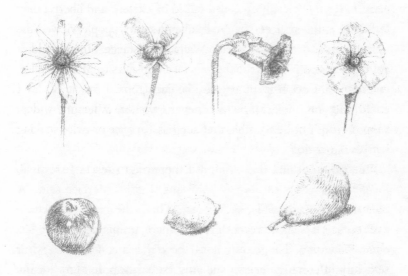

On one of those strange days, in her wax distraction, she left Edmond alone in the courtyard of the Great Monkey House, and I quietly went to him. In the sunlight I saw his blue veins but also a chipped tooth, the mole on the back of his neck. I knew these spots of his: if he was in the sun for any time, freckles would appear on his lower eyelids and on the bridge of his nose, above his dear, uneven nostrils. And then I saw it: his ears began to redden.

'Edmond?'

'Marie.'

'Edmond! Are you there?'

'Marie . . . Here.'

'Are you back? You are!'

And then, so soon, 'Edmond!' called the woman. 'Edmond, where are you? Come at once!' His mother was alert, hollered for him once more, and to her he went. But he turned and waved.

It was during that brief season that Curtius summoned me across into his workshop, almost blushing, some semblance of health upon him. 'Do you know about such things, Little?' he said, shyly. 'Do you have any notion on this topic? Any thoughts? Any advice to give me?'

'What is the subject, sir? You haven't said.'

'I haven't? I thought I had. Well, *love*, Marie. Do you know anything about it?'

'I do, sir, I do. It is my greatest subject.'

'But do you think, Marie, as a person, you *are* a person, do you suppose it might be possible that such as I might love?'

'Yes, sir, I do.'

'But do you think that it might happen that such as I might *be* loved?'

'I do think it possible, sir.'

'You see, since the recent great changes in business, there has come likewise a change over her. I have noted it. Charlotte, dear Charlotte. Before she needed me only for business, but now I think there is a different need. I do not imagine it. No. Love,' he whispered, 'love. What is it? To see that on a face. To capture that in wax. It would be something.'

# Chapter Fifty-Six

*Reductions in the family.*

She did a very stupid thing. Élisabeth did. She tried to get away.
I was so angry with her. To think she'd have left without saying
goodbye. To think she'd have risked her life.

On the night of the twentieth of June, the king, the queen, their
two surviving children, and my Élisabeth — all dressed as assorted
servants and footmen and governesses, roles they could never
convincingly play — fled Paris in a burdensome carriage. At eleven
o'clock the following night, the longest day of the year, the fugi-
tives were apprehended in the countryside and brought back to the
capital. The whole affronted city came out to watch: the people
clogged the streets, filled the windows, climbed the roofs, all watching
the impossible sight of the clumsy royal carriage returning at foot
pace to the Tuileries. The Assembly had mounted signs of warning:

ANYONE WHO APPLAUDS THE KING WILL BE BEATEN

ANYONE WHO INSULTS THE KING

WILL BE HANGED

The crowds kept their hats on as the king passed by. They peered
in the windows of the carriage; they stared so close. I was there
in that crowd; I tried to see her, but I couldn't get close enough.
For just a moment I thought I saw the back of her head, her cap,
a little of her blonde hair. My Élisabeth. She nearly went away, I
told myself, but she's come back, and I shall see her again one day
soon, when she calls for me. She's sure to call now.

The other royal family, my family of wax, were trundled in a cart in the opposite direction, moved from the Palais-Royal to the Great Monkey House. I was so happy to have them, but they were sent now to be exhibited with all the sawn-off heads, with the felons and the guilty. They were no longer displayed in a recreation of the *Grand Couvert*, but rather placed around a simple table with a man in National Guard uniform rushing in upon them as if re-enacting the moment when they were apprehended, at a place called Varennes. There was no time to make a fresh head for the guard, so they found that of a lesser-known poisoner, withdrawn from exhibition long ago, and disguised him with a new black wig. The only royal countenance missing was that of Élisabeth, because I had never modelled her. As if I'd saved her from the scene.

On the seventeenth of July, the National Guard, under the command of Lafayette, fired on a massing of demonstrators, killing fifty. And so the wax Lafayette was brought in to join the criminals on the boulevard, leaving the widow ever lonelier in her dwindling Palais-Royal. The former mayor, Monsieur Bailly, took the same journey, as did Calonne and Mirabeau; all the waxworks were coming home. On the first of April, the widow herself finally abandoned the Palais-Royal. It was almost empty by then, just a smattering of worthies: Voltaire and Rousseau, Gluck and Franklin and the Montgolfier brothers. Edmond was returned to the Monkey House, though kept upstairs.

On the twentieth of April, fearing invasion, France declared war against Austria and Prussia. On the twenty-fifth, the highwayman Nicolas Jacques Pelletier was executed in a very new way, using a machine designed by Monsieur Louis. The Louisette, as it was called, involved a tall wooden frame and a large angled blade; when a lever was released, the blade was dropped from a height directly onto Monsieur Pelletier's neck, causing his head to leap away from his body. Jacques and Émile were there to see it. They came back very disappointed.

'Couldn't see anything,' said Jacques. 'Too fast. Off before you knew it.'

And the shop went about its business, busier than ever. What industry was found within this factory, what a machine for reproducing recent history! None of us had a large understanding of the tides of man; each knew only his little portion. For some it was hair, for others teeth; one concentrated on eyes, another on paint; one mixed the wax, another prepared the plaster. No one could see beyond his own individual station. Only together did we make the anatomy of a city in change; only together did we render things legible to all.

The widow in her office smoked cigars and sucked at quills, wondering if she had missed this or that, fretting over decisions, no longer quite sure which way to turn. She stitched a red Phrygian cap for the head of Louis XVI; when that was over, she worked on the new uniforms for the Cabinet's staff. Once these had been dressed as National Guardsmen, but the guardsmen had lost their popularity after they fired upon citizens in July, so now the boys were to be dressed as sans-culottes, the clothing of the working class: striped trousers and loose shirts and simple jackets. They still wore the Curtius rosette, but to this was added a tricolour cockade: red and blue, the old colours of Paris, and white, the colour of the royal family.

Further down the corridor, I toiled away in the main workshop, opening the moulds and freeing wax heads. With me was Georges Offroy, ready with a palette of pinks and reds. In my old workshop next door was the business of hair implantations and teeth and eyes. On the public floor at the cash box was Martin Millot. We lowered our entrance fees, but the public made up the difference, flocking to us in greater multitudes. Children came quoting loudly from the *Rights of Man and of the Citizen*. Young maids spat at our wax Lafayette, calling him Corrupter. Old men came, speaking only of the fatherland. To visit Curtius's in those days was to be patriotic.

On the night of August the first, no great national event but one of significance in our home, I heard Curtius and the widow upon the landing. My master had hold of Henri.

'It's time to put him away, Charlotte. He's dead! He's dead! Come out with me.'

'I can't!' she said, and there were tears in her voice. 'Be gentle! A little at a time. I'll take away his clothes, but no more. He's my prop. I could have done none of it without him. You never knew him. He's a greater man than you'll ever be.'

'But I am alive!'

'Please, Philippe. I am learning.'

The next morning, Henri was naked upon the landing.

On August the tenth, there was an enormous gathering of citizens demanding the abdication of the king. From the Great Monkey House we heard the shot and cannon of the Swiss Guards defending the Tuileries. Élisabeth! I thought. She is inside there. I went to my workroom and took out the heart and the spleen. 'Be safe, be safe, be safe.'

The Monkey House was locked and shuttered up, like all the other houses around the city. We could not go out; people who did were shot. In the great hall, the hollow people shook a little to the loud report of the guns, Bailly trembled, the members of the royal family tableau jostled in their seats. We lay some of the wax people down upon the ground so that they might not damage themselves should they fall. Everything trembled to the noise of the cannon.

'Please be safe, be safe, please be safe.'

Henri Picot's bell rang out. When the bolts were pulled back and the doors opened we saw Jacques Beauvisage at the gates and with him his Émile. Émile was very slouched, his face very grey, his eyes closed. He was not standing up by himself. And then Jacques Beauvisage, chronicler of the very best murderers, lifted his crop-headed child over the threshold and it was certain that Émile Melin was no longer living. Jacques had at last seen a murder at first hand.

'Jacques, what has happened?' called my master.

'Murder! Murder, murder, murder! Killed my boy. My little boy!'

'Oh, Jacques!' I cried. 'Poor dear Jacques!'

'BOY!' roared Jacques.

By now, the whole city was shut down. Men rode from street to street announcing a penalty of death for harbouring any Swiss Guard from the Tuileries Palace. Searches went on through the night. The whole city was shaken upside down in the hunt. If the Swiss Guards were gone, then the barrier between the common and the royal was dissolved, and all must spill together in a general confusion of flesh. I did not know if Élisabeth was alive or dead.

'Help,' wept Jacques. 'Oh, help!'

In the hot late morning afterwards, in my workroom, it suddenly grew very dark. I went to the window, pushed it open, and there came a horrible buzzing. It was flies on the window glass blocking the light. Thick black clouds of flies moved along the boulevard. There were so many bodies then, all over the city.

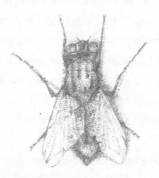

Officers wearing tricolour sashes banged on the door and demanded to know my master's nationality. 'He is Curtius!' the widow yelled. 'Curtius himself.' But the men did not seem to listen. They asked my master again, and he responded that he had been born in Switzerland. Then they asked if anyone else in the building was Swiss, and my master said that yes, his longest-serving assistant, a woman, happened also to be Swiss.

'Two Swiss,' the men said. 'It has been noted.'

'They are loyal citizens of France,' the widow said, 'both of them.'

'They are from Switzerland.'

'This is their home.'

'They are Swiss. Switzerland is their home.'

'They have done nothing wrong.'

'We shall see. Two Swiss. It is noted.'

When they left the widow was shaking. 'You will be safe. I swear it. Even her.'

'Thank you!' I cried. I had expected no such promise from the widow.

'Enough. I don't wish to hear it.'

'But I do thank you. These are the first kind words you have uttered to me.'

'The first? Well. Enough. You have been useful.'

I could not believe it. 'Useful, am I?'

'And, Little,' the widow said, 'one thing further, while I may, you'll want to know. Your Princesse is safe. They're all alive, kept in the Temple. Prisoners, but all alive. This news came several hours ago. You'll want to know.'

'Oh! Thank you!'

'Now, get out of my sight.'

'Yes, I shall, I shall.'

'Then do it.'

To my master she said, 'I don't know the rules any more, they change so fast. I can't guess. She does. She knows more than I! Only she can make anything from these days. Only a creature such as that.'

What had come upon her for her to crack open like this? What danger must we be in, for her wind to be so blown out? She must fear our eviction, I thought. She must fear it very much.

Our welcome on the boulevard, it seemed, was swiftly running out. Florence Biblot, our cook, left us that morning. She said she'd

358

never work for any Swiss. The next day other men came and asked many questions, and wished to see around the building and made many notes, and called my master 'Swiss Curtius from Berne', and no longer patriot or citizen. It was only because Jacques vouched for him that he was not taken away instantly.

Agents returned to the Monkey House daily, searching our rooms, looking for evidence.

'We've done nothing wrong!' cried the widow.

'You harbour Swiss.'

The Great Monkey House was reopened. The Louisette had become the favoured mode of execution throughout the country; an entire factory on the Rue Mouffetard was devoted to producing the machine. By now its name had been changed: when Louisette reminded too many of the disgraced king, it was renamed the Guillotine, after a doctor who had sought for many years a humane device of death-entering for criminals.

To deflect suspicion, the widow and my master put the most reviled figures together in the same part of the hall. The royal family was relegated to the old cage that had once held Lazare, the baboon.

My master, on notice with official Paris, still longed to be seen in the Monkey House. 'She'll come to me, Marie, very soon now. She shall come to me. She needs me. Charlotte. Any day now, just knock, here I am. The walls are coming down.'

'I'm pleased for you, sir. She is most changed indeed.'

Leaving my workshop one night to visit the people who lived silently in the hall, I surprised the widow, kneeling beside the dummy of her late husband, sewing him up. When she saw me she grew agitated, and cursed me for prying; as she got to her feet she jostled the dummy, and it seemed to me I heard him clink.

One morning, I saw André Valentin, the young man with the eyes, back on the boulevard, talking to Martin Millot through the gate. When I approached them, Valentin slunk off.

'What did he want?' I asked.

'Money, of course,' Martin replied. 'Always money.'

'Is he starving?'

'He is hungry.'

'It is best, I think, to leave him alone. He is not entirely to be trusted.'

'He is a Frenchman, nevertheless.'

On August the twenty-fifth we lost five of our staff. They all went off to war, my brave Georges among them, along with thirty thousand others summoned by the Provisional Executive Committee to join the army. We waved them off, so many young men marching out of Paris, drums throughout the city. They never came back.

# Chapter Fifty-Seven

*'Model me.'*

'They're killing them in the prisons.' Mercier had come to give us the latest instalment from the city of Paris. 'This very evening. As I speak to you now, prisoners are being brought forward, and are butchered, without trial, without mercy. These bloodied shoes turned me about and sent me running to you. You will shortly no doubt have many heads, Little.' There was such bitterness in his voice. We were sitting together in the hall, all of us, even Edmond.

'And Princesse Élisabeth?' I asked.

'Not the royal family, no. Priests, mostly, it is.'

'Really?' I said. 'Thank you. I had better make ready.'

Edmond looked at me. I could not tell what he was thinking.

'Sit down, Sébastien,' said my master. 'Drink some wine. We are glad you are here. There has been, in truth, a reduction in visitors of late.'

'Let me tell you about one person in particular,' Mercier continued. 'Upon his body are the bleedings of many men. I do not think even he could say the exact number. He's pulling them apart, hacking into them. Priests and aristocrats. His arms are aching.'

'Mercier, you make no sense,' said the widow. 'Who are you talking of?'

'Doctor Curtius and Widow Picot, may I ask you: where is Jacques Beauvisage?'

'Guarding the district,' said the widow.

'No,' said Mercier. 'I'm afraid not, Widow Picot. Beauvisage is murdering priests who won't submit to the Civil Constitution. He's cutting them open. The life comes pouring out!'

'You must be mistaken,' said my master.

'Your bloody Jacques. I saw him.'

'No, no, I don't think so.'

'He drinks much wine,' he said, setting his own glass aside. 'He's so thirsty, you see. It is hard labour murdering men.'

'I don't think it can be true,' said my master.

'This place,' said Mercier, observing the wax physiognomies, 'is a school for murderers.'

My master blanched. 'We show only what is beyond our gates,' he said.

'But you don't have to show it, do you?'

'We do! We must. The people demand it!'

'These heads will bring on more heads. You must cover them up! Put them all away! You must not show them. You must change this new statuary.'

'They are only what has happened outside, in the city.'

'You cheer it!'

'We observe it.'

'You duplicate it! You hold up the worst and keep it there!'

'There's nothing more honest than wax. Everyone knows that. It can't lie.'

That is truth. Wax never lies – not like those oil portraits in gilt frames I had seen all about the palace. Wax was ever the most honest of substances.

'Cover them up, I beg you!'

'But that would be lying.'

Mercier let out a sorrowful groan. 'This city shall explode.'

Noise outside. The bell rang. A clot of people again. A different clot, but mobs always look the same. Another head had been brought for me, set upon the table, standing upright upon its neck stump. Blonde hair! White skin! Pale-grey eyes!

362

'Oh!' I said in shock. 'This is something else. I knew this head! I spoke to it when it was living!'

'Hush, Little. Marie. Girl,' said the widow as quietly as she could, 'cast it. You don't know it. They'll kill you for knowing it.'

'Is it . . .' said my master, helping me with the plaster. 'Is it Élisabeth?'

'At first, I saw just the blonde hair.'

'Is it?'

'And oh, sir, I thought it was.'

'It is?'

'No. This was – this is some of the Princesse de Lamballe.'

'Oh, it isn't, then. I'm happy for that. That's something surely.'

'Her skin is almost pure white.'

'Think of it then as marble, if that helps.'

'But to know a head, sir!'

'On we go.'

'I've never known a head before! As if we're getting closer and closer to them.'

'Come now, Marie, lift up the head.'

'There's the weight.'

'Good girl.'

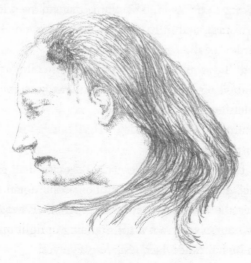

Edmond watched us, busy with the head, and did not look away. His eyes were very wide but he was not crying. He was sitting very upright and holding on to his seat. When our work was done and they'd taken the head out from the Monkey House, I saw Mercier seated in the corner. He was the one weeping.

'I should have left you in Berne,' Mercier said.

'Then I should have never known such beauty,' replied Curtius, looking at the widow.

'Oh, Little,' Mercier said. 'Little cruelty, little knife, little bloodstain. How your face suits the age. How you do come into yourself: little nightmare.'

'Why do you say those things?' I asked. 'Why do you insult so? What have I done to merit it? I didn't cut the heads, did I?'

'Goodbye,' said Mercier. 'I do not think I shall be calling again.'

Mercier was let out through the gates. He stopped, turned back, and kicked the building before he went.

'Happy enough to drink our wine,' said the widow.

'In truth,' said my master, 'I never much cared for his head.'

Later that night, while we sat in the hall, the widow beside my master, Henri Picot's bell was rung again. Jacques Beauvisage was on the other side of the gate, a sabre in one hand and a musket in the other, asking to be let in. The words that follow were spoken in whispers (inside), and in roars (outside).

'He'll murder us all,' said the widow.

'No,' I said, 'he would never hurt us.'

'There's blood on him,' said Martin Millot. 'I see it.'

'Shall we let him in?' asked Curtius.

'He's not himself,' said the widow. 'He'll butcher us all and then weep about it in the morning.'

'Jacques,' I said. 'Our own bloody Jacques.'

'Model me!' Jacques shouted from the gates. 'Model me!'

'It's against the rules,' the widow whispered. 'We don't model ourselves. We ourselves are not for display. We do not take part.'

'I've been busy!' called Jacques.

'He's very drunk,' I said. 'No, he's not himself.'

'Best let him sleep it off on some doorstep,' said Curtius.

'What sleep,' asked the widow, 'can sleep that off?'

'Busy! Oh, busy!' he cried. 'These hands!'

There was a long silence.

'Has he gone?' asked Martin.

'I think so.' But then,

'Oh, help!' Jacques called out at last. 'Help Jacques! Who will help Jacques?'

'I cannot bear it,' said my master.

'Little, help! Little!'

'I want to go to him,' I said.

'Émile! Émile!' Jacques whimpered.

'He is a little quieter. He's calming,' said the widow, 'but we cannot let him in.'

'What to do?' he wailed. 'What to do now?'

'He'll go away soon enough,' said the widow. 'He'll quieten down.'

'Family!' Jacques cried. 'Mother! Father! Sister! Brother!'

'Jacques Beauvisage,' I whispered, 'hush now.'

'I! I! I! Help! Help me!'

He screamed, a long hideous animal howl. All was silent, he was gone.

'Tomorrow, sir,' I said, 'we must look for him.'

'Yes, Marie, he'll be calmer then. I shouldn't be surprised if he comes back later and sleeps by the gates.'

Jacques Beauvisage did not come back that night, or the next morning. Streaked with blood, he had thrown away the softness of his bed, had shaken off warmth and comfort, had cast himself and his agony back upon the streets.

That night the city was a very new place, and the boulevard had lost all its noise. Where carriages and people once coursed up and down in their business, now all was silent. The gates of the city were locked. Patrols of pikemen were in every street, banging on the doors. On the river, boats were positioned at regular intervals, with armed men inside who shot at whatever moved.

In the morning, when the city gates opened again, Curtius and I went out to search for Jacques, calling his name, whistling, shouting. We stopped people in the streets. We offered a reward for news of him. But that day, and for many days thereafter, none came.

'My Jacques,' said Curtius in grief. 'My child! What happens if there are thieves in the night? Who will guard us now?'

# Chapter Fifty-Eight

*No feelings.*

While the gates around the city and all the shutters and all the windows were closed by order of the Commune, while certain essential streets of the city were lined four deep with soldiers, Curtius, the widow, Edmond, and I were sitting in the church of the Madeleine, on the Rue de la Madeleine, summoned early that morning on National Assembly business. Having received the written order to appear, we had been up early, had washed and dressed ourselves carefully. Martin Millot had looked us over, brushed us down, made all our tricolour cockades stand out proud, then stepped back to look us over and sent us off with a wave.

'You'll do,' he said. 'What a day. You have all deserved this.'

Off we went. I turned around to return his wave, but my eye was distracted by a solitary figure on the street nearby, his high collar turned up against the wind.

We spent that long morning at the Madeleine church, so many hours waiting that I nearly forgot why we were there. At last I heard a roll of drums, then a silence, and then a noise that hit the church windows like a massive clap of thunder, an enormous and sudden burst of cheering. We adjusted ourselves a little, sat upright, brushed ourselves down again. Shan't be long now. Any moment now. What butterflies. Curtius's stomach groaning. The widow sweating despite the cold. Edmond holding Edmond in his lap. We kept looking at each other, Edmond and I. But we carried on waiting, just waiting. Not saying anything to each other.

At about ten thirty the gates of the city were opened again, and the day's business could begin. Then shutters throughout the city were pulled back and people appeared at windows, people went about their ordinary business and bought vegetables and meat from the late-opening markets or drank coffee, had a game of chess, went back to bed. At about that same time, just after half past ten, our package arrived for us. We were led outside. The major part was in a barrow; a pit had been dug in the churchyard, and quick-lime was ready in a bucket. We received the parcel in a basket, and were bidden to hurry.

'It's missing most of its hair,' Curtius noted.

'Sold in little bushels,' said one of the men with the barrow.

I had it in my lap, the weight.

'You should hurry,' the barrow man said.

'I think your woman is crying,' said the barrow man.

'I do not think so,' said my master. 'Marie, are you? This is not like you at all.'

'She shouldn't be crying. It isn't right.'

'We are anonymous, Marie,' said my master. 'And we have no feelings at all. We could never afford feelings; they are other people's business. You should know this better than anyone. How many heads have we done? Why this fuss now? We are newspapers. We record only. We are privileged, Marie, to see what we have seen, and this is the pinnacle of that privilege. Kings die, too, in all sorts of ways. History records it so. And now we record it too. Fact. Fact.'

'Thank you, sir. I am better now.'

'And now, this is not right,' said the barrow man. 'The old woman is crying too.'

The Widow Picot, impregnable fortress, had a spot of the king's blood on her lap. She poked at it with her finger. Her eyes, it is certain, were watery.

'The king,' she whispered. 'Oh, the king. What have we done to come to this?'

It was such a head that even the widow was unmoored by it. Edmond, having already lost his breakfast, sat shivering beside his mother, the cloth Edmond in his mouth.

Curtius and I settled down to work. We passed the head between us so that it might be cleaned a little: the width of the severed neck, the slice of the meat, the clots in it, the splinters of bone. I applied the pomade to the face, taking care not to open the eyelids. There was not much expression. A little wrinkling on the brows; the lips had to be pushed into position and held there. Teeth grated down by so much sugary pastry – no, not that, do not think of that.

'*Robinson Crusoe*,' I said, 'was his favourite book.'

'Oil,' said my master.

'If they can do this to him, I think they might do it to Élisabeth, mightn't they?'

'Plaster,' said my master.

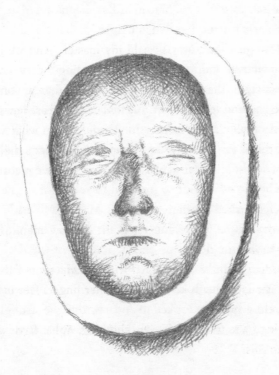

When we were done they put the two parts in the simplest wooden box and covered it with the quicklime. I placed the dried plaster moulds in Curtius's father's case, pending further instruction from the National Assembly. Those empty moulds were more palpable than anything else Curtius had ever made. Then we set off for home, taking turns carrying the heavy bag. I wondered, as we walked, what we would do now with the wax models of the king, the one sitting at table that I had modelled after so many drawings and the one standing that I had cast from life. They were complete models after all, each in one large piece. It was wrong of them to be in one piece still; they should have come apart automatically after the king's execution.

The widow took the bag from me.

'I'll have it now,' she said. 'You've taken it far enough.'

I was part of the family, you see.

When we reached home, I saw that the door marked OUT and one of the gates were open. Martin Millot, I considered, must have left them open for us. I called out to him, but he didn't come. Inside, all was just as before: those heads on sticks, all those personalities thrown over. Curtius put the bag down on the floor, but that didn't seem right; the widow put it on a table. I took the moulds out of the bag and left them on the table with the order from the National Assembly so that everything would be in its place when they were called for. Curtius's bag must always be prepared; I went into the workshop, replaced the plaster supply and the pomade, and left it by the back door so it would be ready for the next time.

When I returned to the great hall, Martin still hadn't come down, so I went to fetch him. He wasn't at his tall stool in the counting room, the desk was empty. I saw that the door of the strongbox was slightly open. That's unlike Martin, I thought, to keep it open; he's usually so strict on such things. I was just going to push it closed when I looked in and saw that the strongbox was empty. There was nothing on the shelves except a single piece of paper.

370

Which I took, and ran back downstairs, screaming as I ran. I screamed as I thrust the paper into the widow's hands. I was still screaming as she took it.

She was seated with Curtius on the bench in the great hall, lottery winner Cyprien Bouchard between them. Her head bent down to read it:

*I have taken 17,675 assignats.*
*I have taken 12,364 Louis d'or.*
*I have taken the 9,000 livres the Widow Picot keeps in her husband.*
*This dirty business is over. I finish it.*
*By the time you return home the gates will be open long since and I will be gone.*
*In signature, Martin Millot*

The widow's head stayed down, reading the note. It stayed down, but I knew it would come rising up again. She always knew what to do. The widow's head stayed down, but any moment now, any moment, it should come up. This was a hard blow, certainly, but she'd fix it. She always knew what to do. We relied on her. The widow's head stayed down. Any moment now, any moment.

The widow's head stayed down.

It stayed down.

It did not come up again.

## Book Six

### 1793–1794

# Quiet House

*My years thirty-two and thirty-three.*

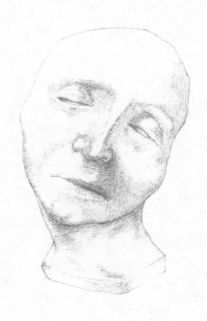

# Chapter Fifty-Nine

*Quiet House on Quiet Street.*

Where were the people arriving in their droves after the end of work? They were not here. They were not coming. Who had money to spend on entertainment, now that bread and candles and cloth had tripled in price? The boulevard entertainers had moved on, packed up, taking entertainment elsewhere. Doctor Graham's establishment had a sign tacked across its door: TO LET. All gone, all gone. What a tumble, what a loss. Not a firework. Not a spark. The Boulevard du Temple had gone out, renamed 'Quiet Street'.

The Great Monkey House appeared abandoned; the front gate Martin Millot had left open, never closed since, now slouched towards the ground. Had Martin robbed us on his own, or did he have help? It seemed so unlike him. Someone surely must have assisted. Weeds grew through the cracks in the courtyard; children played upon the flagstones and no one shooed them away. The rusted bell on the twisted gate was mute. When the widow couldn't raise her head, the Cabinet had simply stopped. It had lost its head.

Not that the house was empty. You shouldn't know it, but there were people inside. Four hearts still beating. One faintly perhaps, but another speeding up, as if in compensation.

'I am a doctor,' Curtius said, 'and you, Edmond, are the son, and you, Marie, are – well, you are Little. Now there shall be nothing but facts, only facts. Nothing but truth, Charlotte. Dear Charlotte: apoplexy.'

Edmond and I gathered straws from the workshop, the same

ones that had been used to help people breathe as they were cast. Now they went into the widow's twisted mouth, to help her feed.

'Apoplexy, I'd almost swear to it,' Curtius said. 'Ligature around the neck, perhaps; a congestion of the brain. Hemiplegia, a fifty-per cent palsy. Or an aneurysm? Are you sensible, Charlotte? Are you understanding what is going on? Will you make a sign? If I could see inside,' he said, lightly stroking her mob cap with the tips of his fingers, 'I'd know instantly. If I could just have a look. Is there clotting? Is there swelling? A crack somewhere? I mustn't look in, though you're keeping the secret from us. Have you had an accident in your head? Help me. I don't know what to do. Charlotte, don't stop. Please, I beg you, do not stop.'

She would only stare at the ceiling. She drank and that was good, though Curtius had to persuade her by holding her nose. She breathed on, and that, he said, was the essential point.

'I'll always be here,' he told her, patting her hand.

A little dribble fell from her mouth down her chin. He dried it.

'Do you need changing?' he said with a sniff. 'You do. I shall change you. Now, Marie, Edmond, off you go please, this is my business. I must shift your mother, Edmond. I must move this great lady, Marie, who has been so much to you. Come back in a little while. I can manage on my own. I'm growing muscles for you, Charlotte. I'm growing very strong. No, Charlotte, I do not miss those other heads. No, I don't care for them at all. I've all I need here. And am much the richer for it.'

Doctor Curtius's new days were days of love. He loved the labour, he loved her sweat and spittle, he loved whatever her body made. Even her groans were not unlovely to his ears, for they were hers. Feeling brave, he would whisper:

'Oh, I love you, I love you. I love you. Did I never say?'

And since no one stopped him, he no longer whispered it, but announced it quite loudly to the right side of her and to the left, so that she might hear. He declared it as often as he could. Sometimes he sat at the broken side of her, looking with sorrow at her drooped face, at the arm and leg that never moved, the slug-shaped portion of the mouth, the eye with the sagging lid.

'Let me tell you about yourself,' he said. 'You're big and moley and hairy, yes you are. There's Charlotte the businesswoman with her cigar, what a success she is; how proud we are of her. You're many shades of wonder. There's Charlotte the mother; what a fine boy. There's Charlotte the head of household; what attentions you give. There's Charlotte the widow too; we must not forget her, a smaller Charlotte than the others. That one can go, perhaps, that one's Charlotte the past. There's Charlotte the present, too, isn't there? After all, here she is in her bed. One side leans backwards, the other, I think, still holds on, doesn't it? A little forward? Yes! There she is, Charlotte the future. Perhaps the best of all possible Charlottes.'

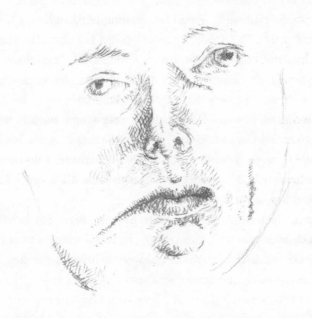

IN and OUT were closed. The plaster mould of the head of the executed monarch awaited its summons from the National Assembly. It never came. No one seemed to want it. There it lay, two halves of a mould tied together. Inside that plaster shell was a hollow space that represented enormous history. We were its guardian.

In those days, Edmond and I were suddenly together. There was no one to stop us. And being together after so long, at first we had no words for each other. We just stood near each other, never leaving each other's side but not knowing quite what to do in this strange freedom. Sometimes we left the Great Monkey House, going out upon Quiet Street for small rations: hours in the bread queue, our former neighbours looking at us, not without pleasure to see us so dishevelled now. Sometimes, when we were nearly at the front of the queue we were sent to the back; sometimes, when we got to the front again, there was nothing left. One day, it was a young man with fishlike eyes who pulled us out, dressed in new clothes, a fine sabre at his side.

'Dead yet?' he asked.

'No, André Valentin,' I said, for it was he. 'She seems a little better today.'

'So much the worse. Where are your papers? I'll see them again.'

'We've already shown them.' In those days, our papers were always with us.

'I'll see them again – I'll see them whenever I choose. Swiss! Do you know what we do with Swiss? We *arrest* Swiss. And we cut off their heads. I wonder how many Swiss there are remaining in Paris these days. The number must be very small, ever shrinking.'

'How did you get your sword, citizen?'

'I earned it. Tell me, how's business?'

'It is slow of late.'

'Yes, yes, I know it is! What a shame for you now that you've thrown poor Valentin out upon the streets. Off with you, back of the line.'

After André Valentin was left on the boulevard the other side of the gates, blood coming from his nose, he had not been idle. He'd shaken his fist at the Great Monkey House, and other people seeing him had joined in. What a deal of fist-shaking there was.

Valentin had turned to his brother and sister fists and told them what a terrible place it was, and they had said, 'Could you tell us more?'

'Yes, much more! How long do you have?'

So they took him in, and for food and wine he told them terrible tales, and in this way André Valentin survived. I believe it was dreams of destroying the Monkey House that kept him among the living.

After Jacques Beauvisage disappeared, Valentin had found himself a job policing the district, looking into other people's things with his eyes, which viewed things at strange angles, and found there evidence that others had overlooked. He pulled open a woman's dress and found dangling from her neck a locket; opened, it showed a picture of the king, and so she was executed. He found a Swiss Guard in the sewers, and he was drowned on the spot. He found a child with a doll of the queen, and the child and the child's mother were imprisoned. And recently, somehow, he had come into money, enough to buy himself advantages here and there; we had our suspicions about that money, but we had no evidence, and no one would support a foreigner's claims against those of a patriotic citizen. André Valentin had grown official, strutting back and forth with a fat tricolour ribbon upon his chest, and we could do little to stop him. He was one of a new tribe of men grown so loud in those days, not in himself longing for liberty but finding such advancement among those who proclaimed it.

Edmond and I came back from the markets with very little, sometimes nothing at all. Once, we returned home to a terrible noise above. Rushing upstairs, we found my master heaving things about.

'Sir! Sir, what are you doing?'

'Help! Give me some help.'

'Oh,' said Edmond.

'I'm moving my bed. We're moving in together.'

'Oh,' said Edmond, desperate. 'Oh dear!'

'If you won't help, go away!'

So his mattress lay beside her bed, on the healthy side.

'This is my happiness, there in that bed. *My* happiness. My life. Prop it up. The left side is weakness, but the right side is sound. I'll have it all, Marie, left and right.'

She lay still in a heap, her eyes fixed on the ceiling, while around us the rooms fell into ruin.

# Chapter Sixty

*The Celestial Bed of Doctor James Graham.*

Some buildings, no matter what befalls them, whether they are abandoned or painted over, whether left alone or leased to new and destructive lodgers, still retain their characters. The establishment vacated by Doctor James Graham was just such a place. Gone from the boulevard was Doctor Graham, fled back to Scotland, and yet some portion, some scent, some essential deposit of this doctor remained. Perhaps it was longing; perhaps it was lust; whatever it was, something of him persisted when he departed, and whatever it was could not get out of the house. DOCTOR GRAHAM'S CELESTIAL BED – TO LET was across the boulevard from us, and in those long mornings and afternoons I took to looking out of the window at the abandoned building.

Upon the outer walls were the flaking remains of two silhouettes, one a man, the other a woman, neither enrobed in any way. I watched those ghostly forms. Edmond came and sat beside me. He was in the light then.

'Edmond,' I said. 'Edmond, I see you very clearly now.'

'Marie,' he said. 'Yes, Marie. I am glad it's you.'

He held my hand. Sitting together at the window, he very close to me, we observed the place of Doctor Graham's. We watched the house opposite. I wondered how it should be to stand inside.

Upon a foggy and scarcely populated evening we approached Doctor Graham's house. We crossed the muddy safe zone between our building and his, led on by those silhouettes. We stood on tiptoes and tried to look in, and at first we saw nothing. Just darkness.

Around the back was a door that we discovered could be easily jemmied open and we stepped inside. We dared to light a candle. Having come in the back way, we entered now the part of the property that we immediately understood was not for the general public. We had come, Edmond and I, upon the dressing rooms of Doctor Graham's house. Cracked mirrors, a frayed underskirt upon the floor, make-up pouches, a stale message inscribed on a piece of yellowing card: 'MEET ME AT RAMPONEAU'S CAFÉ? THE USUAL TIME?' and signed 'FAMISHED VICTOR'.

We travelled along a plain corridor into the belly of the house. Why did the air feel so thick in there? And what was the smell of the place? Some musk or spice I did not know. We reached now the entrance hall and stopped there a while to read a notice painted upon the wall:

Welcome to the temple of Doctor Graham, constructed for the propagation of beings rational, and more beautiful in mental as well as bodily endowment than the present puny, feeble and nonsensical race of probationary mortals, which crawl, fret, and politely set about cutting one another's throats for nothing at all on most parts of this terraqueous globe. Welcome inside, welcome indeed. You shall not be disappointed here, but henceforth be CHANGED. Step in, open yourselves to greater influences. Only step in. Step in.

'Edmond,' I said, 'shall we not take this tour ourselves, step by step, as it is written? Let us follow it as if this place were once again open to the evening's crowd.'

'Yes, Marie,' he said.

'Good,' I said, and read the new words out aloud: 'Proceed, under the new influence of unfettering music and balmy odours.'

We moved into a chamber where the walls were painted with naked figures very close together; illuminated by Edmond's flickering candle, they seemed to be moving. MUSIC SOFTENS THE MIND OF A HAPPY COUPLE, MAKES THEM ALL LOVE, ALL HARMONY, said one banner painted overhead.

'We must imagine that there is music, Edmond.'

'Yes, Marie,' he whispered, 'I can almost hear it.'

Up the stairs we went, holding banisters padded in stuffed silk. At the top of the stairs was a large door, this too with writing upon it:

Inside will be found THE CELESTIAL BED OF DOCTOR GRAHAM. Neither myself nor any of my servants need ever see or know who the parties are in repose in this chamber, which I call the SANCTUM SANCTORUM! The CELESTIAL BED OF DOCTOR GRAHAM. The whole of the apparatus in this apartment, of which I can give little idea in words, has been fitted up at great expense, the result of a long and intense study. Now. Open the door!

Edmond did so. But we stood not before the Celestial Bed of Doctor Graham but before an antechamber. Another door faced us, with another legend emblazoned above it:

THE TEMPLE OF HYMEN.

There were further instructions: 'Do you now, allow my servants to take from you your possessions which shall be returned to you, more sweetly smelling when all is done. HUSH NOW! Do not speak a word!'

Edmond's candle was shaking increasingly, I saw – but as I was about to put out my hand to steady him, I found mine too was shaking. We read on:

'It is entirely sensible and proper for initiates, should they feel the need, which shall always be encouraged, to help the partner with the shedding of society's lent things. No shoes within. No jacket. No bonnet. No wig. No dress. No breeches. No shirt. No corset. No underdress. No underclothes. No thing. No thing at all.'

And the words were of such a commanding nature that, shaking though we were, we obeyed and began, as if in a trance, the business of undressing each other: fumbling with each other's garments, loosening everything and letting it fall to the floor in a pile, all the while gasping for air. The covered part of Edmond was uncovered now. And he whispered to me:

'Marie, your nipples are very small and very pointy. I hadn't thought of that.'

And I said nothing.

And Edmond said, 'They are very nice.'

And then I gently said, 'Ssssh,' for there was another sign: NO WORDS. NO WORDS AT ALL. ONLY MUSIC. LISTEN UNTO THE MUSIC.

But all the music we could hear was the drumming of our hearts.

Now Edmond, moving before me, opened the door to reveal a great silk curtain in front of us on which had been painted the commanding words, PROCUL! O PROCUL ESTE, PROFANI! We found the opening in the curtain, and we went through it, and Edmond whispered:

'The Celestial Bed of Doctor James Graham!'

There was no doubting it, for no other object in the history of objects constructed for horizontal humans ever resembled it. It measured a whole twenty feet by fifteen, and suspended above this considerable surface was a large dome, with a circular mirror inside that reflected perfectly the ruffled silken sheets below. Beneath the dome was the colossal headboard, with yet another instruction from Doctor Graham:

BE FRUITFUL. MULTIPLY AND REPLENISH THE EARTH.

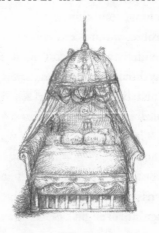

Edmond and I were so small before it. There were not even steps to climb up. Had we been introduced to a simple bed of a quiet and retiring nature, had we entered into an honest, unassuming, and sympathetic location, we might perhaps have been more at ease with one another, but faced with this palatial structure, built for titans, we were very small and uncertain.

I felt watched by that strange chamber, as if I myself were a wax person to be considered from all angles. Thirty-two years old. A diminutive woman. I climbed up onto the bed and pulled the dusty sheets over me. After a moment Edmond followed.

He put his lips on mine, very dry lips at first, and then he kissed me on my cheeks and my neck. Edmond made a sighing noise as if he was very sleepy, and then I was gently pushed onto my back and then he continued kissing from the neck downwards, his lips not so dry now. There was a gentle kissing on my shoulder. I felt him descending still further, and he arrived shortly after at my breasts, which were touched by his fingers and then kissed. 'Your back arched,' he whispered then. 'You gasped!'

Very shortly afterwards, Edmond Henri Picot pushed himself into me, and filled me, and I was held and rocked. I closed my eyes, and in the darkness there was Edmond again.

'I am Edmond Henri Picot,' he said, 'and you are Marie Grosholtz, known as Little, and that is just how it ought to be, and should have been a long, long time ago.'

And so. Once there was an impenetrable girl called Marie Grosholtz, until one afternoon she was cracked open and another Marie Grosholtz was discovered beneath, a painful skinless person, who was existing just beneath the surface. And would not be covered up any more.

That was living. That was such living. I was in love.

In love with Edmond.

Afterwards, we both of us felt our yearnings, at many odd moments, to slip across the boulevard and bring ourselves together upon Doctor Graham's broken bed. Sometimes we were in such a

385

rush for it that I would remain in my dress and Edmond would trip over his fallen breeches and his stockings, all wrinkled around his feet. And it did not matter that we were the only genuine thing in that abandoned property, we made it live again. For me, for my life, it was this body of all bodies, the one that was Edmond Henri Picot, that was mine. I became the greatest expert of Edmond Henri Picot and was enormously proud of my scholarship. We truly fitted together, ulna to radius, fibula to tibia. And always, at the end, there was Edmond, staring at me so intently, laying his head upon my chest.

This life, I thought, goes on and keeps surprising.

This little box, this chapter, ends here, sealed tight from those others that surround it, so that those other people of different chapters may not come in here and disturb, so that its vault may be sealed up, never spilling beyond its boundaries but kept tight shut and precious, and godly and triumphant, and wonderful too. But remain only itself. Wax, also, is privacy. Wax seals letters. Wax keeps all the world's words where they should be, until the right hands come to let them out.

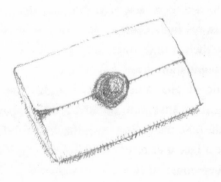

# Chapter Sixty-One

*Sixth heads.*

In the line for bread, I said to some confused stranger, 'Edmond Picot's unpeeled me.' Walking home, I stopped an old man to announce with joy, 'I am unbuttoned!' I told a young mother, 'I am loved! *I* am!' Those were our days, Edmond's and mine, with occasional interruptions from my master. When we were not considering ourselves, when we had my master's company, we looked about us and considered everyday things – windows and shutters, lintels, doors and their handles – and were grateful for them. Buildings kept upright, so that we might live inside them. We said our good mornings and good evenings to each other. These days we sat at table not in the dining room, for we had seen a rat opening a cupboard there, but in the old kitchen. A setting for the widow was always laid. Children played outside on the broken paving stones, their sounds disturbing our brittle home.

The wax population grew dusty. The king's severed head remained made of air. When we visited the figures, removing certain among them that were no longer safe to display, our feet left tracks in dust. So many likenesses had become dangerous. You must not have a face that resembles Mirabeau; you must not have a Lafayette; there must be no evidence that such a person ever had a face. The royal family – most of all the royal family – were not to be at your home, not at dinner, not even in a cage.

Like her king, the queen was executed; we stayed inside that day, though we still heard the cheers. But Élisabeth was still alive, kept prisoner in the Temple. And I knew I must not visit her, for such a thing would threaten all our lives. I satisfied myself by walking by the building once a week. I must wait, I thought. They'll be satisfied now they've taken the queen. They'll be quite full up now.

Our footprints in the dust of the great hall resembled a history of the French people, as we dragged the forbidden ones into back rooms and there undressed them – first of their clothes, then of their heads. The bodies remained in one piece; only the heads were dangerous. We lifted the forbidden heads, Edmond and I, high above our shoulders and then we hurled them to the floor, smashed them one by one, until they all were mixed in together. Edmond handed me the heads of the royal family. It was my privilege since I had made them. And down they tumbled. A nose of the queen muddled up with the ear of her husband or the chin of her brother-in-law, or with a piece of Mirabeau's pitted cheek, or Bailly's empty eyesockets. (Eyes were saved because they could be used again.) We walked upon all those yesterday heads, crunching them underfoot, then swept up all those fractions and dropped them, every last crumb, in our great brass bowl. Then we lit the fire and melted them all together.

Once they had liquefied, and we'd put out the fire, Curtius stood over the bowl with great dignity to perform the rite. Putting his hands over the cooling substance, feeling its last heat, he muttered:

'Man that is born of wax hath but a short time to live.'

Half an hour later, we upturned the big pan and, with a little help from a palette knife, freed the contents. With a thump it fell upon the table, a large half-sphere of melted time, utterly illegible. Heads lost. Surfaces forgotten.

I sat down next to my master, quiet now. The widow was sleeping upstairs.

'So much work,' I said.

'Some fine work, some not so fine.'

'All gone. Lost forever.'

'And yet,' he said.

'And yet, sir?'

'We have the moulds. Not quite forgotten after all. Only invisible.'

388

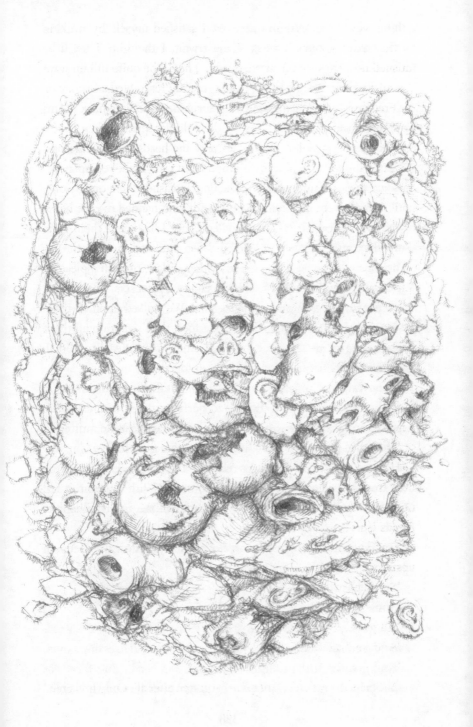

There we were, Edmond and I, holding hands in the back rooms of the Great Monkey House. There was Doctor Curtius, busying himself around the Widow Picot, whose merest noise would prompt him to marvel: 'Listen to her! What spirit!'

But our life could not continue undisturbed. Late one night, near midnight – we had been asleep – a sound rang through the hall. We barely understood it at first; we had forgotten what it was.

Someone was ringing Henri Picot's bell.

Ten men. Coming past the rusting fence, banging upon IN, banging upon OUT.

'They won't go away,' I said. 'I'll tell them we're closed.'

'I can't go down,' said Curtius. 'I mustn't leave her.'

'Perhaps they've come for the king at last.'

I went down. Edmond came too.

'Is it only you?' they asked.

'Yes,' I said quickly, 'just us here.'

'Where's the master?'

'Not available,' I said.

'Do you have equipment?'

'Do you mean for casting?' I asked, surprised. 'Yes?'

They said we had better come at once, that we should bring our equipment. They took us across the river. Hurry, hurry, they said. To a small house with a great crowding around it. People weeping. Our escort pushed us through. We went up to the first-floor apartment, where we were led along a corridor filled with men all gathered around a single woman in a striped dress, slightly ripped, whom they would not let go.

'What has she done?' I asked.

'Murder,' was the reply.

We were ushered into a crowded bedroom. The crowd parted, revealing a man upon the bed, naked save for an old dressing gown, a sort of white turban wrapped around his head. The face was moon-shaped and very pitted, the large eyelids were not quite closed, the wide mouth was open, the tongue sticking out a little from the corner, the skin was diseased, sores, scabs, broken wheals. There was a great hole in the chest, a deep, dark mouth; you could see right down its throat. The man had begun to congeal; the liquids inside had steadied and started their darkening.

'Are you all right, Edmond?' I asked.

'Yes thank you, Marie,' he said. 'Do not worry about me. I'm very strong. I'm made of tough stuff. You tell me what to do, and I'll be doing it right beside you. There, I quite surprise myself! There, I looked at him again. A dead, murdered man.'

A deafening roar outside: the girl from the corridor had been taken down.

Beside the body stood a tall curly-headed man with a sketchbook. He put his pencil down and turned towards us. I'd thought him very beautiful at first, but when he turned I saw his left cheek: a swollen, twisted thing, a bit like the widow's, that stretched the left side of his mouth into a gash. He spoke in strange, stammering words.

'Whaa-whoooo?' he asked.

'We are from Curtius,' I said. 'We have been trained. I've done heads before, dead ones, living ones. Edmond Picot does the bodies.'

'Currrrtiasss?'

'Could not come.'

'Mussht make the whole b-bady in wacks.'

'Yes, sir,' I said. 'We can do that.'

'And kwuck!'

'Yes, sir, right away.'

'It phades, the bady. It is ratting.'

'Yes, indeed, it has certainly begun to decompose.'

'And I musht pain it.'

'Paint it, sir?'

'Pain the mardured heerow fah the Cunnnvunshan.'

'You are a painter, sir?'

'I yam Daffeeeeed.'

He was. Jacques-Louis David. The painter.

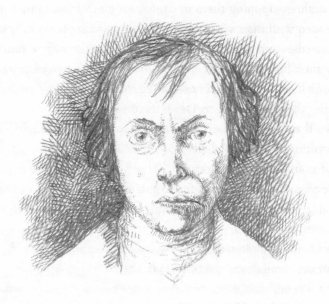

'Oh yes, sir?' I had never heard of him. 'And who, if I may ask, is the unfortunate victim?'

'MARRAAAAHHHH!'

He was Doctor Jean-Paul Marat. Seething Doctor Marat, who daily called for more people to be guillotined so that the country might be saved. Rabid Doctor Marat, who called himself the Rage of the People. Ailing Doctor Marat – his illness no doubt increasing his temper – who, while sitting in his slipper bath to cool his infected skin, had had a bread knife put through his left lung, his aorta, and into his left ventricle.

We must be quick, we must be careful, we must preserve the horrible body.

We were the first at Marat, first of many. We took casts, Edmond and I, busy together. Only the head and a portion of the chest; the rest was too delicate. Marat's face was caving in, his eyes as murky as oyster flesh. When we had our casts, other men opened the body up; they threw some pieces out, but were more careful with others, wrapping them in dampened cloths. It was their job, these men with their vinegar and arsenic and mercurial salt, with their needles and thread, to prepare the body for a state funeral. They took his heart, his real heart, and put it in a porphyry urn. We took his head, its plaster cast, and brought it home, with orders to bring the death mask to David at once.

'We'll do this together, Edmond,' I said as we hurried home. 'Everything together. I shall need your help.'

'Of course,' he said. 'I know that.'

First we swept the floor of the large workshop. Then we scrubbed the table and polished the instruments. We laid everything out: measures, plaster dust, soft soap. Only when all was neat and ready did we bring the plaster mould onto the table.

Curtius came down. 'What is this?'

'It's a head,' I said.

'Business?' he asked, shocked. 'Is it business?'

'Yes, sir,' I said, 'a little business.'

'No, no more. The shop is shut.'

'We must, sir. We have been ordered.'

'Who is it?'

'Someone has been murdered.'

'No more death. Just life now. I want everyone living. Mustn't touch death. Might spread.' With shaking hands he gave me the key to the wax cupboard. 'Take it. I'm done with it. I must go back. Don't wake Charlotte, she's sleeping. I must go back.'

Our first casting of the plaster death mask was placed in the window of Marat's apartment, looking down on the street for all the hundreds of mourners.

'Yasssh! Yassh!' said David when I delivered it. 'Greyed paytreeottt!'

Great patriot, he called me.

In two days we were able to substitute the death mask for a bust of the murdered man. David instructed us to make a full body in

393

wax of Marat for public display. The actual body was rapidly decomposing in the summer heat and the huge funeral preparations were not yet ready.

'Hish hall baddyyy; harry, do pleeesh harry!'

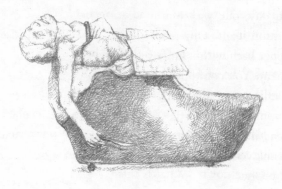

We went back home, and to work, the two of us. The wax Marat came in twelve different sections. Where it had been impossible for us to take a cast of his actual flesh – chest, shoulders, back of the neck and head – we had had to reconstruct a replica of clay, relying on my notes and Edmond's measurements taken at the source. We must fit the death mask onto the clay body and then make fresh moulds of the whole; from those new moulds would come the wax figure. We added the dyes to the Chinese wax, carefully turning it in a water bath, heating it to the right temperature, and pouring it slowly into the moulds. Then we freed the wax and joined all together, then painted the sores, adding small flakes of wax for the broken scabs.

'You're making too much noise,' Curtius said.

But we barely spoke a word, Edmond and I. Locked in our work.

On the third day of Marat's death, the fifteenth of July, when I came to David to report on our progress, the corpus Marat had turned green. On the fifth day, the heavy exhausting weather broke, rain fell, and the girl who had murdered him was executed.

On the sixth day, the body of Doctor Jean-Paul Marat was at last removed from his home and taken to the church of the Cordeliers to lie in state. The fatal wound was on show. People got up close so that they might look in, and the body was constantly sprayed with perfumes. All was venerated. On the seventh day, our wax Marat was ready and was taken to the Convention itself. Our Marat in his death-breath, the figure in the slipper bath with a knife in his breast, in an agony of frozen movement. You could put your hands out and touch him. Marat not smelling, not decomposing, fresh and shining slightly. It would remain there until David finished a vast painting of the man dead in his bath, a martyr, a saint, a god.

'Thennk yoooou, cittttissunns,' he said, tears running down that twisted cheek.

People longed for souvenirs of the murdered man. Where could such things be got? They saw the death mask in the window. Where could one of those be had?

Without exactly meaning to, we had become the principal source of Marat.

# Chapter Sixty-Two

*A new business.*

In those weeks, in those months, we found we had stumbled into a most successful cottage industry. We made plaster heads of the radical Marat: in the morning Marat, throughout the day only Marat, into the night just Marat. We put a message beneath the words IN and OUT:

FOR MARAT

PLEASE CALL ROUND THE BACK

'Now, Edmond,' I said, 'it is for us to manage this business.'

'We are the ones?'

'Only us. Curtius devotes himself to the widow. It's all down to us.'

'How we come on, Marie, you and I!'

We heaved the ticket desk around the back, and Edmond and I sat there together taking the money: seventy assignats per Marat head. In those days I discovered what it was to be totally with another person, to share days and space and bodies, to sit tight together at a bench, hands touching under the desk. We were a shop frozen in time, paused, hovering for months, above the thirteenth of July 1793, the day of Marat's death.

'Just one head?' asked Doctor Curtius. 'Only one?'

'Yes, sir, just one.'

'But can it be right? One head. What if it's the wrong one?'

'I don't understand it either, sir. It does seem strange. But we have always been a Monkey House filled with the most popular of people, and today they come for Marat.'

The cloth Edmond was larger now than he had ever been, wound round with brilliant colours, threads of turquoise and vermilion and magenta, small patches of lavender and indigo and sienna, all plucked from his mother's abandoned workshop. The cloth Edmond was as bold and brilliant and handsome as flesh Edmond was formerly reserved and aloof and plain.

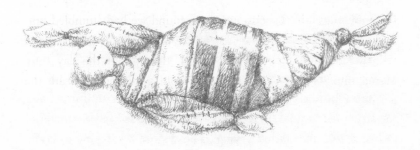

'I measured your Marta,' he said.

'Go on, Edmond,' I said.

'I remember that.'

'What else?'

'I visited you at night. I've thought of it so often.'

'Yes, oh yes.'

It might have been the unaccustomed sound of Edmond talking so much. It might have been the people calling for Marat heads. Or perhaps it was the constant presence of Curtius about the bed, his adoration and attention, his thousand tales of the human body. Whatever the cause, something began to stir inside the remainder of the Widow Picot.

Doctor Curtius said she was making more noises, that he'd seen her looking at the walls and not the ceiling. Poor Doctor Curtius, we said to each other, poor man, she looks just the same, he's so fond. But one morning when Edmond came in to see her, her eyes moved from the ceiling to the wall, and then – he swore it – they

397

fixed upon him, and once they were on him they did not leave him. He went over to one side of the room; they followed. He went over to the other; they followed. Edmond screamed. We came running.

'Look! Look!'

By the time we had arrived, she was asleep again. But the next day, when I came in, Curtius was talking to her, and her sounds had some new intelligence to them.

'Wuuuuuuur,' she said.

Come again.

'Wuuuuuuuuuurrrr,' she said.

'Oh, yes we were, we were indeed,' he said, 'but not any longer.'

'Work, Widow Picot?' I asked. 'Do you mean work?'

'Wuuuuuurrrrrrrrrrrrrrr,' she said.

I brought her some old clothes, some old staff uniforms, and she struggled to hold on to them. When I pressed the old material to her cheek, she started crying. The widow was trying to come back – perhaps not all of her, but a part. We heaved her out of the bed. We put her in a barrow and pushed her around the upstairs rooms. We gave her things to play with; often she threw them to the floor, as if for the pleasure of watching us fetch them back. One morning Doctor Curtius leaned over her and, with a quick swipe of scalpel, severed the cord of her cap. The cap fell away, but the hair did not. A smell was instantly in the room. There was too much privacy in that smell. A vast hair knot of brown and grey and white, not pleasant colours, but colours of neglect. The widow's hair had grown solid, it had turned almost into bone. Curtius hummed, hovering above it with an ivory comb, not knowing where to strike first. He tried here and there, put the teeth in, pulled a little, and the widow's whole head went back. Edmond watched in trauma. Next Curtius took up a pair of long-necked clamps with two forked heads, designed for surgery of the uterus; with this he managed to puzzle out some of the hair, to unravel some of those old plaits. Some of the hair then fell away of its own accord. How Curtius trembled when he held the widow's terrible tangled, thick, matted, strangled, bumpy, fettered, time-gnawed, rat-tailed, stale and lifeless hair in his hands. While her cap was off all her love was out again, and how strange the love had grown; what a feeble, rickety, odd person that love was. Curtius attempted to straighten it all out.

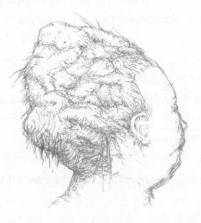

She bit him.

He stood in front of her aghast. And then he clapped. 'How you come on, Charlotte, how you come on! Bite again. Bite now!'

She had indeed come back. But she was not her former self. She suffered Curtius to pick at her hair, sometimes let him trim it; he carefully, lovingly, pruned her. Edmond showed her the old account books; she, using her working hand, ripped some pages out. We carried her down into the great hall, but it was so broken now, full of empty seats where wax people had once sat, empty plinths. We passed her in front of the remaining wax people, but she gave no sign of caring. I showed her the new work, the many shelves of Marat in plaster, but she couldn't be made to understand. I showed her the money we made, but it was the new money, the assignat, and each time we placed it in her hand she let it fall. Then Edmond grasped her under her armpits, my master and I each cradled a leg, and we carried her back upstairs. She preferred, I think, to be in her room.

It was Edmond who brought up the dummy of Henri Picot, very drab now, bottomed out after Martin Millot – and any fellow thieves – had had at him, a very shrunken chest.

'I want you, Mother, to remember Father and to remember me. I am Edmond, your son. It may be that I look different from how I once was, that may well be, and you might struggle to recognise me. But I want you to know me as I truly am. Your son, grown strong at last.'

Curtius chewed on his knuckle, doubled up, looking away. Edmond set his deflated father in front of his mother, and she looked at it, and she looked at it, and she looked at it, but she saw nothing there.

'Father,' remembered Edmond, 'spoke in a very quiet voice, a whisper almost.'

Curtius ducked, terrified of the widow remembering her husband.

The widow looked at the ceiling.

'Father,' remembered Edmond, 'sometimes nodded when he talked.'

Curtius nodded repeatedly, furious at himself. He had got so used to mimicking the faces he modelled – trying so hard to understand them – that it had become a habit with him. And now, as Edmond recalled his father, my master involuntarily imitated him.

The widow looked at the ceiling.

'Father,' remembered Edmond in triumph, 'would sing hymns as he worked.'

'No! He didn't!' whispered Curtius, but he hummed a very little.

The widow looked at the ceiling.

'Father,' shouted Edmond, my Edmond so strong, 'was pigeon-toed!'

'Oh, God!' said Curtius, turning his toes inwards.

And the widow looked at the ceiling, but frowned.

'Father . . .' yelled Edmond, 'Father's ears stuck out.'

'Help! Help! Help!' screamed Curtius, cupping his own ears.

But the widow had fallen asleep.

Back at our small business, each time I opened the mould, I wondered if it would be someone else this time, if someone different might be lurking within, but it was only ever Marat. Sometimes, when I opened the mould, I could not help myself: I was sick.

'It's the head,' I said. 'It's only the head. I feel better when I look away.'

So far had we come along in this domestic life that the following mundane, everyday conversation could be had, containing the sort of information that might occur in other houses where ordinary people went about their lives.

'No,' said Edmond, looking very serious, 'I do believe I've worked it out. It's not the head, Marie.'

'Is it not?'

'No. No. You're pregnant.'

# Chapter Sixty-Three

*Edmond keeps company.*

On August the twenty-third, a declaration called the *Levée en Masse* was made. The male population was required for military duty. Men were rounded up and marched off. Young men about their daily business were seized in the streets.

In the Monkey House, Edmond began to exist only behind closed shutters. Then even that was not enough. He must return to the attic.

'No, Marie. I'll not go back up there again.'

'For your safety you must.'

'I hate it there.'

'But it is safest.'

'Is it? How can you say that? Have you stayed up there? That place has a terrible hold on a person. It dominates so.'

'No,' I said. 'Not any more, not now. Not who you are now.'

I came up to see him whenever I could, but he must stay hidden. If anyone should catch a glimpse of him, if anyone should hear him, he would be taken away and all would be lost. Edmond stayed upstairs, and downstairs no one called for him yet. In the meantime, the visitors purchasing Marats told me everything.

'Mercier has been arrested – did you not hear?'

'Poor Monsieur Mercier! I hadn't heard,' I said.

'Then you don't know who it was that arrested him?'

'No,' I said.

'It was Jacques Beauvisage.'

'Have you seen Jacques? Do you know where he is?'

'It's what I was told. I was only told it was him.'

Edmond resigned himself to the top, with the wooden doll of me and his cloth people. He put all the shop dolls in one room, all in a grouping. Sometimes he would stand himself among them, as if they had all been convened for a meeting of a guild of mannequins. We stored dried food up there, just in case we were taken away. So that in our absence he could ration himself.

With Edmond upstairs, Doctor Curtius hastened the disintegration of Henri Picot. When no one was looking, he nonchalantly tugged upon the seams; he snipped off pieces; he used little patches of Henri Picot to block a hole in a wall. One day I saw that the former tailor's dummy had now shrunk to no more than a pitiful rag which he kept in his pocket and occasionally used to wipe the widow's brow. 'Who's this, who's this now?' he asked her, holding up the rag, but she could not say and he nodded at that.

Another time, Curtius said to me, 'I know anatomy. I'm acquainted with the human form. There were parts of mothers brought to me with puerperal exhaustion. I have seen heavy torsos come in. One I remember very well; she had not been so busied with as the others. I opened it up' – his voice now a whisper – 'little person inside. What, Little, what, Marie, have you got there?'

'Baby,' I said.

'A real one?' he said.

'Yes,' I said, 'I hope so.'

'How did it get in there?'

'The usual way.'

He looked very confused. I pointed up at the ceiling.

'Oh!' he said.

'Yes, sir.'

'It's very dangerous,' he said. 'It's not safe.'

'People have babies.'

'You're old. You're too old! You'll die!'

'Perhaps, sir,' I said, 'perhaps I won't.'

'No, oh no. You will.'

Now my master had two women he must look after. He would listen to my chest and belly several times a day, demand that I lie down. He would wash my face, and shake his head. He even came to help me with the Marats. By then our own wax Marat had been returned to us; in its place at the Convention hung the painting by David. That began the decline in demand for Marat casts; though ours was taken from Marat's own face, it was ugly next to David's. He had made Marat beautiful and holy, as if he'd come out of the Bible, but he hadn't really been like that at all. The painting was a lie.

Edmond stitched himself a simple sackcloth suit, one very like a shop doll's.

'If anyone comes up here,' he said, 'they won't know me from one of them.'

'It is not forever, Edmond,' I said. 'Remember who you are. You must not forget. Look out of the window, at Doctor Graham's. I shall come to you tonight.'

'We shall have a child.'

'I hope so, Edmond, if we are lucky.'

'There's one there, inside you, growing.'

'Yes, but that does not mean it shan't suddenly stop.'

He started crying.

'But we shall do our best for it.'

'Yes, our very best.'

It was in those shadowy half-lived days when we moved so slowly in the darkness of our home, making such little noise, that news from outside came to us. Someone from another life. I hadn't thought of her. I'd forgotten to think of her. If I'd been thinking of her, then perhaps she'd have been safe, she'd still be alive, she'd still be breathing.

I was going out for bread, but the back door was locked. Doctor Curtius was standing by, as if to block it. 'Best not go out today,' he said. 'We don't need bread today.'

'We do,' I said. 'We do need bread.'

'It is better,' he said, 'that we don't go out today.'

And at first I didn't think of it.

Doctor Curtius insisted I sit with the widow for a while. Then Edmond showed me a papier-mâché mask he had made himself: it covered his face, with just holes for nostrils. The mask even had crudely painted eyes to cover his own.

'Don't do it, Edmond, it's too much.'

'No, no, I feel much better now. Much safer.'

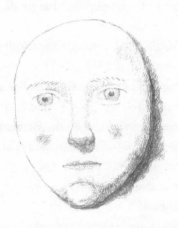

He would put it on whenever he heard someone creaking up the attic stairs. Curtius wanted me to tell him all over again about our days in Berne. Curtius said, 'Let us talk of our first heads. Put that blanket around you.' And so, wrapped in blankets, we sat by the fire and remembered all that old wax of no consequence.

I worked it out in the end.

My thoughts went like this: the shutters are all shut up, just as they were when the king died and the queen, so perhaps someone big was killed off today. I wonder who. But when I cracked open one shutter and looked across at the remaining occupied houses, I saw that ours was the only house bolted and shuttered, and then the panic began to start. Perhaps it's her, I thought. Maybe it's her. Perhaps it is. Why else would they all be looking at me that way? Why would they be stroking and patting and petting so?

'Mmmmmmm,' said the widow.

'Élisabeth?' I asked.

'Marie?' said Edmond. 'Let me stroke your belly.'

'Élisabeth?' I asked.

'Marie,' said my master, 'sit by the fire with me.'

'Élisabeth?' I asked.

'Tell me of those Berne heads.'

'Élisabeth?' I asked. 'Élisabeth? Élisabeth?'

At last he nodded, 'Élisabeth,' and then, 'come sit by the fire.'

And I, so help me, I did.

The twenty-seventh of May 1794, or the eighth of Prairial, Year II, in the language of their new calendars. Perhaps she had her plaster Jesus with her, the wretched thing. I should have been there. All stuffed in the tumbrel, so many of them. Praying, no doubt, all the way. She went on that journey bareheaded, so they say, after the wind blew her kerchief away. She was number twenty-four. There were twenty-three before her that session. My Élisabeth. My Élisabeth, off to death without heart or spleen. My Élisabeth. She never called for me.

Why did you not call?

The next morning I went out to buy the bread.

# Chapter Sixty-Four

*Gone away.*

On the tenth of June 1794, the Law of the Twenty-Second of Prairial was passed. 'The Tribunal must be as active as the crime and conclude every case within twenty-four hours.' And so people, ordinary everyday people, were herded from their gaol places to the courtroom sometime in the morning, their verdict was given by two o'clock in the afternoon, and by three they were in the tumbrel on their way to the guillotine. The public prosecutor pointed and declared: 'You are guilty by dint of your dress. You are guilty because of your name. You for your moustache. You for your hair. You shall be killed because you were born with more money than others. You because you have less. You because you once whispered an opinion. You because you went out without your cockade. You because your neighbour was heard speaking about you. You because you have not been heard shouting loudly enough. You shall be killed for we do not like your countenance. You shall be killed to make up the numbers. You shall be killed because we say so. We know you inside your head; you threaten our liberty; you are not safe.'

We stood in the mould room, Curtius and I, shelves on shelves of heads in negative.

'We must break them all up,' I said. 'We must, sir. These moulds will be our execution if they are found. Every day André Valentin is upon the boulevard. He'll never leave us in peace. We must break them, sir. They'll kill us otherwise.'

He looked bleak.

'Here is my life built with the widow,' he said. 'To throw it all away!'

'It must be done, sir.'

'Only wait! Wait! Perhaps there is a chance. What if, Marie, we should fill the whole mould room, from floor to ceiling, with plaster? Fill it all in until there's no room at all, only plaster. All plaster, right through plaster. And later – if there is a later – we come very carefully with hammer and chisel and chip it out. We put the moulds in first, at the back of the room, cover them with a tarred canvas, then fill the rest with plaster. Whoever frees this room will know when they come to the canvas that they have reached the moulds, safe and sound.'

And so we did. The moulds were all stacked and covered over. Bucket on bucket of plaster was poured, and planks were secured against the doorway to keep the rising level in, until there was no room left in the room. A room has space in it; here there was no space, only a few head-size gaps, waiting for another time. I even put in the king's head. No one had ever called for it, and those who had ordered it were no longer alive. We ripped away the lintels and put in a skirting board where the door once was. A no-longer door to that no-longer room.

We kept to the Great Monkey House, listening quietly as the people marched outside. Sometimes André Valentin appeared at our broken gates, smiling. Once he came in, pushing things over, even rapping his knuckles against the widow's head. He demanded to know where Edmond was. We told him he had gone away, back to his wife. He did not believe us and set his eyes looking all over the Great Monkey House, even in the attic, especially in the attic, but even though he must have looked directly at Edmond among all those shop dolls there, his squinty eyes did not see him. He came back again, and he looked again, and he left again. And perhaps, we dared wonder, perhaps André Valentin shall just bully us in this way, perhaps he enjoys the game, and it shall only be that, just a game. But then Valentin was downstairs once more, kicking up the dust, upturning the chairs. Florence Biblot, former cook, was with him, a tricolour sash across her big body.

'Well, Citizen Biblot, are these the people?'

'Ddddd,' she said.

'And they are loyal to the overthrown king?'

'Ddddd,' she said.

'And they are Swiss?'

'Ddddd,' she said. '*Rösti. Fleischkäse.*'

'Anything else?'

'Ddddd,' she said, 'They are sorry for the king. I heard her. Dddd. Heard them over the years, trying to get a portrait of the queen. Loved them. They all did. That one even lived at Versailles.'

She spat.

'Thank you, citizen,' said Valentin.

'Ddddd.'

He blew his brass whistle.

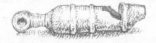

'You are arrested under the act of the twenty-second of Prairial,' he said, unable to look at us exactly. 'You will follow these men. Shut up this house.'

We were taken away.

All except for Edmond. He stayed in the attic, in his sackcloth suit and his mask. If they came for us, we'd agreed, he'd hide himself away with his brothers and sisters.

I never had a chance to say goodbye. And I dared not look back.

## Book Seven

### 1794–1802

# The Waiting Room and the Cardboard Property

*From thirty-three years to forty-one.*

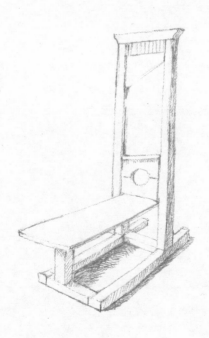

# Chapter Sixty-Five

*Life and death in a room.*

We were taken first to the prison of La Force, where we were formally charged. There the widow and I were separated from Doctor Curtius, dispatched to different prisons until we were called for our trials, though neither of us understood that this was the parting moment until my master was pulled away. Then another journey, watching the streets and houses through the carriage slats as if seeing them for the first time, finding beauty everywhere, then to the monastery of the Carmelite Friars and to darkness. Here, on one of those September nights, it was said that Jacques Beauvisage had done some murdering of priests. That night we had been free, with Edmond beside me; now I was with his failing mother in a room with twenty other women, cattle like us, waiting and weeping on old straw.

*Carmes,* they called that prison. It sounds so peaceful.

Our little room may as well have been at the bottom of the ocean. Time was heavy in there, filled with the last living of twenty women, all in together. In that room you took every breath seriously. One of us might say to another, 'I'm so glad your dress has yellow in it. Otherwise yellow should not be here with us at all, and that would be a pity.'

Here were women, in this little room with its thick walls and doors. The youngest was a girl of twelve, the eldest an old countess in her seventies. I think some of the women, on behalf of the twelve-year-old, resented the seventy-year-old.

What a smell, all those women together.

Women came and women went. It was always certain where they were taken: to the Conciergerie, antechamber of death, from there to the Place du Trône, and then that final journey of all, onto the sliding planks and through the National Window. I kept hold of the widow's hand. She couldn't understand where she was, having lost what little sense she had left. Our bodies can be so kind to us.

They did not guillotine pregnant women. Girls yes, old mad-women certainly, but the pregnant were safe, for a while. After I had given birth, in all likelihood I would be taken away. So long as my baby remained inside me, so long was I safe. We kept each other alive. I should live then, by my calculation, another three months.

The room measured, I estimated, twenty by thirty feet. The floor was stone, but bundles of piled straw were offered as bed arrangements. There was not quite enough – sometimes you had to fight for a bed – but mostly people took turns. We were allowed to clean out the room once a week. There was a single horrible little window that looked out only onto a grey, mean-spirited wall. You could not see the sky. One of the walls had a bit of moss on it. I liked to look at the moss. Moss has colour.

Our shared bucket was not regularly taken away. Some of the women were very nonchalant about using the bucket; some conversed loudly as they sat there; to others it was a daily humiliation, a profound torment. One mother had her daughter hold up a piece of clothing in front of her while she was at it, but that sorry cover was no wall, it hid none of the noises, merely drew attention to them. Some of the women could not understand the modesty of others. There was no solitude there. Or perhaps the only little solitude was inside the head of old Mother Picot.

I had never been with so many people. The younger women sat together and talked of men. There were fights, of course, over big things, over little. All the little relationships in that room were the last efforts of life. Sometimes we were cruel to each other, sometimes kind. Everyone wanted a little human warmth. I recall one woman, a former lottery-ticket seller, who would move around the room all day, asking one person and then another, 'May I hold your hand now, please,' or 'It is your hand that I should like to hold next,' or, 'Could I hold on a little longer yet.'

On occasions we were allowed to move around Carmes. There were men there, too; the whole place stank of human waste and ammonia and damp. Everyone there moved about in thick still air. In those moments outside our cell, pushed about among the others, seeing men as hopeless as we were, people whispered about who had been taken, how many yesterday, how many today. At Carmes I heard more stories of Jacques Beauvisage: he'd been seen here and there in the worst of the atrocities, waist-high in blood, murdering whole families, setting fire to villages. But in all these reports there was nothing of substance about Jacques, no solid fact: no mention of his limp, no talk of his tremendous grief for a dead boy. I believed none of them.

Giving form to our lives at Carmes were the lists, published nearly daily, of the people who would be next. Often, after a new list was published, there were twenty-four hours before those people were called for. The pain of those hours! And then the sounds of people being ushered out, goaded upstairs, the screams, the begging, the struggles. But out they went. At night we all sweated, and many cried. If only we could get some air, some new air.

We had so much time.

We had no time at all.

One by one, the women disappeared. No, that's not true; sometimes three or more went at a stroke. And time somehow went on. And we were alive still, the widow and I. Sometimes a woman could not control herself, would scream or sob, but it made no difference, it only upset everyone else. We tried to live with what dignity we had, to behave well, to be civil and proper and nice. Sometimes we even laughed. For some there was even relief in being there; our lives out in the city had been lived under pressure,

415

waiting for the banging on the door, so that when it actually came there was some comfort, a little peace: we had been taken, we could be ourselves again. Our minds were never far away from the door. Some tried never to look at it, but none of us could stop herself from contemplating the door.

There was one very handsome woman, utterly sensible and kind, who had such dignity that she inspired us all to bravery. The night before her name appeared on a list, I heard her whispering, 'I know that I shall be next.' Before leaving she kissed us all goodbye and gave away everything she had left. I thought I would like to go like that.

Our days were punctuated by hard food, bread and peas and beans, which broke old teeth and made the jaw ache from sucking on the stiff food. My baby hurt with hunger. How like Élisabeth's poor suffering people we all were, I thought. As if the misery were a type of mandatory uniform we had all been given. She'd mistake me for one of them if she saw me now, if she weren't already dead.

We were all in that room together, and everything was precious. There was so little to love. All that noise of Paris people trapped, living with it day and night.

We had so much time.

We had no time at all.

The cast kept changing.

At first my time was occupied by the widow. We played together, and I talked to her of Edmond and of Doctor Curtius. Keeping her calm. Washing her. Wiping her. Holding her to me, letting her rest her wrinkled head on my shoulder. Trying to unpick the twisted nest of her hair with my fingers. Making her look pretty, and telling her so. She was softening so in her illness; I couldn't hate her any more. I tried to love her instead. She couldn't understand the idea of being a grandmother, but she stared at my belly and looked very sad and was always upon the brink of remembering something, but was never quite able. How strange that it should end with us two together.

'You've a son. Remember? Edmond, he's called. He's alive and well. He is hidden and safe. No one shall find him.'

'Wooooooo.'

Edmond skirted her consciousness, a misty figure, gone again soon enough. I so wanted her to remember him. Once I thought she recognised me, a rage showed on her face, but afterwards tears flooded her vision; she had lost me again. From behind she didn't look like a real person at all, poor old child, but a collection of sacks.

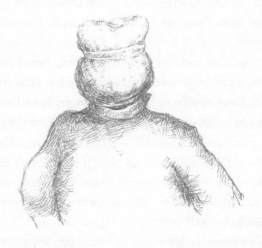

She didn't understand, when her name came on the list. I didn't tell her; how could she possibly understand? I kept very close the whole day. I sang to her. I never let her out of my sight. She slept a couple of hours with her head in my lap. I stroked her broken hair. Someone would be cutting it soon, before the final journey. Hair was always cut short around the neck. I hope she broke the shears. When they called her name, she did not understand that that name was hers. I had to answer for her. She was happy enough at first, but she couldn't understand why I wasn't coming with her. She started crying when I said I wasn't allowed. It's a terrible thing when old women cry. I hope she'd forgotten me by the time she was taken up the stairs. I hope she understood nothing of that cruel process called her trial. I hope someone was kind to her in the

417

tumbrel. I hope she was the first in her batch. I hope she didn't understand that she would lose her head. Perhaps she thought all those people were being made into tailor's dummies; perhaps she did not mind that she would be made into one too. I think the blood on the planks would have upset her. I hope it didn't. I hope it was sunny. I hope it was warm. Big mad old lady. Oh, help me, help me, help us all.

We had so much time.

We had no time at all.

The cast kept changing.

Afterwards, when she was gone, I would lie down with Marta very stiffly in the straw and pretend there was only sawdust inside me. For days I didn't care to be spoken to. I ate for my baby, not for myself. I could only face Edmond again if I kept his child. I hadn't kept his mother. There was a life inside me, and so I went on.

I began to speak to people again.

We told each other our stories. Again and again. You always knew the true ones from the false ones, for the false ones changed at every telling. The true ones remained constant. What is a life? This is what we were left with: stories. They were our clothes.

After one woman, the wife of an already executed deputy, had been called away, I heard another woman tell her story as her own the following night. The story thief was an actress from the Comédie-Française, arrested after she was heard quoting from a play about a king – not the beheaded locksmith, but some other king from long ago. It didn't matter. A king was a king. She had listened to the story of the deputy's wife, and now she repeated it, almost word for word, to two unsuspecting new ladies. We were furious. We called her a thief. But she just shook her head sadly. She was not a bad woman, she said. She merely wanted to collect all these stories, all that was left of these people, and to keep them safe in her prodigious memory. This was why she had become an actress, she saw now: so that she might tell other people's tales,

418

not the fictional people she had supposed but the real people of this one room, so that when they were dead they were not forgotten. Surely this meant it was her fate to survive, so that all the stories should be saved with her. But her name was called, too, and her library left with her.

After I had been there a month, I too began to recite the lives of those other people who had gone before – not as my own, but pointing them out to newcomers. Over there, in that corner, there used to be an Élodie, and this is her story; over there was a Madame de Grenlin from Marseilles; there by the window all day was a Mademoiselle Cossé, see the marks she made there with her finger-nails. There were marks all over the walls; the whole place was crowded with poignant little messages, the sole remaining evidence of a life. Sometimes the women screamed at me to shut up, but many so feared being forgotten that they would come and tell me their stories, then question me in detail about what I'd learned. I had to remember freckles and dimples and a set of chairs, the flowers in gardens, old men and young men, boys in wigs and stockings, girls who loved strawberries and women who had faith, young backs, journeys to relatives, games of cards, soft-boiled eggs, monies earned and little houses and first wallpaper, babies being born and children lost and deceased parents, all of it, so many stories, favourite dogs, favourite horses, an old song, who saw the king when, jewellery and splendour, family heirlooms, poems, the fairy tales 'Cendrillon' and 'Persinette', my son at the guildhall. Remember, will you, Marie? Do you remember now? Have you got that? Who was my first cousin? Where did I meet Pierre? What is my coat of arms? The little scar by his eye. What a lot there was. Slow down, slow down, or I'll lose it.

There were too many stories to remember, I could not keep them all in. Little pieces from one story would get muddled up and appear somewhere else: Madame D.'s love of daffodils would be given to Mademoiselle P., whose great passion for a soldier

419

named Augustin would surface in the confused biography of an elderly matron from the Faubourg Saint-Marcel, whose sister, her companion, would suddenly be found in the little history of a woman who sold refreshments on the Place de la Révolution during the executions.

I began to fear those stories. They came to me when I slept. They pushed themselves into my dreams. They were bad for my baby. I was certain of it. I stopped listening to the tales. I no longer wished to hear about anyone else. There was only me, my baby, Edmond. I tried to keep myself myself.

Now I have lost those stories; they come back to me in little pieces. At times my sleep is troubled by a great chorus of dead women, in various costumes, calling out their names and the names of the people they loved, their own little details. One woman told me she could never abide people who didn't like the Brussels sprout. 'Weak people, characterless people,' she said. One woman told me she had once danced with a bear at a country fair. The bear had been a tolerable dancer. A girl told me about an imaginary people and an imaginary island she'd made up herself, had drawn maps of and written laws for. Books' worth of stories, they gave me.

Within that almanac of loss, one story is told by so many still that it shall not be forgotten yet. At Carmes, two months after I arrived, came a Creole woman from Martinique who'd grown up on a slave plantation. Her husband had also been at Carmes, but his name had been listed already. She was born Marie Josèphe Rose Tascher de la Pagerie, but she went by Rose then.

She was a solid woman. Slightly sullen, handsome but no astounding beauty, sloping shoulders, dark hair, thick eyebrows, large eyes and mouth, and the nose too, come to think of it, was not small either. Weeping was her usual state; later she would say she'd been brave, that she'd gone from woman to woman, comforting, but that was not how it was. She was terrified. Who could blame her? She sat with me and wept upon my shoulder.

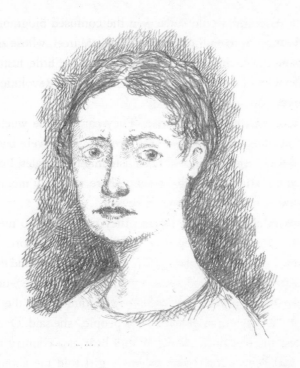

'I'll tell you, Mademoiselle,' she would begin. 'I will not call you citizen; that's done with for good and all. I shall tell you who it is I miss most. It is not my husband, though I'm sorry for him, but he wasn't always fair; he wasn't loyal. I'm sorry he died, but I cannot bring him back. It is not my son or daughter; I love them both with a mother's love, but they are being looked after beyond the city walls. I had them apprenticed, for their protection – Hortense with a needlewoman, Eugène with a cabinetmaker. They are safe enough, but how changed will they be afterwards? Who will they become? No, most of all, I shall tell you who I miss: it's my pug dog. Nothing's better than Fortune. I like to see him scratching his ears, shifting his bottom, sleeping, barking, catching his breath, sneezing. It's Fortune I miss most, my darling pug.'

Having no dog with her, it was not long before she took to calling me Pug. Small-nosed canine. What a joke that was, how she amused herself. She called out for me in the night. Inconsolable

421

until I was with her, until she could pet me and stroke my hair. I didn't mind. Sometimes she gave me food. I needed food.

I even got to meet Fortune myself. Rose charmed one of the guards, and he arranged for Fortune to come to us for weekly visits. His arrival gave us back a little life. He was a jolly little fellow, devoted to his mistress, and we were all pleased to see him. Here was innocence again. Little harmless thing with a sad black face and worried eyes, as if he understood our plight. He did us such good. His little noises. His openness. His blamelessness. We were sad to see him pad off again, and hoped that we would live to see him next week. Let us last at least till then, we said.

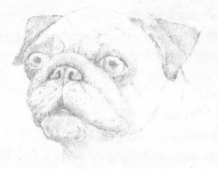

I was patted by Rose, my belly stroked by her. She did not help me with the mucking out, but she talked to me while I and the other women were about it. I suppose I fell in love with her a little. She in her turn fell for a military man imprisoned at Carmes, handsome with an impressive sabre scar. She spent a good deal of her time trying to look after herself, trying to keep herself pretty for the scarred man, whose name was Lazare Hoche. He was certain he wasn't going to die by the guillotine, and his confidence was comforting to her. How she preened herself for him.

I was older than her by two years, but did not seem it. I've outlived her too. She died of complications of abdication in 1814, aged only fifty-one. I thought she had more stamina than that. She provided much diversion to my last days in prison.

On July the twenty-eighth 1794, the tenth of Thermidor, Year III, the door opened and the guard called out, 'Anne Marie Grosholtz.' I am pregnant, I said. Look at my belly, I said. If they placed their hand down upon it, soon enough they'd feel a little kick. But they called my name again and said I must go. Now, I supposed, even pregnant women were no longer safe. It doesn't come as such a shock in the end, I thought. It is not so surprising. Why, after all, should I be spared? What makes me so significant? Baby, off we go; I shan't leave you. I can't leave you.

I was taken upstairs to ground level again, the air so much thinner, my lungs shocked by the change. My hands filthy, my dress filthy, my hair filthy. I thought I'd been looking after myself; I supposed it didn't much matter anyway. Holding my belly, apologising to it. Up the stairs, out of the monastery entrance to a Parisian street, and there the National Guardsman said to me:

'This way please, citizen.'

'I am pregnant.'

'Yes,' he said. 'Do not worry.'

'But I *am* worried!'

'You are not going to trial.'

'No?'

'No, citizen, not at all. Something else.'

# Chapter Sixty-Six

*The shattered jaw.*

I heard people on the Rue Saint-Honoré cheering, such holiday noise. What a sound! 'It's over!' I heard someone calling. 'The Tyrant is no more!' 'The Tyrant's dead, and they're rounding up all who were close to him!'

They took me to a room near the Place de la Révolution. People were crowded around certain objects there, on tabletops. Objects like at the butcher's. Only these would not be weighed and eaten.

'Heads,' I said. 'I do heads. I'm only called for at the end of people's lives. Here's heads.'

'Yes,' they said.

'Who's this one?' I asked.

'This,' they said, giving the tour, 'is Couthon the cripple. The angle of his cut is like that because they had to do him sideways. He'd been trodden upon by the other people in the cart, trampled over.'

'And here?' I asked.

'This mess was called Augustin Robespierre, the brother. When he knew all was up for him, he threw himself from a high window onto a courtyard. Must have hurt. Shattered himself, but did not kill himself – no, we did that later on, little nick in his neck; you might see that there. Beside him is the neat one, Saint-Just. So clean next to the others.'

'And here? Here?' I asked.

'The Incorruptible himself.'

There upon the table was the particular sphere of Maximilien

424

Robespierre. That's when I met Robespierre – never before. The mess upon the head was not merely from the trauma of the neck stump. This history of mine began, a country ago, with a jaw, a family property that had gone missing, misplaced by a backfiring cannon. Here, towards its end, was another shattered jaw. This one was not absent, it was still connected, this lower jaw hanging down from the upper, ripped by a bullet. Robespierre had tried to shoot himself and had missed, a suicide botched.

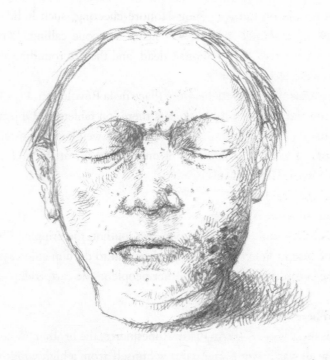

I had not been released from prison as a special privilege to observe the day's basketfuls. I must work. Plenty of plaster was ready. There was wax – ordinary candle wax, of the worst quality, but it was all they had – from hundreds of gathered-up candle stubs. I must make casts to be placed in the Convention. I did it.

It took me two days.

'Many people,' I said, 'shall wish to see these heads. Many people will come to be sure he is dead. Don't you think so? I think so. I'm certain of it. People will come for decades to see such things.'

When my work was done, I asked them what would happen now.

They told me I was free to go.

Free to go where? I asked.

Go home, they said. Why don't you go home?

'Home,' I whispered. 'I hadn't quite thought of that.'

I took the long way, through circuitous streets. I didn't want to hurry. I couldn't be sure what was waiting for me there.

# Chapter Sixty-Seven

*Little black list.*

I wish I were hollow. But I'm filled up. I wish I were hollow. Someone should tip me out. I must make a list. Set it all down. Bodies come and bodies go; you should not get too attached. While I was in prison, people went away. I must make a list.

*Picot, Charlotte, aged sixty, an old lost woman.*

It's not finished, my list. I'm small. I'm a snail. No, I'm made of leather. I'm black and broken. I'm very small and very robust. I was making my list; I haven't finished. There's a man in the Bible called Job. He loses his family, and when that doesn't crush him he's covered in boils and beaten and smashed, but still he goes on. He probably doesn't know why. I was writing down my list. It doesn't always hurt so much any more. My list. Do it then.

I came home to half a house. Half had tumbled to the ground; the crutches had given way or been tugged free, bricks and timber in the dirt, toppled like a house of playing cards. The Great Monkey House, ambition fallen. Two whole walls of bricks had collapsed, revealing the old rumpled wooden structure underneath. The flag-stones had been pulled up and taken away; there was no longer any fencing, nor any bell that had belonged to Henri Picot. Once there was hope around this place; so many people had laboured here; so many attended. Once the greatest show on the boulevard, the greatest in Paris.

I stood silent before it.

'Edmond,' I whispered, 'I'm home.'

No, no answer.

'Edmond.'

None.

What had happened? While I was away? I learned it all later, from a record at the Préfecture du Département de la Seine. Fill in the pieces. Get it over.

Those of our district, section leaders, National Guardsmen, old natives – André Valentin, I presume but can never prove – came upon the Great Monkey House. They had hated it for so long. They surrounded the house and they began to pull it down. It did not need much help. The crutches came away easily enough; the whole house yelped and moaned, as if all the monkeys were inside again. Section leaders wrecked high and low, every cupboard, every trunk, every drawer, every room, upstairs, downstairs, in and out, up and down. They went about our doll's house, breaking it, for they wanted to hurt our wax people. They hauled some out, danced drunkenly down the street with wax partners, then left them broken upon the ground. They pulled and upturned everything. But the plaster room was still safe. They did not know it existed. And higher yet?

At the foot of the stairs I discovered the doll Edmond had made of me, collapsed in doll-hopelessness, legs bent impossibly back, skirt pulled up, a crack one side of the head, a hand twisted behind as if for protection, as if it couldn't bear to look.

On I went. The attic, or what was left of it. Much of the roof had collapsed.

As they searched on, drunk and furious, as they rummaged through the Great Monkey House, upstairs were still the many brothers and sisters Picot. Quiet gentle folk. Suddenly bleak and bitter men were among them, knocking them down, pulling them about, laughing, such fun. Tugging on the beams. They started to throw the Picots out through the windows. Mannequins broken on the ground, toppling one after the other, the upstairs walls groaning, the timbers failing. And then a warm mannequin.

'Ssssh,' he said, to the section leader. 'I'm a shop doll.'

428

The section leader stared at him.

'Sssssh,' he said. 'I keep very quiet.'

The section leader took a handful of sackcloth. The attic called out.

'I'm made of wood and canvas and stitching. My head's painted papier-mâché. I'm cloth. I've sawdust for guts.'

The timbers were giving way.

'Then this shan't hurt you, shall it?'

Did it happen like that? Was it, I wonder, his ears that gave him away? He could have been the pattern for a thousand more. He didn't call out, I'm sure he didn't. No, perhaps he did. Perhaps he called to them when they were downstairs: 'My name is Edmond Henri Picot! Edmond Henri Picot! I do not forget!' Or perhaps in the end, by dint of concentration, he had turned completely into a shop doll. Broken brothers and broken sisters. And among all those bits and pieces, shattered limbs and heads, collapsed torsos, one that was heavier than the rest. Perhaps he never said a word, and they never knew it was a living person they were throwing from a high window – not until he struck the ground and they saw the red. My life spilled out of the house. And he could not be fixed again. I fill in the gaps. Was that how it happened? Or was it only that the attic, long distressed, had begun to fall apart, and Edmond, traumatised, had leapt?

I was given the record at the Préfecture du Département de la Seine. *Man fallen out of building, five foot five inches, one eighth. Name unknown.* Edmond had practised for disappearance all his life. Here it was, and here ended my private life.

*Picot, Edmond Henri, aged thirty-nine, master of mannequins.*

The house was left a fraction of its size. All the property built upon the grounds of the chess café had collapsed. And my list. I haven't finished my list. I have to do it.

I went to the Salpêtrière hospital. There, among crowded beds, my baby was born. But she did not make a sound. There was a rush inside me and I suddenly knew that I'd fallen in love. I've an object, I said, what a miracle. Little hands, and little legs, and little belly. The lips so thin and red. She had the Grosholtz chin, there it was again, but not the Waltner conk. In its place she had Edmond's insubstantial nose. My dear daughter. She never had a chance. A little creature I made. Born without life. Stillborn. She didn't move and they took her away from me.

*Marie Charlotte Grosholtz, baby.*

The world is broken, I said, cracked. Some things are missing from the world and they will never be replaced. They can never be. Only then did I truly understand, as the widow had always understood, that the world is full of gaps, and these were mine. Perhaps I couldn't make anything living. I'm sure it's my fault I can only ever create life*like* and life-*size*. What do you expect from a father who was more mannequin than man? What do you expect from a mother who spent more time with imitation people than real ones?

I went back home.

# Chapter Sixty-Eight

*There's not a bone.*

I stayed deep inside. All angles, all crooked. There was a knock on the door. I thought it was the local children come to taunt me again, so I didn't answer, but the knock kept on. It wasn't a loud knock like the children gave; it was a little gentle knock, an apologetic knock. It wasn't like the little knocks of industry that Louis the locksmith made at his forge; it was a knock, I began to understand, of sympathy. A loving knock. I went to the door. I opened it a crack.

My master Curtius.

Doctor Curtius and his pupil together again. We stood there, at opposite ends of the wooden plank I'd laid down after the steps had come away. Looking at each other, just looking, he by the broken stones of the old courtyard, me on the threshold of the ruin I lived in. Perhaps only for a few seconds, perhaps longer, perhaps minutes, tens of them. Such food for eyes! He'd been at the hospital of the Hôtel-Dieu, a place that Mercier had told me of during our kitchen walks of Paris; that was why it had taken him so long. He'd been so ill they'd taken him away from the prison for fear he should infect the other prisoners, lest they should die before they could be guillotined. He was removed to the Hôtel-Dieu, where he rotted with other starving men, but, contrary to all expectations, he did not die. Day after day he did not die. At last, very slowly, as others died beside him, he began to recover. And when he was well enough to walk a little he was sent home, a free citizen. My dear old man, very thin of course, not well at

431

all, but *living*; a shrivelled, stretched root, juiceless, but able to make movement and sound.

'Hello, sir,' I said.

'Can it be . . . my Little? I so hoped it would be.'

'Yes,' I said, 'it's she. Surely.'

'Here we are then: you and I.'

'Will you come in, sir?'

'Yes, yes, I think I will.'

He came in. I closed the door. It did not shut properly.

'It's very dark, Marie,' he said.

'I'll fetch a candle.'

'Ah, light! Light in the darkness.'

Something else was on his mind; I saw the panic upon his face; but he did not ask it then. We sat down together, and we talked of nothing much to stop the silence. After half an hour, he had courage enough to ask, very quietly, the important thing:

'Little, Marie, where's everybody else? Have they gone out? When will they be coming back?'

I shook my head.

We were silent a very long time.

'Where is Edmond, surely . . . upstairs?'

'No, I wish that he was. That would be something indeed.'

'Oh dear,' he said, and sighed. 'An excellent mannequin maker.'

'Yes, sir.'

'My poor girl.'

'Yes, sir.'

'And you, Marie? What about you? There was to be . . . a new life.'

I shook my head.

'There's no bone,' he said, his expressive fingers moving on their own, 'not a bone that can be comfort enough.'

There was a silence. Then:

'Not her, then, too?' he said very, very quickly. 'At least not her. Tell me, not the widow, tell me.'

432

'Yes. Yes, even the widow.'

He closed his eyes.

'But she was cracked, she was broken.'

'I'm so sorry.'

'I thought she might have. I didn't like to wonder . . . I thought she might not . . . What a thing, oh what a thing it is.'

He sat hunched over in his chair. There was a slight tremor in his face, a wave of nervous reaction, a twitching of an eye, his lips pursed. And then what followed I can only describe as the noise of a whole building collapsing, floors falling in upon floors, a great heaving of rubble, a crashing, a sliding of heavy material, tumbling in a heap; only these sounds were coming from inside my master. But he stayed sitting, and though there was sweat on his forehead and a little black liquid coming from one of his ears and though one eye seemed to lose its sight, still the ruin breathed on. It may have been the cold in that room, but when his mouth opened it seemed to me a strange cloud of dusty air came out.

There we were, in the wretched Monkey House.

'Was it good for us, in the end, Little? The body bits, I mean. Not our models, not our wax, the human bits. Did we live with them too long? Perhaps they're calling to us.'

But that is not the end. Not quite. We went on, Curtius and I, just a little further. We kept very close to one another. We didn't like to move alone, lest singly we come across some ghost of our lost people, here in this house where they had all been. We went on, and we stumbled, but we went on. We tidied, we swept up, buttons there among the rubbish. Where there were holes in the house, we made canvas walls. After a while, we felt brave enough even to open some of the shutters. We started work upon the plaster room, which, being so solid, had survived well enough; we chipped into it until we reached the tarred canvas, all those moulds safe and sound. Even then, the king's head, taken from death, would remain uncast.

It had begun with Curtius and me, it continued that way. Two months after my master returned, we opened again for business with a handful of mangy wax likenesses. We were given permission to use the moulds of the heads of Robespierre and his followers. Doctor Curtius had a hunger for people; he always had; it kept him going.

'You have been with me all this way,' he told me. 'What companions we are. You do the widow's work, and almost as capably as she. It is not right that you call me sir, not any more. I'm ashamed of it. And so perhaps, if it suits, Little, if it doesn't repel, Marie, if it wouldn't stick in the throat, since after all you've no mother but a doll of pegs, nor any father but a metal jaw piece – perhaps you might come to consider me an uncle. And even address me as such.'

'Uncle?'

'Yes.'

'No, sir, I don't think I could.'

'No, well, perhaps in time.'

'Sir, shall I be paid now?'

'Well, I should like that.'

The busts of Marat were smashed; people were ashamed to have them in their homes. Marat's body itself was disinterred from the Panthéon and thrown upon a dungheap. We still exhibited our wax man, murdered in the bath; Edmond and I had made him. We painted a large sign:

YOUR MONSTERS WITHIN

Not so many people came. We could not blame them. Everyone had had enough of monsters. We invented a new name for ourselves:

JUSTICE HOUSE

Still, only a few came every day. 'Why,' they asked, 'should we pay to see the head of Robespierre, when it was Robespierre who had our mothers, fathers, sons, daughters put to death?' We were not certain how to answer that, so my master let many people in without charge, a gesture the widow would never have allowed. We no longer had a guard dog, so we had no shield when people jeered at us on the street; all we could do was keep going; children threw stones at me, Curtius was tripped up. It seemed that some people considered us not without guilt.

Yet my master never lost his faith in his work. 'Only mirrors, Marie,' he said. 'Only mirrors. That's what we do. That's what the shop has ever been. They do not like the look of themselves. They are ashamed of what's in the looking glass.'

Our business crawled on until the last hours of September the twenty-fifth. In the first hours of the twenty-sixth, I heard Curtius clapping in the night; otherwise the event should have been as quiet as Father's. He didn't come down in the morning. I sat on the steps for a while, just as I had when Mother died. Finally I went to him.

'Up you get, sir, up you get. Don't you know the time?'

He wasn't listening.

'Open your eyes at least. You could do that, couldn't you? It's not so much to ask. Let me see your eyes again. They're blue, I know.'

Stubborn man.

'A sound. A little noise, sir. That's all I require, then I'll tiptoe out and leave you till later. Did you say something? Try again. I think you moved. Didn't you? Don't leave me alone, sir. You must not leave me alone. It's not a kind thing to do. What if I shook you a little? Oh, sir, sir! To be so still! What am I going to do?'

But all along I knew. I washed his face, combed back his remaining hair, put on the soft soap, mixed the plaster, no need for straws. How odd it was, the head still connected, the body rather in the way; I'd forgotten that. Death mask of Philip Wilhelm Mathias Curtius, born in Berne in 1737, died in Paris in 1794, greatest of Parisian showmen, chronicler of history, maker of people, lover of a widow, who knew the human body better than almost any other, but never shared his own with anyone. Great Curtius.

'I shall call you uncle after all,' I said. 'Uncle.'

The funeral, under revolutionary law, was held at midnight, without any religious ceremonies. It wasn't well populated. Just a few sodden mourners. One man came pushed in a wheelbarrow, it was Louis-Sébastien Mercier. After Robespierre's death, Mercier, like so many others, had been released from prison. The light of Paris shone on him, but the poor man was blind to it. His eyes worked well enough, but they could see only the past; he could no longer make sense of Paris. This new place, he said, was not known to him.

Throughout his long imprisonment, Mercier had never removed his beloved shoes. At first he had walked them around his cell floor every day, but after a while he took to sitting in corners, and neither he nor his shoes had any exercise. The room was damp; it dripped; his straw was never properly cleaned out. And over his long indolence, when his past walks grew increasingly confused in his mind, and he got lost in his thoughts, his shoes began to fester. The skin of their leather grew into the skin of his feet. His swollen ankles spread over the tops of his shoes, and over time shoes and feet became one. The pain he felt when they touched the floor of Paris was excruciating. He had to be carried from his prison cell.

The doctors had called for surgery to remove his shoes from his feet, he told me, but he wouldn't allow it. He had come to see Curtius off. He invited me to live with him, to be his shoes, tell him what I saw walking about the new Paris. I thanked him but declined.

My master's lawyer, Gibé, a vole of a man, was the person who told me that there was a will, and the details written therein. 'Everything to one person,' he said, 'to you.'

To me? To Little? To Anne Marie Grosholtz? Are you sure? All of it? No, that is not right. Let me see the paper again. It cannot be. Tell me, now, are you not lying? I am very easy prey; you should not lie to me. It would be no great victory. Read it out, will you?'

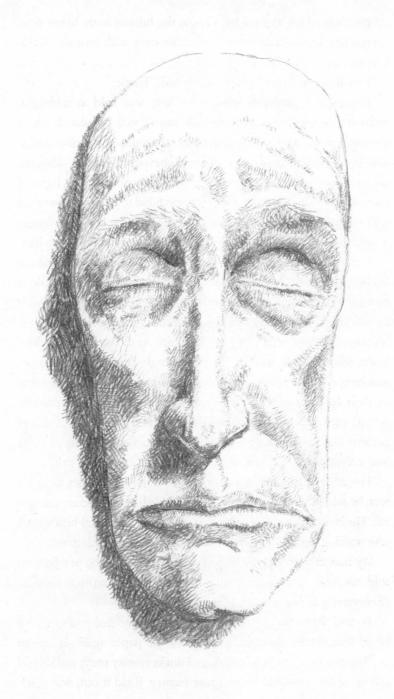

'To Anne Marie Grosholtz, my equal in art.'

Hand to my mouth.

'That's me! I'm her! I've been paid! I've been paid at last!'

I had a home. Uncle gave me one.

'There are,' said Gibé, 'debts.'

My master owed a doctor-surgeon, two tailors, a locksmith, wax wholesalers; he had not paid his previous year's tax; a debt of fifty-five thousand livres in all. Such a sum, it didn't seem possible. Such a sum you could drown in.

# Chapter Sixty-Nine

*Portrait of A. M. Grosholtz (by Louis David, Year III).*

I am nearly at the end now, with small business to attend to. I looked around for anyone I knew; they were all gone. Once, it's true, a pie was left upon the broken doorstep of the Monkey House. I knew Florence Biblot had left it there. Was that an apology? I kicked it into the mud. I never saw her or her pies again. I was the owner of a business, a person of note. I even had my portrait painted, by Jacques-Louis David, while he was imprisoned at the Luxembourg Palace.

I was one of his few visitors; there was very little else for him to paint. I didn't mind. A little woman dressed in black. I had Marta on my lap; it should have been little Marie Charlotte, but Marta would have to do. I insisted that I be shown with my hand over my face; I wasn't quite ready to be looked at yet.

He protested that he could not see me properly, that my face was covered up.

'Ppppleashhhh!'

I insisted. As blank as that doll on my lap. Any number of faces underneath it.

So then: how to fill in the blank. Fifty-five thousand livres.

I borrowed money. From the plaster wholesaler; his business was, after all, my business. It was not enough. I must be clever. I was thirty-four, with a business. It seemed that I should lose everything if I did not move fast. The Monkey House, crooked place, was not attractive to look at. I sold back the land either side of the old house; they hauled the rubble away. Given time, I

A.M.GROSHOLTZ          AMICUS LUD. DAVID

thought, I could probably display some of the old people again; given time, their popularity might come back.

I sat on my own, with a shop doll in Edmond's shape. I thought, I shall keep this way. With my own cloth cap done up. But then, in the end, I am not like the widow. There was too much to be done; I was on my own. I could not keep still. Desperate people make bad decisions. And so.

To save myself, I committed a common enough union: I married.

Word had got about. People still supposed that Curtius must have been worth several fortunes. It wasn't true, but he was worth one Monkey House, and now so was I. Men called for me; people were starving, opportunities scarce. One showed me figures in a notebook, and little architectural drawings spidered in ink. Perhaps.

On the fifth of October 1795, there was fighting on the streets again. On the twenty-sixth, Jacques-Louis David was given amnesty. On the twenty-eighth, at the Préfecture du Département de la Seine, Ville de Paris, in a dirty little room without any decoration, with lines of benches where the witnesses, the unadorned brides, and the unadorned grooms waited to be called upon to be registered, here were married Anne Marie Grosholtz and François Joseph Tussaud. 'This is a business matter,' I said to Citizen Tussaud, and Citizen Tussaud, tucking his notebook inside his breast pocket, agreed.

Citizen Tussaud, my husband. It is not a happy story. His parents are perhaps to blame. As a child they had taken him to the theatre, and he had fallen in love with it. It made François dream, and François as he grew up did not manage to forget his dream. Like countless others who are taken in by stage landscapes and stage characters, he was slowly smashed by the prettiness and light. He never really knew what it was like backstage. He'd never troubled himself to go beyond the door marked PRIVATE. He loved cardboard theatres and played with them. A nice enough man, perhaps, but useless.

441

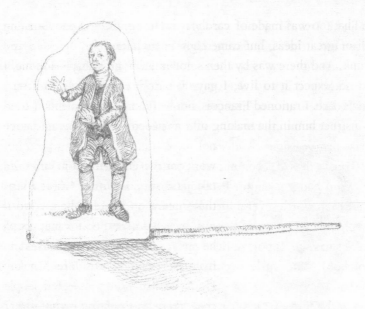

I do not recall the feel of his moustache; I do not recall the sound of him on the corridor; I do not recall his knocking at my room door, the door of the room that once belonged to my master. I do recall viewing his bank figures and the horror of that. Simply he had lied to me and I had been stupid enough to believe him. A most unfortunate marriage.

I lived through it somehow. I got up every day; I had to. Citizen Tussaud and I did not sleep in the same bedroom, but he lived in the Monkey House with me, and he came to me every now and then and, so help me, I did not send him away.

He expected me to earn the money. He expected me to have money all the time. I gave him pocket money as parents do their children. He spent it on elaborate business cards. 'Now,' he said, 'all will go well, you'll see.'

*François Joseph Tussaud*
*L'architecte des théâtres*

*Grand atelier, 20 Boulevard du Temple*

That too was made of cardboard. He went out in the morning full of great ideas, but came back in the afternoon defeated and drunk. And there was by then someone new growing inside me. I did not expect it to live; I gave it barely any thought at first; I didn't dare. I rationed François, but he ran up further debts. I tried to instruct him in the making of wax people, but wax people were

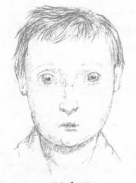

not interesting to him. He would not work for the Cabinet; he would only take its money. He found where I kept that money, no matter where I hid it – if he had a talent, that was it – and he spent it and wept or bellowed in front of me afterwards. The Monkey House needed more people, but people cost money. Perhaps I thought I should grow my own army. It was dangerous certainly at thirty-four to

Little F.

have children, but then it was dangerous at seven to have been left with Doctor Curtius, and it was dangerous of Doctor Curtius to come to Paris.

And then the new flame, the new incredible great luck. The new fire.

One, and then, in time, two!

Little François was born in 1798, Little Joseph came in 1800. They both had unmistakable Waltner noses and Grosholtz chins. Here was company

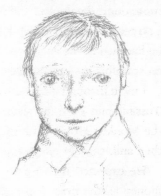

Little J.

again! I taught them, as Edmond and Curtius had taught me, what I knew of the world, what the widow taught me too. Citizen Tussaud wept and cooed at them; he was in love too. They moved, those little boys, and they made noise, and I nursed them in front of wax people.

We were even happy for a little while with such new and splendid company. But the business was failing.

The Monkey House had to be secured, and the children too. By the age of four Little François was already working for me, inserting hairs into wax heads, mixing plaster dust and water, setting up the fire as I had for Curtius.

'He is only four,' Citizen Tussaud said.

'He has to work,' I said. 'You don't mind, do you, Little F.?'

'No, Mama, let us get to work, please.'

Good little boy.

'Where are we going, Mama?'

'To the Tuileries Palace.'

'Where Princesse Élisabeth was?'

'Yes, for a short time, that is right. Well done, Little F.'

'But it's five in the morning,' Citizen Tussaud complained. 'The child needs to sleep. Come, little man, back to bed.'

'No, Citizen Tussaud,' said the little fellow to his father, 'I'm going with Mama.'

If he'd stayed in bed, he'd never have met Napoleon.

# Chapter Seventy

*My last French figure.*

I had a great plan, a plan as dangerous as the widow's had been when she moved us to the Monkey House. I had not yet told anyone of it, but kept it growing inside me. Moving to the Monkey House was an inspired and outrageous thing to do; so was collecting all those people, famous and infamous. Be bold or be bankrupt. I started collecting again. I wanted the very best example of French people. And so I looked about me. There was only one name on my list – on anyone's list. I called in favours to get Napoleon.

The First Consul, for that was his title then, had married an acquaintance of mine, Weeping Rose from Carmes. I had written her a note, signing it affectionately 'Pug'. It would not be easy, she replied; he had no time for such things. But he so loved Rose, though he preferred to call her Joséphine.

Rose kissed me and tapped Little François fondly on his nose. Fortune ran around us. And there was Consul Bonaparte.

'Approach,' he said, and I did.

'Not you,' he said, 'the other one. The future of France.'

I pushed Little François forward. He advanced, wrinkling his little beak. Napoleon Bonaparte came very close and put his hand on my son's shoulder and looked down into him, and Little François stood very still, and then squealed, not with fear but with mirth. Little François found the strangest things funny.

François, my first son though not my firstborn, would tell this story often. It is part of his mythology. He would boast of it to his classmates, though they wouldn't believe a word.

445

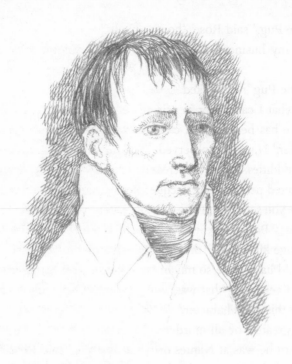

'Are you the mother?' Napoleon asked me.

'I am, sir,' I said. 'Isn't it obvious?'

'He is brave. We need brave people. Get to your work.'

I laid everything out. I explained exactly what would happen. His face should be completely covered in plaster. Little François came forward with the straws. He nodded.

We went to our work.

When it was done, he said, 'You have me, in the plaster there?'

'Yes, First Consul, an exact likeness.'

'Be careful with it. It is a fine head.'

'I never make any judgements on heads, First Consul,' I said. 'I was taught not to. Some heads last forever, but that's unusual. We never melted Franklin down, or Voltaire. But people have even forgotten the murderer Desrues. You never can tell, there's no guarantee. But we keep at it, First Consul, we don't stop; there's always someone to make, there's always someone to melt down.'

'Little Pug,' said Rose, 'how you talk.'

'It *is* my business. I know my business. I don't mind talking of it.'

'"Little Pug"?' he asked.

'It's what I called her in prison, between visits from Fortune.'

'There has been such a cast of exaggerated personages, Lady Face-taker,' Napoleon observed. 'The Revolution has produced all sorts of oddities. Roux, the screaming monk; Marat, the doctor who only wanted people dead; Jacques Beauvisage, the executioner.'

'Have you seen him, First Consul? Jacques Beauvisage?' I asked.

'Jacques Beauvisage is a story. Have you heard how Jacques Beauvisage killed him? they say. How he dispatched her? No one man could have done so much. He'd be the greatest monster ever known. Everything that was worst about the Revolution has been given to this one character.'

'The greatest of all murderers,' I said.

'I heard he was at Nantes drowning people,' said Rose.

'I heard he sentenced people with Fouquier-Tinville,' said Napoleon.

'I also heard,' said Rose, 'that after the September Massacres, miserable with regret, he took himself to the Place de Grève, screaming and cursing, and a large crowd gathered around him, and when they were several hundred strong he murdered himself in front of them, a pistol shot to the head. Wild dogs, so the tale went, slept on the spot for many nights afterwards.'

'Is that true? Was that what happened?' I asked. 'Poor Jacques.'

'None of it is true,' said Napoleon. 'All legend. A ridiculous name, "Jacques Beauvisage". There never was such a person.'

'Oh, but there was, sir. I knew him. He was with us first, sir, at the Cabinet of Curtius. We used to call him our guard dog. We grew up together.'

'This story,' said Napoleon, 'is a new one to me. Don't expect me to believe it.'

'We've looked for him so long. But he hasn't come home.'

'Another tale made out of the Revolution, to frighten children and adults. To add mystery, no doubt, to your business. Do you have proof of him? Was he cast in wax?'

'No, he was not. Though he asked to be.'

'Well. Are you done then, citizen?' said Napoleon.

'Since the world is still interested in heads, I've still work to do.'

'You have what you came for, then. Good day to you.'

'Thank you, First Consul, I shall not need to come back. Goodbye, Rose, thank you. Goodbye, Fortune.'

A year later, Fortune would be killed by Napoleon's cook's English bulldog.

And we were out again. Others were waiting in the corridor; it seemed to be Consul Bonaparte's morning for receiving artists. There was David, and Houdon, the old sculptor, looking very impoverished, and a young and handsome man I had never seen before. I wondered which of these would be admitted next.

In time Houdon would make Napoleon into a life-size bust, and that was nothing much. In time David would paint him crowning himself emperor on a canvas twenty feet by thirty-two feet: they were born for each other, David and Napoleon. The young man in the corridor would sculpt him in the finest marble, more than fourteen feet high, as Mars, god of war. That artist's name was Antonio Canova.

It was those two, David and Canova, among others, who made five foot seven into a colossus. And by then every artist in the city of Paris had only that one head to make, over again, the whole city one large factory of adoration. Who would come to a wax house filled with Napoleons when just such a head was seen all over the capital, from every angle, in every street, in every room, both public and private? They used to say, at his peak, that there were seven million people living in France and five million were sculptures of Napoleon. What waxworks could thrive under such circumstances?

448

# Chapter Seventy-One

*And never come back.*

With Napoleon cast, I could at last reveal my plan. Not a new Monkey House. Something even bigger. A new country. A new city. London was the place to go. Paris was fragile; London was full of promise. In Paris the people were skin and bones; in London they were stout. In London there was future, in Paris past only. In London, I had learned, magic-lantern men from the boulevard were making money showing slides of the guillotined.

I had something better: I had heads. Tangible heads. And now Napoleon.

I wrote letters, I transferred funds, I rented a room at the Lyceum Theatre. I'll live again. Little François and Little Joseph will grow up with those snouts of theirs. They'd sniff something good of their lives. They'd last.

'London,' I announced. 'Lon-don. Say Lon-don, Little F.'

'Lon-don,' he said.

I told Citizen Tussaud I'd be back, but I didn't believe it; why should he? He was a man built only of negative figures, a subtraction, a leaking pocket. I'd leave him the Monkey House, a chance to prove himself. It was up to him. I was saying goodbye to that house: goodbye to the widow, Doctor Curtius, Edmond. To Jacques Beauvisage, too, who never came home, and whose story is never complete, but whose myths are never forgotten. They whisper tales of him in the boulevard even now, I'm told. Go to sleep, children are warned, or Jacques Beauvisage shall get you. Goodbye to it all.

449

'I'm taking the children to England,' I said. 'I'll earn us some money.'

Citizen François Tussaud, husband, not inhuman, had fallen in love with his children and fought for them. Torn with pain, he spent his pocket money on lawyers. The judge in our case – how our fortunes do climb and fall – was André Valentin. Still with one eye set eastwards and the other west, getting on in the world, ascending the ladder.

'Swiss. Still here?'

'Leaving now.'

'Where to?'

'To London,' I said. 'Foreigners are always welcome there.'

Looking at me and Tussaud simultaneously, he declared that one child could go with the mother, but the other must stay with the father. There was nothing I could do. I still had a heart in there, choking up, spluttering and kicking. I was forced to leave Joseph with my husband, forced by the man who may have killed Edmond. But what could I do against a judge? André Valentin, still thieving.

'Were you there?' I asked. 'When Edmond fell? I think you were. Were you?'

'I do not know what you are talking about.'

'What happened, please?'

'Shall I impound your papers?'

'Did you? Edmond?'

'Now, citizen, there are other cases than yours. To conclude: one child here, the other there.'

The ship was called the *Kingfisher*. Later it came apart, breaking up against the Isles of Scilly, but first it took us to England; there are no waxwork personalities with seaweed beards in the deep dark of the Channel. On deck I held Little F., most precious, my future. Below were the people of my past, a lifetime of things, my history, my people, my wax loves and hates, shifting in their crates. Edmond's portrait of me in wood and hair and glass. A shop mannequin in his shape. I'd not leave them behind.

450

I brought the history of France, carefully padded and crated, to the British Isles. Voltaire broke his nose on the journey, and Franklin lost an ear, and Jean-Paul Marat's chest caved in. But these things could be fixed. I had the moulds.

I waved goodbye to Paris and all it held. I'm going to an island, I said. We shall be separated by the sea. Don't follow me, don't ever follow.

Here I was, speeding across the English Channel, with love all about me, to tell the English our stories. You've heard of 'Bluebeard' and 'Sleeping Beauty' and 'Puss in Boots'? Here's another: the little woman who carried history on her back. You want blood? That I have. Palaces? Of course. Hovels? Certainly! Oh, and monsters? Yes, yes, I have monsters! Come and see, only come and see, let me show you how it was all done, let me tell you, how I can, what a human being is.

But do you have love in there?

Yes. Oh yes.

Away we went, Little F. and I. France was there behind us, getting smaller and smaller, until there was no more France at all. Never any more André Valentin to wreck my heart. I turned my back upon it, and directed Little F. to look forward. Over there is Great Britain, I said. What shall it do for us? What shall we do for it? They speak English there – do we know any English? *George le third. Doover. Lyceum Theatre, Lon-don.*

'Will we be coming back home, Mama? Will we ever be coming back?'

'We'll make a new home, F., a whole new one. And we'll never want to leave it.'

## Afterwards

### 1802–1850

# At Home

*I am eighty-nine.*

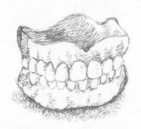

# Chapter Seventy-Two

*Seventh heads.*

Here I am. Upstairs. With all my things. There on the wall is the portrait of me that Jacques-Louis David painted. There in its glass case is the death mask of my Uncle Curtius; there is Edmond's wooden doll of me still, and beside her a mannequin in the likeness of a man I once knew; there is a wax heart and beside that a wax spleen, and there my head in wax, aged seven, modelled by Curtius; and there is Father's jawplate, not forgotten these long years, and last and first of all, my faceless doll Marta, gift of my mother. There they all are and here am I. And where are we all?

We are in London. Are we in the poorhouse? No. No one has things in the poorhouse. We are in our own home; we own it; we've done very well. We've climbed to the top of London, which is the greatest of all dungheaps ever laid by man, an excrescence of appalling dimensions. I must confess, however, that I am not all here. I come now in three pieces. My teeth have all gone, replaced by other teeth: I put them in, upper and lower rows, snap my jaw like Father. When I take them out, my face collapses, and my nose comes so close to my chin they almost touch. I wear ever thicker spectacles, round wire-framed ones. I can see no one, observe nothing, without their assistance.

My home is in Baker Street, which is only fitting, for in our way we also cook people. It is a large building we live in, a massive elephant, a great monster. This building is where history is kept. We show our people, our dolls, on the first and second floors and in the cellar. We have a gallery for royalty and other worthies, all the greatest latest people. On the third floor is our workshop factory; there every day people are melted down or poured out, people grow, people go. I watch them all, the circus of life. All those people so desperate to do well. I'm safe at last. I remember the Widow Picot thought that behind her gates. No building is ever safe, but all long to fall apart.

Down below, out of the sunlight, in the cellar, in the dark, we keep other people, the disgraceful ones, the ones who didn't behave well. There are always such people. Today's villains, mixing with yesterday's. A chamber of horrors. Only yesterday, when I went down to the cellar, a boy there, a cockney lout, was standing before Jean-Paul Marat bleeding in his bath, the wound still appearing so fresh, his sad body built by Edmond, and this boy was munching away upon a pork pie.

I do my rounds, visiting them all, moving about the old people. Looking sometimes at the new, but I belong to the old. I outlive everyone. I brush down Napoleon, smooth the brocaded jacket of Louis XVI. In his pocket I have put a map of the island of Robinson Crusoe. I can see his sister in his face.

People come to touch me, too. The History Lady some call me, others Mother Time. Many call me Madame Two-Swords. I am rather a public building. I used to tell my visitors the story of my life. Is it all true? they wondered. Wax, I told them, does not know how to lie.

I cannot sit at the desk any more taking admission fees. I'm too fragile, I might break. Others collect the money in my stead. François and Joseph have made me in wax, keeping my post. Sometimes I go and join her of an afternoon; how the public enjoy that, two of us together. It has inspired Mr Cruikshank to make a cartoon labelled MADAME TUSSAUD BESIDE HERSELF. In truth, it is not an especially brilliant likeness. But I do recognise myself in the wax model, in that shrivelled crumb of human existence, that corrugated, leathery old creature, something like a spider, something like a beetle, a wingless moth, a hunched form made of dust and dirt, all in black from boots to bonnet. Widow Picot, a man comes once a quarter

456

to pluck my chin. Frightened children shriek when they see me. They dream of me and wake up screaming. Those same children are told fairy tales now – not the adults any more; these days those stories are kept in the nursery. Those same children sing 'Twinkle, Twinkle, Little Star', a tune first written down in the year of my birth. I am as old as that noise.

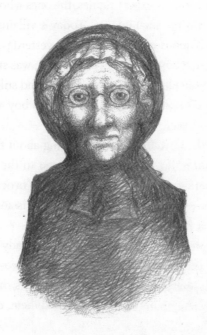

One by one, some in a hurry, some taking their time, everyone has died. Louis-Sébastien Mercier in his sleep, his shoes still stuck upon his feet. Jacques-Louis David, in disgrace, in exile. Joséphine, Weeping Rose, ejected from the empress's throne. Even Napoleon, on his rock in the Atlantic. François Tussaud senior, husband, amidst debt. And André Valentin at last, having risen to high service, sliced into two pieces, one falling this way one falling that, for crimes of embezzlement against the emperor.

The Monkey House, long vacated, gave one final baboon shriek, coughed a cloud of dust, then fell to rubble and was towed away. New buildings there now.

No one left living understands me. Only my dolls.

The novelist Mr Dickens comes to me. A thief, of course. I tell him everything. He takes notes. I have Burke and Hare downstairs, near Marat, Scottish bodysnatchers, one taken from life, the other from death. The Duke of Wellington used to come to visit my wax Napoleon. Now I have Wellington in wax.

There is a state between life and death: it's called the waxworks.

I live at the top of the house, in our rooms, with my family. Past the door marked PRIVATE — STRICTLY NO ADMITTANCE — KEEP OUT — STAFF ONLY. This is my bedroom. In here are my own things, never to be displayed, kept private. My personal collection, my personal history.

And here he comes every day, my seventh and final doctor, Doctor Marcus Healy. A balding man, corpulence setting in though he tries to hide it, to busy himself about me. He moves me as if I can't move myself, fusses over me like a child with a toy.

This world has turned mechanical. The new world is made of iron. Life now is heavy, propelled by steam and pistons. In place of candles, people illuminate themselves by gas, which gives off a light without mystery. Here's a sign of my great age: people don't look the same as they used to. Men grow whiskers, until they look more like spaniels than men, and use what wax they have to shape their enormous facial hair. And there is something else new. François is worried that it may hurt our business. This newest thing is called a daguerreotype. It traps an image of a life, captures people on polished silver. It's much quicker than wax. It can be guaranteed not to make mistakes. They want to take my image with their machine. I intend to die before they do it.

Here I am, breathless in bed. I can see the end, clearly enough, in this room. I'm eighty-nine years old. I shall not see ninety. I am Anne Marie Tussaud, née Grosholtz. Little.

Who shall never go away.

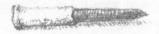